CRITICAL ISSUES IN PSYCHIATRIC DIAGNOSIS

Critical Issues in Psychiatric Diagnosis

Edited by

Robert L. Spitzer, M.D.
Chief of Psychiatric Research
Biometrics Research Unit
New York State Psychiatric
* Institute*
New York, New York

Donald F. Klein, M.D.
Director of Research
New York State Psychiatric
* Institute*
New York, New York

Raven Press ▪ New York

Raven Press, 1140 Avenue of the Americas, New York, New York 10036

Made in the United States of America

Library of Congress Cataloging in Publication Data

Main entry under title:

Critical issues in psychiatric diagnosis

  Includes bibliographical references and index.
  1. Mental illness-Diagnosis. 2. Psychiatry,
Transcultural. 3. Psychodiagnosis. 4. Mental
illness-Genetic aspects. 5. Psychiatry-Philosophy.
I. Spitzer, Robert L. II. Klein, Donald F ,
1928- (DNLM: 1. Mental disorders - Diagnosis-
Congresses. 2. Psychological texts-Congresses.
3. Genetics, Behavioral-Congresses. 4. Electro-
diagnosis-Congresses. 5. Neurohumors-Congresses.
QM141 A512c 1977)
RC469.C74   -16.8'9'075   77-72812
ISBN 0-89004-213-6

Preface

The very concept of psychiatric illness has been under considerable attack in recent years. This attack has largely depended upon studies derived from the social sciences. Some have taken the stand that what are called mental illnesses are simply those particular groups of behaviors that certain societies have considered deviant and reprehensible. This viewpoint has been aided by the fact that no generally agreed upon definition of mental illness has been propounded that is not open to the criticisms of cultural relativism.

The first section of this volume on "Definition of Mental Illness and Labeling" attempts to deal with this complex issue. Murphy deals directly with the issue of cultural relativism by speaking to the universality of the recognition of psychotic states in non-Western societies. Spitzer and Endicott, and Klein, in their respective contributions, attempt to develop systematic definitions of mental illness that would be of value throughout the range of human cultures. Salzinger presents a critique of traditional diagnoses and offered behavioral analysis as an alternative model for understanding so-called "sick" behavior. Moore raises a number of problematic examples and indicates that these definitions would not be of importance only to psychiatry but would have forensic and institutional impacts beyond the narrow confines of the medical profession.

A classificatory system is valid insofar as it allows correct statements that extend beyond the defining characteristics of the class, about the members of the class. The second part of the volume deals with the relative strengths and weaknesses of psychological testing as a basis for clinical psychiatric diagnosis. Singer focuses on the utility of projective testing, Gittelman on the special area of psychodiagnosis in children, and Chapman on the issue of spurious correlations derived from stereotyped social attitudes as a basis for apparently reliable diagnostic conclusions. Zubin, from his extensive background in both testing and diagnosis, offers an overall critique and prospectus for future work.

Although family history and the genetic approach has been a mainstay of scientific psychiatry, it is only in recent years that methodological advances have allowed for a careful dissection of the nature-nurture components of the class of behaviors under review. The studies of Crow with regard to antisocial personality, hysteria and alcoholism, Kety, Wender and Rosenthal with regard to the schizophrenic spectrum, and Goodwin with regard to alcoholism, demonstrate the power and complexities of adoption study methodology. Certainly, this has been the most frontal attack upon the nature-nurture controversy. Tsuang utilizing the remarkable resource of the Iowa 500 records amplified by blind behavioral assessments at follow-up, has once again indicated the utility of the well studied pedigree in discriminating some subtypes of psychiatric illness. Gottesman presents a wide ranging and critical discussion of the strengths and weaknesses of these various approaches pointing out the difficulty in reconciling some findings with specific genetic models.

A relatively new approach to the validation of psychiatric diagnosis is derived from the electrophysiological and biochemical laboratory. In particular, the burgeoning of computer technology has allowed for detailed studies of EEG and cerebral evoked potentials as discussed respectively by Fink, Sutton and Tueting.

One of the major problems in biochemically contrasting differing diagnostic groups is that the contrasts may not reflect the underlying diagnostic difference as much as the correlates of these differences, that have resulted in varying life experiences with regard to hospitalization, diet, physiological treatment, etc. Goodwin and Murphy, in their respective contributions, present an up-to-date description of the remarkable range of biochemical differences between specific psychiatric diagnostic entities, in a critical framework that specifically deals with the issue of artifact. Two of the foremost contributors in the area of applying advanced biochemical techniques to psychiatric problems, Wyatt and Lipton, critically review this material and give valuable leads for future endeavors.

The importance of psychiatric diagnosis both for the behavioral professions and society at large is becoming clearer. The recent efforts towards the development of the Third Diagnostic and Statistical Manual of the American Psychiatric Association had been focused on the problem of criterion reliability. Contributions to this volume, which are mainly focused on the area of validity have not extensively dealt with the question of reliability. Without reliability you can have no validity, but without substantive validity, reliability remains fruitless. To complicate matters one can have reliability with only trivial validity. The chapters of this volume focus on progress towards substantive validity that should pay off both for knowledge and practice.

The Editors

Contents

Definition of Labeling and Mental Illness

1 The Recognition of Psychosis in Non-Western Societies
Jane M. Murphy

15 Medical and Mental Disorder: Proposed Definition and Criteria
Robert L. Spitzer and Jean Endicott

41 A Proposed Definition of Mental Illness
Donald F. Klein

73 A Behavioral Analysis of Diagnosis
Kurt Salzinger

85 Discussion of the Spitzer-Endicott and Klein Proposed Definitions of
Mental Disorder (Illness)
Michael S. Moore

105 Discussion: Definition and Labeling of Mental Illness

109 Delusional Disorder (Paranoia)
George Winokur

The Role of Psychological Testing in Psychiatric Diagnosis

123 Projective Testing and Psychiatric Diagnosis: Validity and the Future
Margaret Thaler Singer

141 Validity of Projective Tests for Psychodiagnosis in Children
Rachel Gittelman-Klein

167 Psychological Tests and Psychodiagnosis
Loren J. Chapman and Jean P. Chapman

177 Discussion: Role of Psychological Testing in Psychiatric Diagnosis
Joseph Zubin

189 Discussion

Genetics as a Tool in the Validation of Psychiatric Diagnosis

193 Genetic Studies of Antisocial Personality and Related Disorders
Raymond R. Crowe

203 Familial Subtyping of Schizophrenia and Affective Disorders
Ming T. Tsuang

213 Genetic Relationships Within the Schizophrenia Spectrum: Evidence from Adoption Studies
Seymour S. Kety, David Rosenthal, and Paul H. Wender

225 Familial Alcoholism: A Diagnostic Entity?
Donald W. Goodwin

237 Exploring Psychiatric Taxa and Their Validity with Genetic Family Studies
Irving I. Gottesman and Robert R. Golden

249 Discussion

Laboratory Approaches to Psychiatric Diagnosis

253 EEG Response Strategies in Psychiatric Diagnosis
Max Fink

265 Evoked Potentials and Diagnosis
Samuel Sutton and Patricia Tueting

281 Amine Neurotransmitter Studies and Psychiatric Illness: Toward More Meaningful Diagnosis Concepts
Rex W. Cowdry and Frederick K. Goodwin

305 Neurotransmitter-Related Enzymes and Psychiatric Diagnostic Entities
Dennis L. Murphy and Monte S. Buchsbaum

323 Discussion
Morris A. Lipton

327 Diagnosis and Psychiatry
Richard Jed Wyatt

331 Discussion

335 Subject Index

Contributors

Richard Abrams, M.D.
University of Chicago
School of Medicine
Chicago, Illinois 60680

Nancy Andreasen, M.D.
Department of Psychiatry
University of Iowa
College of Medicine
500 Newton Road
Iowa City, Iowa 52240

Monte S. Buchsbaum, M.D.
Adult Psychiatry Branch
National Institute of Mental Health
Bethesda, Maryland 20014

Jean P. Chapman, Ph.D.
Department of Psychology
The University of Wisconsin
Charter at Johnson
Madison, Wisconsin 53706

Loren Chapman, Ph.D.
Department of Psychology
The University of Wisconsin
Charter at Johnson
Madison, Wisconsin 53706

Paula J. Clayton, M.D.
Department of Psychiatry
Washington University
School of Medicine
4940 Audubon Avenue
St. Louis, Missouri 63110

Raymond R. Crowe, M.D.
Department of Psychiatry
The University of Iowa
500 Newton Road
Iowa City, Iowa 52242

David Dunner, M.D.
New York State Psychiatric Institute
722 West 168th Street
New York, New York 10032

Jean Endicott, Ph.D.
Biometrics Research Unit
New York State Psychiatric
 Institute
722 West 168th Street
New York, New York 10032

Max Fink, M.D.
Psychopharmacology-EEG
 Laboratory
State University of New York
 at Stony Brook
Department of Psychiatry and
 Behavioral Science
Health Sciences Center
School of Medicine
Stony Brook, New York 11794

Rachel Gittelman-Klein, Ph.D.
Child Development Center
Long Island Jewish–Hillside Medical
 Center
271–11 Union Turnpike
Glen Oaks, New York 11040

Robert R. Golden, M.D.
Department of Psychiatry
University of Minnesota
School of Medicine
Minneapolis, Minnesota 55455

Donald W. Goodwin, M.D.
Department of Psychiatry
The University of Kansas Medical
 Center
College of Health Sciences
 and Hospital
Rainbow Boulevard at 39th
Kansas City, Kansas 66103

Frederick K. Goodwin, M.D.
Section on Psychiatry
Laboratory of Clinical Science
NIMH
9000 Rockville Pike
Bethesda, Maryland 20014

Irving I. Gottesman, Ph.D.
Department of Psychology
University of Minnesota
Minneapolis, Minnesota 44344

Seymour S. Kety, M.D.
Department of Psychiatry
Massachusetts General Hospital
Fruit Street
Boston, Massachusetts 02114

H. E. King, Ph.D.
Department of Psychiatry
University of Pittsburgh
Pittsburgh, Pennsylvania 15219

Donald F. Klein, M.D.
New York State Psychiatric Institute
722 West 168th Street
New York, New York 10032

Gerald L. Klerman, M.D.
Department of Psychiatry
Massachusetts General Hospital
Fruit Street
Boston, Massachusetts 02114

Morris A. Lipton, M.D.
Department of Psychiatry
University of North Carolina
School of Medicine
Chapel Hill, North Carolina 27514

Dennis L. Murphy, M.D.
Section on Clinical
  Neuropharmacology
Laboratory of Clinical Science
NIMH
Bethesda, Maryland 20014

Jane M. Murphy, Ph.D.
Department of Health Services
Division of Behavioral Sciences
Harvard University School of
  Public Health
677 Huntington Avenue
Boston, Massachusetts 02115

David Rosenthal, Ph.D.
Laboratory of Psychology and
  Psychopathology
NIMH
9000 Rockville Pike
Bethesda, Maryland 20014

Edward J. Sachar, M.D.
New York State Psychiatric
  Institute
722 West 168th Street
New York, New York 10032

Kurt Salzinger, Ph.D.
Biometrics Research Unit
New York State Psychiatric
  Institute
722 West 168th Street
New York, New York 10032

Charles Shagass, M.D.
Department of Psychiatry
Temple University
Eastern Pennsylvania Psychiatric
  Institute
Philadelphia, Pennsylvania 19129

Margaret Thaler Singer, Ph.D.
University of California
Berkeley, California 94705

Robert L. Spitzer, M.D.
Biometrics Research Unit
New York State Psychiatric Institute
722 West 168th Street
New York, New York 10032

Samuel Sutton, Ph.D.
Biometrics Research Unit
New York State Psychiatric
  Institute
722 West 168th Street
New York, New York 10032

Ming T. Tsuang, M.D., Ph.D.
Department of Psychiatry
University of Iowa
500 Newton Road
Iowa City, Iowa 52242

Patricia Tueting, Ph.D.
Biometrics Research Unit
New York State Psychiatric I
  Institute
722 West 168th Street
New York, New York 10032

Paul H. Wender, M.D.
University of Utah
Medical Center
50 North Medical Drive
Salt Lake City, Utah 84132

George Winokur, M.D.
University of Iowa
College of Medicine
500 Newton Road
Iowa City, Iowa 52240

Richard J. Wyatt, M.D.
National Institute of Mental Health
5600 Fishers Lane
Rockville, Maryland 20852

Joseph Zubin, Ph.D.
New York State Psychiatric
Institute
722 West 168th Street
New York, New York 10032

Critical Issues in Psychiatric Diagnosis,
edited by Robert L. Spitzer and Donald F. Klein.
Raven Press, New York © 1978.

The Recognition of Psychosis
in Non-Western Societies

Jane M. Murphy

Harvard School of Public Health, Boston, Massachusetts 02115

THE ISSUE OF CULTURAL RELATIVITY

Ruth Benedict went to Zuni in 1924. This event has become a landmark in studies of personality patterns and forms of mental illness in non-Western societies (26,27). Yet at the time, the fact that a Columbia University anthropologist undertook to study a group of Pueblo Indians in New Mexico was a little known and scarcely noticed event.

Ten years later Benedict (3) finished the book *Patterns of Culture.* Few books from the social sciences have been so widely read; few translated into as many languages; and few destined to influence the history of humanist ideas more profoundly than this one. Even those who have no associations to the name of Benedict and no idea where the Zuni Pueblo is located are nonetheless conversant with the idea of cultural relativity.

Patterns of Culture concerns the thesis that the meaning attached to human behavior is relative to the cultural context in which the behavior is enacted. What is thought to be abnormal in one cultural setting is the normal, everyday, automatically engendered behavior of another cultural setting. In view of the attention Benedict directed to distinguishing between normality and abnormality, it is not surprising that her influence on psychiatry was particularly strong. For a time she was an editor of *Psychiatry,* and had a close affiliation with the William Alanson White Foundation.

In many regards, Benedict is the symbol of cultural relativity. She stands for something which is much larger than her own work, a tradition of social research and social philosophy which began before her experience at Zuni and which has continued to flourish since her death in 1948. Yet when a person—whether anthropologist, psychiatrist, sociologist, psychologist, or philosopher—tries to give the quintessence of cultural relativity, the name of Benedict and the imagery of *Patterns of Culture* appear.

The sedate and ceremonial Zuni whose moderation and quiet restraint appealed so greatly to Benedict are one of the three groups which constitute the basis for comparisons in *Patterns of Culture.* The following excerpt indicates something of the role filled by the Zuni Indians in her thinking:

In the psychiatric records of our own society, some . . . impulses are recognized as bad ways of dealing with the situation, some as good. The bad ones are said to lead to maladjustments and insanities, the good ones to adequate social functioning. It is clear, however, that the correlation does not lie between any one bad tendency and abnormality in any absolute sense. The desire to run away from grief, to leave it behind at all costs, does not foster psychotic behavior where, as among the Pueblos, it is mapped out by institutions and supported by every attitude of the group. The Pueblos are not a neurotic people. Their culture gives the impression of fostering mental health. (3, p. 257)

The point of *Patterns of Culture* emerges not from the descriptions of Zuni alone, however, but rather from comparison to other groups: the Dobuans whose ethnography had been reported by Fortune (13) and the Kwakiutl who had been studied by Boas (4). The Dobuans are presented as displaying paranoid suspiciousness and carrying out endless acts of sorcery to protect their South Pacific gardens. The Kwakiutl Indians are described as rivalrous and megalomaniac in their Northwest Coast Potlatching.

The imagery concerns similarity within cultural groups and great differences among them. The *similarities* are based on the strength of cultural influence. Benedict wrote:

Most people are shaped to the form of their culture because of the enormous malleability of their original endowment. They are plastic to the moulding force of the society into which they are born. It does not matter whether, with the northwest coast, it requires delusions of self-reference, or with our own civilization the amassing of possessions. (3, p. 254)

The *differences* among cultures are based on the fact that each cultural group arbitrarily selects certain themes for elaboration. The theme which provides integration for one society may be diametrically opposed to that of another. The competitive, flamboyant Kwakiutl is normal in his own environment but would be abnormal among the Zuni, just as the Zuni would be abnormal among the Dobuans.

The continuing influence of Benedict is revealed in such new work as that of Scheff (36), a sociologist who in 1966 formulated a theory of the relationships between social labeling and mental illness. Scheff suggests that "the culture of the group provides a vocabulary of terms for categorizing many norm violations" (36, pp. 33–34). These designate deviations such as crime and drunkenness. There remains a residual category of diverse kinds of deviations which constitute an affront to the unconscious definition of decency and reality uniquely characteristic of each culture. Although Scheff believes that the "culture provides no explicit label" for these deviations, they nevertheless form in the minds of societal agents as "stereotypes of insanity." When other people around a deviant respond to him in terms of these stereotypes, "his amorphous and unstructured rule-breaking tends to crystallize in conformity to these expectations." Scheff suggests that these cultural stereotypes tend to produce uniformity of symptoms within a cultural group and "enormous differences in the manifest symptoms of stable mental disorder between societies" (36, pp. 82–83).

In the 50 years under purview from Benedict's field work at Zuni to the present, a main change in the trend of thought about the relativity issue has been rejection of the notion that whole cultures may be pathogenic and a focusing rather on the relativity of deviant behavior within different cultural settings. Interest in relativity has shifted its base from anthropology to sociology and psychology; and it plays a crucial part in theories about the influence of labeling as exemplified not only in the work of Scheff but also Goffman (15), Lemert (24), Rosenhan (34), Sarbin (35), and others. In psychiatry its influence is clearly perceptible in the writings of Szasz (39) and Laing and Esterson (22).

These recent formulations involve two fundamental positions. One is that the definition of the kind of abnormality we call mental illness is essentially arbitrary. The other is that mental illness is the product of learning and of experience in responding to the social cues and responses which behavior engenders in "significant others."

PURPOSE AND METHOD OF STUDY

The purpose of this chapter is to employ anthropological information about the non-Western world with its marked contrasts to our own society and to describe my work and that of others concerning definitions of abnormality and the recognition of insanity.

The focus will be on individuals in cultural settings rather than on cultures as wholes, and the main concepts to be employed are those of deviance and social roles. The point I will make is that my observations as an anthropologist and my interpretation of other contemporary ethnographic studies lead to the conclusion that cultural relativity has been much overemphasized and that what is remarkable is that human behavior is so similar, and so similarly evaluated, despite wide variations in cultural practices and beliefs.

The field work I bring to these questions concerns mainly two non-Western groups. One is a group of Siberian Eskimos who live on an island in the Bering Strait (28,31). The other is a group of Yorubas living in Nigeria (23,30). These are exceedingly different groups in terms of cultural and environmental considerations. The island is icebound much of the year and is located just under the Arctic Circle. The area in Nigeria is tropical and somewhat above the Equator. The Eskimos are a hunting and gathering group, while the Yorubas live in settled agricultural villages. The Eskimos are Oriental, the Yorubas are Black. I have also had some opportunities for checking my observations in other areas—the Gambia, the Sudan, and

South Vietnam. There was no design in the choice of these areas, merely the happenstance of history, opportunity, and the desire to compare contrasting groups.

The Arctic has generated some of the liveliest and most colorful literature on the topic of deviance and psychopathology. The long winter darkness and the endless brightness of summer have fascinated travelers and ethnographers. Many people have wondered what influence these environmental conditions have on human behavior and functioning. The literature includes reports on Arctic hysteria (14), ritual suicide (19), and most of all the psychotic and sometimes transvestite shaman (5,8). "Shaman" is, in fact, a Siberian term, but it has come to be used generally for the healer who employs possession or trance as part of a curing seance. The Siberian shaman more than any other has been cited as demonstrating that a psychotic person can fill an extremely useful and valued role in a society which accepts him (38).

The kind of field work I carried out is traditional to anthropology. It is basically the ethnographic method involving participant observation, interviewing key people, and voluminous daily recordings of events, comments, and observations. It does, however, represent one difference from the kind of ethnographic work carried out by Benedict and anthropologists of the first half of the century. Traditionally, ethnography has concerned descriptions of ceremonies and customs. The goal has been to describe the regularities and uniformities of cultural beliefs and practices. My work is like that of the newer anthropology, represented among those concerned with personality formation and psychiatric illness by, for example, the Whitings (42), Edgerton (11), Levy and Kunitz (25), Caudill (7), Graves (16), and others. This kind of anthropology has been influenced by the need to sample time, place, and persons in order to strengthen the base for generalization.

I organized my data gathering around a known universe of individuals: a census among the Eskimos, and samples among the Yorubas. What I brought back from the field were dossiers on individuals, a compendium of observations by Eskimos about specific other Eskimos, by Yorubas about specific other Yorubas. It is useful to find out what Eskimos or Yorubas *in general* do in regard to housing, clothing, diet, hunting, burials, and marriages. Insofar as I was interested in variations regarding what people feel and believe and how they interact with each other, I found it much more meaningful to deal with the specific rather than the general.

The people I talked with are a wide selection of individuals—healers, shamans, *bales* (the village headman in Yorubaland), men, women, old people, and young people. These conversations occurred in a variety of interviewing and observation settings: from using a census and going over it completely during a period of 5 months with an Eskimo; to using rather specific questions about their patients with a group of Yoruba healers; to numerous less structured approaches.

QUESTIONS TO BE ADDRESSED

Three questions serve as a means of presenting what emerged from these procedures:

1. What kinds of behaviors do these peoples think are abnormal in their own terms? I will focus on the abnormalities with which healers deal and not those with which native courts deal.

2. Are there roles in these cultures which can accommodate and make use of psychotic disorders which would be socially disabling in another?

3. If a person is abnormal or deviant in these cultures, is his behavior highly specific to the beliefs and values of that culture?

Definitions of Insanity

Regarding the first question, the way I began to get a handle on it was in the census work among the Eskimos. I began with the simple question, Can you tell me about such and such a person? This led to hearing about what kind of a hunter the person was, who he married, who his children were, whether he had spent much time in Siberia, and whether or not he had ever had a healing ceremony. Gradually the question was concretized in my mind, What behaviors and events lead Eskimos, and later Yorubas, to go to a healer?

Among other things, the Eskimo shamans take care of people when they have been lost in the snow and are frozen, when they have pains in their stomachs, when they cough, and when they have been wounded. The Yoruba healers do much the same. They help women who are trying to have children but who cannot conceive; occasionally they deliver children. Mainly, however, their patients have pains and aches. Another question then was, Do the Eskimos and Yorubas have any idea of ills that may not be in the flesh and bones?

The first indication of an answer was when one Eskimo woman who had died some years before was described as "getting wild" and "going out of her mind," but it was added "she might have had sickness in her body too." "Getting wild" in this instance meant running out in the winter at night to the lake near the village and struggling with her son when he found her and tried to bring her home. "Going out of her mind" meant not knowing where she was and accusing her family of things they did not do. As the pieces began to fit together, it seemed to me that there was indeed a distinction between mind and body in the conceptions of the two groups. To an Eskimo, one of the main phenomena which happens to the mind is *nuthkavihak,* a word which is translated as crazy. The Yorubas have a similar word, *were.*

Clearly, for the Eskimos the notions of "getting wild" and "being out of mind" were two components of their concept of *nuthkavihak.* There were other attributes as well: screaming at somebody who does not exist; believing oneself to be an animal; refusing to talk; getting lost; hiding in strange places; drinking urine; or going on a spree of killing dogs. For the Yorubas, *were* referred to behaviors such as: hearing things other people do not hear; laughing to oneself; talking all the time; asking questions and then answering them oneself; tearing off one's clothes; setting fires; and defecating in public and then mushing around in the faeces.

When a person behaved in these ways or indicated that he believed these kinds of things, the course of action was to take him to a healer and have a curing rite performed. The explanation of these behaviors was that something had gone wrong inside the person. His soul, his spirit, or his mind was out of order.

Let me emphasize that these catalogues of behaviors are not a case history. They do not refer to one person, but rather to the several who were described as *nuthkavihak* or *were*. Perhaps the most important attribute I discerned was that when any one person was described, he was said to exhibit more than one of these behaviors. I understand this to mean that some *pattern* of behaviors was in mind. No single person suffering from *nuthkavihak* fit the total pattern perfectly, but neither did any have only one component. The idea that *nuthkavihak* was conceived of as a pattern and a process rather than as one specific kind of bizarre act seemed to be borne out when one Eskimo defined *nuthkavihak* in these terms: "the mind does not control the person, he is crazy."

Although I started this work with the expectation that the Eskimos and Yorubas would have a very different concept of abnormality from ours, I now think that their idea of insanity is much more striking for its similarity than for its difference.

The expanding ethnographic literature on this topic indicates that the concepts I have presented as reflecting Eskimo and Yoruba beliefs are common throughout many parts of the world. Important among the recent studies is that of Edgerton (10) who worked with four tribal societies in East Africa. He provides a list of 24 behaviors ascribed to psychosis by these groups, including such patterns as "serious assault; arson; abusing people verbally; shouting, screaming, crying; running wild; going naked; talking nonsense; wandering aimlessly; and eating and smearing faeces." Edgerton noted that "the most obvious aspect of the many behaviors ascribed to 'psychosis' is the agreement between the four tribes." Comparing the African view of psychosis to that of the West, he wrote:

> It is remarkable how alike these African conceptions of psychosis are to the Western European psychoses, particularly to the constellation of reactions known as schizophrenia. The Africans of these four tribes do not regard a single behavior as psychotic which could not be so regarded in the West. That is, they do not produce symptoms which are understandable as psychotic only within the context of their own cultures. What is psychotic for them would be psychotic for us. (10, p. 415)

Another contemporary study which provides similar evidence is that of Selby (37) who worked among the Zapotecs of Mexico. He found that insanity was recognized and that the condition was defined as having "something to do with the soul and was symptomized by agitated motor behavior, ataraxia, violent purposeless movement, and the inability to talk in ways that people could readily understand" (37, p. 41). These investigations along with such other studies as those of Prince (33), Field (12), Beiser et al. (2), Kiev (21), and Kaplan and Johnson (20) point in the same direction. They do not bear out the view propounded by Benedict and taken up in the labeling orientation that what is abnormal in one context is normal in another.

Roles Played by Individuals Identified as Insane

Given that insanity appears to be recognized by comparable indicators in many cultural settings, it can now be asked if people so identified play roles in their societies which are useful and which are accorded prestige and respect so that little social disability is associated with insanity. Because shamanizing has been described as such a role, I shall draw mainly on my experiences among Eskimos to formulate a response.

When a shaman undertakes a curing rite, he becomes possessed with the spirit of an animal. He believes himself to be something which he is not. Further, he says that he sees and hears things relevant to the causes of illness which other people cannot hear or see. These two features, "believing something which appears not to be true," and "seeing and hearing things which others do not" were mentioned in the descriptions of *nuthkavihak*. They are similar to what we call delusions and hallucinations.

To illustrate possession, I will quote from my field notes a description of a shamaness at work.

> When my brother was sick, my grandmother who was a shamaness tried her best to get him well. She did all her part, acting as though a dog, singing some songs at night, but he died. While she was singing she fell down so hard on the floor, making a big noise. After about fifteen minutes later we heard the tapping of her fingers and her toes on the floor. Slowly she got up, already she had become like a dog. She looks awful. My grandfather told me that he used to hide his face with his drum just because she looks different, changed and awful like a dog, very scary. She used to crawl back and forth on the floor, making big noises. Even though my brother was afraid of her, he tried not to hide his face, he looked at her so that he would become well. Then my grandmother licked his mouth to try to pull up the cough and to blow it away. Then after half hour, she fell down so hard on the floor again. (29, p. 59)

The attempt to pull up the cough by licking the mouth was an extension of the old Eskimo practice of sucking on the part of the body which was painful and then blowing the pain into the air where its force would be rendered impotent. The boy was found later to have tuberculosis and he died. The shamaness was not, however, numbered among those who were said to be *nuthkavihak*.

Compare this to a case, reported by Teicher (40), of a Baffin Island Eskimo who believed that a fox had entered her body. This was not associated with shamanizing but was a continuous belief. She barked herself hoarse, tried to claw her husband, thought her feet were turning into fox paws, believed that the fox was moving up in her body so that she could feel its hair in her throat, lost control of her bowels at times, and finally became so excited that she was tied up and put into a coffin-like box with an opening at the head through which she could be fed. This woman was thought to be crazy, but the shamaness was not.

The most renowned shaman on the island where I lived had a walrus as his spirit familiar. As an overture to a seance when the group was singing and drumming, he carried out a series of acts perceived to demonstrate power. For example, he wound a thong of walrus skin around his neck and gave each end to men standing on opposite sides of him. After they pulled for a while, his head appeared to fall off onto the ground in front of him. Then a voice told the group that someone should go down to the shore and there he would find a bundle wrapped in a parka which he should bring back to the shaman. When this was done and the parka given to the shaman, the shaman's head would reappear on his shoulders. With these and other acts, the shaman worked up to a spectacular pitch of frenzy, at which time he became possessed of the walrus spirit and began curing procedures.

This shaman was called many things by the Eskimos who knew him. He was called "smart," "mean," "full of tricks," "powerful," and a "miracle worker," but no one ever called him "crazy." In describing the seance, an Eskimo said, "The shaman is out of his mind when he is curing, but *he is not crazy.*"

It seems to me that this reflects a sense of the difference between a part and a whole. In a specific situation, the shaman exhibited a component of the pattern of *nuthkavihak,* but, failing to show other aspects, he was not thought to be crazy. There can be no doubt that the Eskimos value the ability to see things, special meaningful things. I do not think they consider this phenomenon to be abnormal. Further, many Eskimos try hard to achieve this. Some people do achieve it, and some do not. Insofar as this is true, the cultural relativity idea applies. Clairvoyant phenomena are valued and respected by Eskimos, as they are by many other non-Western groups. Such experiences tend not to be valued in Western societies. This is, however, quite different from saying that the pattern of abnormality as seen by one group will be thought of as the normal pattern elsewhere.

Among the 500 Eskimos who constitute the study population of my investigation, 18 were said to have shamanized at some point in their lives. None of these was called *nuthkavihak,* whereas four other Eskimos were described as insane at some period in their lives. There was no overlap between this sample of people who played the role of shaman and this sample of people identified as *nuthkavihak*. It is important to note that this does not mean that a madman has never become a shaman. I am sure this has happened sometimes. What seems noteworthy is that it did not occur among an Eskimo group where the shamans outnumbered the psychotics by better than 4 to 1 and where the group partakes of a cultural tradition which has been described as making extremely good use of its disordered members. Even in this society where a role exists which seems well suited to the characteristics of an insane person or a schizophrenic and where the role is common enough to be open to a range of personalities, the fit between individual psychopathology and useful social role did not take place.

I have focused on the Eskimo shaman because the Yoruba healers have not been described in the literature as likely to be insane. Further, none of the healers I know were thought to be psychotic. If, then, people exhibiting *nuthkavihak* and *were* do not become shamans and healers, what roles do they play in societies such as Eskimo and Yoruba? First of all, many of them become patients. If they do not recover, they fill roles which elicit caregiving in some instances, and control, extrusion, and restraint in other instances. Just as the Eskimos used the coffin-like box for the fox-possessed woman, other groups in the Arctic have tied insane people to poles or put them in barred igloos. Selby (37) reports a similar use of a barred hut among the Zapotecs. In Yorubaland, patients are shackled and not infrequently sedated with herbal concoctions.

One of the Eskimos described as *nuthkavihak* was living in the village while I was there. She was said to be considerably improved as compared to past periods of her life; yet she moved from home to home more than anyone else. It seemed to follow a pattern of being accepted by a relative and then after a while being extruded from the family; accepted, and then extruded. The role she played seemed to be that of the wanderer. Her situation was similar to that of the vagrant psychotics in Nigeria described by Asuni (1).

A case which illustrates ambivalence of social response involving both the provision of care and extrusion from the group concerned an insane man I encountered in Gambia. This man lived on an abandoned anthill just outside a village. The anthill was about 8 feet long and 5 feet high. The top had been worn away to fit the contours of his body. Except for occasional visits into the village, the insane man remained on this platform day and night and through changing weather. His behavior was said to have become odd when he was a young man. When I saw him, he was called insane and had not spoken for years, although he sometimes made grunting sounds. The villagers put food out for him and gave him cigarettes. The latter act was accompanied by laughter because the madman had a characteristic way of bouncing several leaps into the air to get away from anyone who came close to him. This was considered amusing. Once a year, however, someone forcibly bathed him and dressed him in new clothes.

Although there may occasionally be exceptions, insanity appears commonly to be associated with social disability rather than with social useability in these traditional cultures. In this regard, as in the definition of psychosis, there appears to be much in common between modern and traditional societies.

Cultural Patterning of the Psychotic Process

A number of researchers in the field of cross-cultural psychiatry take the position that the underlying process of insanity is the same everywhere but that the specific content varies among cultural groups (9). A psychotic person, it is thought, could not use the imagery of Christ if he had not been exposed to Christian ideology; he could not believe himself to be Napoleon if he did not know about the Napoleonic Wars; and he could not elaborate ideas about the *wittiko* cannabalistic monster if not exposed to Cree and Ojibwa Indian traditions. This position makes use of relativism in a modified fashion. There have been several attempts to study phenomena such as *wittiko* (32,41) and *pibloktoq* (17), the former being thought of as the culturally defined content of a psychotic process in which the person believes himself to be a cannibalistic monster and the latter as a culture-specific form of hysteria found in the Arctic. The evidence of their existence comes from early ethnographies. It has been difficult in the contemporary period to locate people who have these illnesses. There are no recent reports of individuals exhibiting *wittiko,* and even the existing documentation from early investigations is open to question. After an extensive review of these materials made in 1967, Honigmann wrote, "I can't find one [case] that satisfactorily attests to someone being seriously obsessed by the idea of committing cannibalism" (18, p. 401).

Pibloktoq is a pattern of episodic and transient alteration of consciousness involving running away, jabbering in neologisms, making faces, and, lastly, having a seizure. Scattered cases have been reported from Greenland across the Canadian Archipelago to Alaska. Among the Eskimo group with whom I worked, I found only one description that was anything like the classic description, and it did not involve seizure. One woman was described as "once in a while having her face go every which way for short moments." People thought she might be on the verge of becoming a shamaness. She did not achieve this, but neither was she thought of as ill.

Foulks (14) has carried out a much larger and more comprehensive study of Arctic hysteria. His conclusions are similar to mine in that he found very few cases which could be said to match the prototype. Among the 10 located, there was great heterogeneity; some appeared to have epilepsy, some were diagnosed as schizophrenic, and one was possibly alcoholic. Thus it appears that these highly particular, culturally patterned phenomena are exceedingly rare. If they ever did exist, they represent a kind of cultural patterning which has not been sustained in the way which labeling theorists suggest that a stereotype molds and maintains behavior. It is possible that the stereotype of the *wittiko* psychosis is in the minds of Western observers and not in the culture-carriers themselves.

Prominent in the descriptions of the images and behavior of people labeled *were* among the Yorubas and *nuthkavihak* among the Eskimos were cultural beliefs and practices as well as features of the natural environment. Eskimo ideation concerned Arctic animals and Eskimo people, objects, and spirits. The Yoruba ideation was based on tropical animals and Yoruba figures. The cultural variation was, in other words, general. There was no evidence that if a person were to become *were* or *nuthkavihak* he would reveal one specific delusion based on cultural mythology. The lack of cultural specificity was borne home to me when I was introduced to a psychotic Sudanese. He thought he was Napoleon, an idea which represents his knowledge of history but which was not tightly linked to his own cultural tradition. Thus in this regard I agree with Brown (6) when, as he set out to see how far labeling ideas would aid his understanding of hospitalized schizophrenics in this country, he said: "Delusions are as idiosyncratic as individual schizophrenics or normals. . . . There seems to be nothing like a standard set of heresies, but only endless variety" (6, p. 397).

CONCLUSION

I began this discussion by describing Ruth Benedict's experience at Zuni and her comparative analysis of psychopathology in different cultural groups. She concluded that:

> There can be no reasonable doubt that one of the most effective ways in which to deal with the staggering burden of psychopathic [sic] tragedies in America at the present time is by means of an educational program which fosters tolerance in society and a kind of self-respect and independence that is foreign to . . . our urban traditions. (3, pp. 273–274)

The conclusion I draw from research that has been carried out in the years since is different; in fact, it is opposite. Psychosis, especially a process such as schizophrenia, is widely distributed around the world suggesting that the causes of insanity are ubiquitous in human groups. Insanity appears to have content manifestations which are colored by cultural beliefs and knowledge but not to be inextricably bound to them in any standard way.

Everywhere, insanity seems to be a serious and troubling affliction, troubling to those who exhibit it and troubling to those in the families and communities who must respond to it. Further, there appear to be few if any experiments of cultural tolerance which have solved the problems posed by these afflictions. Surely, social attitudes and societal reactions have considerable influence on what happens to people so troubled as they progress through life, but that tolerance alone will cure the trouble is exceedingly doubtful.

ACKNOWLEDGMENTS

This report draws on materials presented in "Psychiatric Labeling in Cross-Cultural Perspective" by Jane M. Murphy which appeared in *Science,* 191:1019–1028 (1976), and is adapted here with the permission of the publisher. The Eskimo and Yoruba studies which form the core of this chapter have been carried on as part of the Harvard Program in Social Psychiatry directed by Alexander H. Leighton and supported by funds from the Social Science Research Center of Cornell (for the Eskimo study), the National Institute of Mental Health, the Ministry of Health of Nigeria, and the Social Science Research Council (for the Yoruba study).

REFERENCES

1. Asuni, T. (1968): Vagrant psychotics in Abeokuta. In: *Deuxième Colloque Africain de Psychiatrie,* pp. 115–123. Association Universitaire pour le Développement de l'Enseignement et de la Culture en Afrique et à Madagascar, Paris.
2. Beiser, M. Burr, W., Ravel, J. L., and Collomb, H. (1973): Illness of the spirit among the Serer of Senegal. *Am. J. Psychiatry,* 130:881–886.
3. Benedict, R. (1934): *Patterns of Culture.* Houghton Mifflin, Boston. (Sentry Edition with a preface by M. Mead, 1959).
4. Boas, F. (1921): *Ethnology of the Kwakuitl.* Thirty-Fifth Annual Report of the Bureau of American Ethnology, Washington, D.C.
5. Bogoras, W. (1909): *The Chukchee.* Memoir of the American Museum of Natural History, New York.
6. Brown, R. (1973): Schizophrenia, language and reality. *Am. Psychol.,* 28:395–403.
7. Caudill, W. (1972): Tiny dramas: Vocal communication between mother and infant in Japanese and American families. In: *Transcultural Research in Mental Health,* edited by W. P. Lebra, pp. 25–48. University of Hawaii Press, Honolulu.
8. Czaplicka, M. A. (1914): *Aboriginal Siberia.* Clarendon Press, Oxford.
9. deReuck, A., and Porter, R. (1965): *Transcultural Psychiatry.* Churchill, London.
10. Edgerton, R. B. (1966): Conceptions of psychosis in four East African societies. *Am. Anthrop.,* 68:408–428.
11. Edgerton, R. B. (1967): *The Cloak of Competence.* University of California Press, Berkeley.
12. Field, M. (1960): *Search for Security.* Northwestern University Press, Chicago.
13. Fortune, R. F. (1932): *The Sorcerers of Dobu.* Dutton, New York.
14. Foulks, E. (1972): *The Arctic Hysterias of the North Alaskan Eskimo.* American Anthropological Association, Washington, D.C.
15. Goffman, E. (1962): *Asylums.* Aldine, Chicago.
16. Graves, T. (1974): Urban Indian personality and the *Culture of Poverty. Am. Ethnol.,* 1:65–84.
17. Gussow, Z. (1960): "Pibloktog" (hysteria) among Polar Eskimos. In: *Psychoanalysis and the Social Sciences,* edited by W. Muensterberger, pp. 218–236. International Universities Press, New York.
18. Honigmann, J. (1967): *Personality in Culture.* Harper & Row, New York.
19. Hughes, C. C., and Leighton, A. H. (1955): Notes on Eskimo patterns of suicide. *Southwest. J. Anthrop.,* 11:327–338.
20. Kaplan, B., and Johnson, D. (1964): The social meaning of Navaho psycho-

pathology and psychotherapy. In: *Magic, Faith, and Healing,* edited by A. Kiev, pp. 203–229. Free Press, New York.
21. Kiev, A. (1972): *Transcultural Psychiatry.* Free Press, New York.
22. Laing, R. D., and Esterson, A. (1964): *Sanity, Madness and the Family.* Basic Books, New York.
23. Leighton, A. H., Lambo, T. A., Hughes, C. C., Leighton, D. C., Murphy, J. M., and Macklin, D. B. (1963): *Psychiatric Disorder Among the Yoruba.* Cornell University Press, Ithaca, New York.
24. Lemert, E. M. (1962): Paranoia and the dynamics of exclusion. *Sociometry,* 25: 2–25.
25. Levy, J., and Kunitz, S. (1974): *Indian Drinking.* Wiley, New York.
26. Mead, M. (1959): *An Anthropologist at Work, Writings of Ruth Benedict.* Houghton Mifflin, Boston.
27. Mead, M. (1974): *Ruth Benedict: Leaders of Modern Anthropology.* Columbia University Press, New York.
28. Murphy, J. M. (formerly Hughes) (1960): An epidemiological study of psychopathology in an Eskimo village. Ph.D. dissertation, Cornell University, Ithaca, New York.
29. Murphy, J. M. (1964): Psychotherapeutic aspects of shamanism on St. Lawrence Island, Alaska. In: *Magic, Faith, and Healing,* edited by A. Kiev, pp. 53–83. Free Press, New York.
30. Murphy, J. M. (1973): Sociocultural change and psychiatric disorder among rural Yorubas in Nigeria. *Ethos,* 1:249–262.
31. Murphy, J. M., and Leighton, A. H. (1965): Native conceptions of psychiatric disorder. In: *Approaches to Cross-Cultural Psychiatry,* edited by J. Murphy and A. Leighton, pp. 64–107. Cornell University Press, Ithaca, New York.
32. Parker, S. (1960): The Wittiko psychosis in the context of Ojibwa personality and culture. *Am. Anthrop.,* 62:603–623.
33. Prince, R. (1964): Indigenous Yoruba psychiatry. In: *Magic, Faith, and Healing,* edited by A. Kiev, pp. 84–120. Free Press, New York.
34. Rosenhan, D. L. (1973): On being sane in insane places. *Science,* 179:250–258.
35. Sarbin, R. (1969): The scientific status of the mental illness metaphor. In: *Changing Perspectives in Mental Illness,* edited by S. Plog and B. Edgerton, pp. 9–32. Holt, Rinehart & Winston, New York.
36. Scheff, T. J. (1966): *Being Mentally Ill.* Aldine, Chicago.
37. Selby, H. (1974): *Zapotec Deviance.* University of Texas Press, Austin.
38. Silverman, J. (1967): Shamans and acute schizophrenia. *Am. Anthrop.,* 69:21–31.
39. Szasz, T. (1961): *The Myth of Mental Illness.* Hoeber-Harper, New York.
40. Teicher, M. I. (1954): Three cases of psychosis among the Eskimos. *J. Ment. Sci.,* 100:527–535.
41. Teicher, M. (1960): *Windigo Psychosis.* American Ethnological Society, Seattle.
42. Whiting, B., and Whiting, J. (1975): *Children of Six Cultures.* Harvard University Press, Cambridge, Mass.

Critical Issues in Psychiatric Diagnosis,
edited by Robert L. Spitzer and Donald F. Klein.
Raven Press, New York © 1978.

Medical and Mental Disorder: Proposed Definition and Criteria

Robert L. Spitzer and Jean Endicott

American Psychiatric Association Task Force on Nomenclature and Statistics; and Biometrics Research Unit, New York State Psychiatric Institute, New York, New York 10032

It is rather remarkable that classifications of mental (psychiatric) and other medical disorders have existed for decades despite the lack of any agreed on definition for what constitutes a medical disorder in the first place. In fact, the official classification of the World Health Organization (the *International Classification of Diseases*) and of the American Psychiatric Association (the first and second editions of the *Diagnostic and Statistical Manual of Mental Disorders*), made no attempt to address the issue. Nor, with a single exception (17), do the standard textbooks of medicine and psychiatry.

As Kendell (7) has noted, physicians rarely concern themselves with defining what is a medical disorder and instead spend their time, as best they can, diagnosing and treating individual patients. If questioned, they readily acknowledge that much of their work actually involves conditions which are generally not considered medical disorders, such as pregnancy or childbirth, or preventive medicine, such as giving advice to mothers of children attending a well-baby clinic, or advising middle-aged men regarding diet and exercise.

A review of some of the literature regarding definitions of illness, disease, and other related conditions indicates that the problem has been of more interest to sociologists, psychologists, philosophers of science, and members of the legal profession than it has been to medical professionals (2,8,9,12). Of the medical specialties, psychiatry has shown the most concern because of its difficulty in defining its own professional responsibility (13).

Our own preoccupation with defining medical and mental disorders grew out of our involvement with the American Psychiatric Association's Task Force on Nomenclature and Statistics, which is responsible for developing the official classification system of the mental disorders in this country. The initial impetus grew out of the controversy as to whether or not homosexuality, *per se,* should be deleted from the psychiatric nomenclature (18). This led to an initial attempt on our part to delineate criteria for mental disorders

(17), without any consideration as to how it related to a definition of the more general rubric of medical disorder.

Our conviction that there was a need for a definition of mental disorder grew as we became involved in the preparation of the Third Edition of the American Psychiatric Association's *Diagnostic and Statistical Manual* (DSM-III). Decisions had to be made on a variety of issues that seemed to us to relate to the fundamental question of the boundaries of the concept of mental disorder. We believed that without some definition of mental disorder, there would be no explicit guiding principles that would help to determine which conditions should be included in the nomenclature, which excluded, and how conditions included should be defined. As we considered the many conditions traditionally included in the nomenclature, we realized that although the definition of mental disorder proposed at the time of the controversy regarding homosexuality was suitable for almost all of them, a broader definition seemed necessary.

With the help of our colleagues, particularly other members of the Task Force on Nomenclature and Statistics, we eventually came to believe that mental disorder should be defined as merely a subset of medical disorder, and that our attention should therefore be directed toward defining the broad rubric of medical disorder. We developed such a working definition which we believed could serve many functions. With the recognition that any proposed definition is tentative and likely to change with further knowledge, the Task Force (with a few dissenting members) was initially convinced that such a working definition was not only of value in developing the revised classification, but that it should be included in DSM-III as a formal statement.

This initial definition of medical and mental disorder was presented at a special session of the 1976 annual meeting of the American Psychiatric Association (15). The definition was critiqued by a panel of discussants representing many disciplines and points of view, as well as by members of the audience. For the most part, to our chagrin, the reaction was negative. Some questioned the need and wisdom of having any definition. Many argued that the definition proposed was too restrictive, and if officially adopted, would have the potential for limiting the appropriate activities of our profession and would redefine the major educational activities of psychiatry; they also felt that it was out of keeping with trends in medicine that emphasize the continuity of health and illness. Furthermore, some questioned our claim that the definition that we proposed was actually helpful in making decisions regarding the nomenclature. Rather, it was argued, decisions were made and then the definition tinkered with to justify them.

With the wisdom of hindsight, we now acknowledge that many of these criticisms were warranted. It now seems unlikely that any proposed definition will be found generally acceptable to the profession. Without such acceptance, there would be little justification for its adoption by the Task Force as part of DSM-III. We also recognize that it is not possible or useful to sharply define the boundaries between disorder and "normality," as we had originally intended, and that the definition that we had proposed was, indeed, too narrow (even though some of our critics thought it was too broad).

Perhaps as evidence of our failure to learn from experience, we have continued to modify the definition to meet some of the criticisms received. We are still convinced that some working definition of medical and mental disorders is of value. This chapter describes our current definition of and criteria for medical and mental disorders with the hope that many of the deficiencies of the initial attempt have been corrected. Surveying the literature of previous attempts to grapple with these difficult issues indicates that the approach taken here is unique in providing not only a definition of medical disorder, but detailed operational criteria. Furthermore, these criteria avoid such terms as "dysfunction," "maladaptive," or "abnormal," terms which themselves beg definition.

We believe that the definition offered here helps clarify the goals of medical classification. It helps delineate the areas of responsibility of the medical system from those of other societal systems which also have as their purpose improving or otherwise changing human functioning, such as the educational or criminal justice systems. It provides a rationale for decisions as to which conditions should be included or excluded from a medical classification. In addition, it provides guidelines for determining the boundaries of those disorders which are seemingly continuous with variations in "normal" functioning. Furthermore, since the definition of mental disorder proposed here is merely a subset of the definition of medical disorder, it contributes to the continuing debate concerning the appropriateness of the medical model as applied to psychiatric disturbance (14).

KEY CONCEPTS IN THE DEFINITION OF MEDICAL DISORDER

We believe that there are several fundamental concepts in the notion of a medical disorder: negative consequences of the condition, an inferred or identified organismic dysfunction, and an implicit call for action. There is no assumption that the organismic dysfunction or its negative consequences are of a physical nature. Therefore, throughout this chapter we use the broader term "disorder," rather than "disease" (which often denotes a progressive physical disorder with known pathophysiology) or "illness" which often refers to the clinical manifestations of a disorder (5).[1]

The purpose of a classification of medical disorders is to identify those conditions which, because of their negative consequences, implicitly have a *call to action* to the profession, the person with the condition, and society.

---

[1] We note with pleasure that in the text of the World Health Organization's *International Classification of Diseases,* the term "disorder" is used in the same sense as we use it.

The call to action on the part of the medical profession (and its allied professions) is to offer treatment for the condition or a means to prevent its development, or, if knowledge is lacking, to conduct appropriate research. The call to the person with the condition is to assume the patient or sick role (9). The call to action on the part of society takes several forms which may include giving various exemptions from certain responsibilities to those in the sick role and to provide a means for the delivery of medical care.

Implicit in the call to action is the assumption that *something has gone wrong with the human organism* which has led to negative consequences. On the other hand, this does not imply that conditions which are not considered disorders are equally desirable or represent optimal functioning or should be ignored by the profession. For example, although the medical profession recognizes that it is generally better to have the physical stamina needed to participate in active sports, its absence when due to simple lack of sufficient regular exercise is by itself not considered a disorder. Similarly, although a high degree of intellectual curiosity is generally viewed as desirable, its absence in an individual who is not mentally retarded is not usually viewed as a manifestation of a disorder.

There is no implication that it is inappropriate for the medical profession to be interested in conditions that are not disorders. For example, the study of genius, longevity, and normal coping mechanisms may be of interest in and of itself, and may provide knowledge which, in the long run, will be of value in preventing or treating disorders.

PROPOSED DEFINITION OF MEDICAL AND MENTAL DISORDER

The proposed definition of medical and mental disorder is presented here in a highly abbreviated form. The rationale for the definition is to be found in the discussion of the operational criteria which follow.

A medical disorder is a relatively distinct condition resulting from an organismic dysfunction which in its fully developed or extreme form is directly and intrinsically associated with distress, disability, or certain other types of disadvantage. The disadvantage may be of a physical, perceptual, sexual, or interpersonal nature. Implicitly there is a call for action on the part of the person who has the condition, the medical or its allied professions, and society.

A mental disorder is a medical disorder whose manifestations are primarily signs or symptoms of a psychological (behavioral) nature, or if physical, can be understood only using psychological concepts.

OPERATIONAL CRITERIA FOR MEDICAL DISORDER

The operational criteria discussed in the following sections can be viewed as providing sufficient evidence for both an organismic dysfunction and justification for societal recognition of the appropriateness of the sick role.

A condition must meet all four criteria to be considered a medical disorder. The criteria with examples of both mental disorders and other medical disorders are shown in Table 1. Each of the criteria follows with explication of key concepts.

Criterion A. The condition in the fully developed or extreme form, in all environments (other than one especially created to compensate for the condition), is directly associated with . . .

A *condition* is any set of facts about an organism which has correlates. Liking pistachio ice cream and being an American are both conditions, although the correlates of these conditions (liking ice cream in general, speaking English) are not of any relevance to medical disorder.

The phrase *in the fully developed or extreme form* is used because in medicine many conditions are recognizable in an early form, frequently with the aid of laboratory tests, before they have any undesirable consequences. For example, an X-ray examination may reveal a carcinoma of the lung before the patient has any clinical sign of the illness. The condition is still regarded as a medical disorder because the natural history of carcinoma is such that in the fully developed form there are inevitably undesirable consequences of the condition. As Feinstein (6) has noted, this was not always the case. Early in the history of medicine, disorders were not recognized unless they were clinically manifested by signs of illness. Unfortunately, in psychiatry we rarely have laboratory procedures which permit us to diagnose mental disorders before they have clinical manifestations. However, sometimes our knowledge of the clinical course of psychiatric disorders, such as mania, alcoholism, or schizophrenia, does permit us to detect the disorder prior to the development of obviously negative consequences.

In defining the boundaries of a disorder, it is essential to exclude related conditions which may seemingly appear to be milder forms of the disorder. Thus, a useful definition of alcoholism excludes social drinking because the correlates of the two conditions are extremely different. Defining alcoholism to include social drinking would greatly weaken its power as a diagnostic category. Thus, alcoholism is conceptualized as a different condition than social drinking and not merely an extreme form of it.

The phrase "in all environments (other than one especially created to compensate for the condition)" is used to operationally assure that the negative consequences of the condition are intrinsic to that condition, rather than a result of an interaction between the condition and a specific environment. If the negative consequences occur in all environments, the condition is a disorder. If they occur only in special environments, then the condition is considered a vulnerability. For example, sickle cell trait is a vulnerability because in environments of oxygen deprivation the disorder of sickle cell

TABLE 1. *Proposed operational criteria for a medical disorder*

All four criteria, A through D, must be met for a condition to be designated as a medical disorder. It should be noted that if criterion A is met only by virtue of A.3, disadvantage, the designation of the condition as a disorder is heavily dependent on social definitions of the degree of the disadvantage or undesirableness, as well as other considerations, as to the consequences of considering the condition a medical disorder.

Criteria	Examples	
	Medical (nonmental)	Mental
A. The condition, in the fully developed or extreme form, in all environments (other than one especially created to compensate for the condition), is directly associated with at least one of the following:		
1. Distress—acknowledged by the individual or manifested.	Trigeminal neuralgia	Phobic disorder
2. Disability—some impairment in functioning in a wide range of activities.	Pituitary dwarfism	Antisocial personality disorder, manic disorder, alcoholism
3. Disadvantage (not resulting from the above)—certain forms of disadvantage to the individual in interacting with aspects of the physical or social environment because of an identifiable psychological or physical factor.		
The following forms of disadvantage, even when not associated with distress or disability, are now considered, in our culture, as suggestive of some type of organismic dysfunction warranting the designation of medical disorder:		
a. Impaired ability to make important environmental discriminations	Color blindness, lack of pain perception	
b. Lack of ability to reproduce	Sterility	
c. Cosmetically unattractive because of a deviation in kind, rather than degree, from physical structure	Fused toes Port wine stain	
d. Atypical and inflexible sexual or other impulse-driven behavior which often has painful consequences		Sexual sadism, kleptomania, pathological gambling
e. Impairment in the ability to experience sexual pleasure in an interpersonal context		Anorgasmia, fetishism
f. Marked impairment in the ability to form relatively lasting and nonconflictual interpersonal relationships		Narcissistic personality disorder, hysterical personality disorder

B. The controlling variables tend to be attributed to being largely within the organism with regard to either initiating or maintaining the condition. Therefore, a condition is included only if it meets both of the following criteria:

  1. Simple informative or standard educational procedures do not lead to a reversal of the condition.

> Thus, anxiety regarding physical health unrelieved by negative laboratory tests suggests hypochondriasis, and illiteracy despite adequate standard reading instruction suggests a specific reading developmental disorder or mental retardation.

  2. Nontechnical interventions do not bring about a quick reversal of the condition.

> Thus, pain of foot while caught in door suggests a medical disorder only if it is not quickly relieved by opening the door.

> Thus, inattentiveness and hyperactivity which persist in a child despite changes in school and other environment suggest attention deficit disorder.

C. Conditions are not included if the associated distress, disability, or other disadvantage is apparently the necessary price associated with attaining some positive goal.

> Thus, wanted pregnancy and childbirth are not medical disorders even though they cause pain and some disability.

> Thus, simple grief is not considered a mental disorder but is seen as the natural consequence of psychological attachment to others.

D. Distinctness from other conditions in one or more of the following features: clinical phenomenology, course, response to treatment, familial incidence, or etiology.

> Tuberculosis (but not cough)

> Panic disorder (but not nervousness); depressive disorder (but not unhappiness)

crisis may develop, although in all other environments it has either no negative consequences or in environments in which malaria is endemic, it actually has some advantage. On the other hand, sickle cell disease is a disorder because it has undesirable consequences in all environments.

The distinction between a vulnerability and a disorder is recognized in other fields of medicine. Much of medical practice is directed toward preventing the development of conditions rather than treating disorders. For example, the use of antigens to desensitize an individual who has a vulnerability for the development of hay fever is clearly different from the use of antihistamines to treat the symptomatic disorder, hay fever. Some psychiatric practice is also directed toward reduction of vulnerability for the development of a disorder, for example, counseling all freshmen to detect and possibly reduce the vulnerability of those who appear to have a high likelihood of the development of a mental disorder.

The phrase "(other than one especially created to compensate for the condition)" is used in recognition of the fact that occasionally it is possible to create a special environment that will prevent the negative consequences that would result from the interaction of a disorder with all naturally existing environments. For example, an individual without the normal immune mechanisms can be placed in a germ-free environment to avoid the otherwise inevitable consequences of such a disorder. Similarly, an individual with a phobic disorder may be able to organize his immediate environment to avoid exposure to the phobic situation and the negative consequences of such avoidance. Nevertheless, in both instances, the condition should be regarded as a disorder.

The phrase "directly associated with . . ." recognizes the distinction between a predisposing condition and a condition which is a disorder. A predisposing condition increases the probability of developing a disorder but may not itself have the negative consequences required in the definition of a disorder. Thus, social drinking predisposes to alcoholism, and skiing predisposes to fracture. Some disorders are also predisposing conditions. Thus, tobacco use disorder (as defined in DSM-III) and hypertension are both disorders and predisposing conditions because they increase the likelihood of developing other disorders.

Whether a predisposing condition should be prevented depends on an evaluation of all of its consequences, some of which may be desirable. Thus, although social drinking does predispose toward alcoholism, it also has some positive correlates, such as relief of tension and increased sociability, which mitigate against a medical policy of discouraging all social drinking. On the other hand, being overweight predisposes to the development of a variety of medical disorders and would seem to have no redeeming features. In such a case, it is reasonable for medical intervention to be used to prevent the development of the predisposing condition.

There are three undesirable consequences for the individual with the condition, at least one of which is required for criterion A. Fortunately, for mnemonic purposes, they all begin with the letter *D:* distress, disability, and disadvantage.

1. Distress—Acknowledged by the Individual or Manifest

This means that either the subject complains about the distress that he experiences or distress is inferred from his manifest behavior. The distress may be in the form of physical pain or any dysphoric affect such as anxiety, depression, or anger. An example of a nonmental medical disorder which causes distress is trigeminal neuralgia. An example of a mental disorder which causes distress is phobic disorder.

2. Disability—Some Impairment in Functioning in a Wide Range of Activities

This means that there is impairment in more than one area of functioning. The reason that a wide range of activities needs to be affected is to avoid *a priori* decisions as to what areas of human activity are "basic," or "essential." Pituitary dwarfism is an example of a nonmental medical disorder resulting in disability as defined here, as are antisocial personality (as defined in DSM-III), manic disorder, and alcoholism. Some disorders which ordinarily result in disability may occasionally result in immediate death (the ultimate disability) without passing through a stage of impaired functioning, as, for example, a suddenly rupturing aortic aneurysm.

As a consequence of the requirement of generalized impairment, it is possible for a condition to be associated with impairment in a single function and not be classified as a disorder, providing that the condition does not result in any of the other two *D*'s. Thus, homosexuality *per se,* which represents an impairment in functioning in the area of heterosexual relationships, is not considered a mental disorder because the area of impairment is often limited, and this condition does not qualify for either of the other *D*'s, as we have defined them.

Before proceeding to the third and most controversial *D,* it is important to recognize that almost all of the conditions traditionally regarded as medical disorders (including the mental disorders) meet the inclusion criteria of distress or disability as defined here. All of the major psychiatric disorders, such as the organic mental disorders, schizophrenia, paranoid disorders, personality disorders, affective disorders, and anxiety disorders, in their extreme or fully developed form are almost invariably associated with impairment in functioning in many areas.

3. Disadvantage (not resulting from the above)—certain forms of disadvantage to the individual in interacting with aspects of the physical or social environment because of an identifiable psychological or physical factor.

There is an extremely small number of conditions generally regarded as medical disorders which are not directly and intrinsically associated with either distress or disability. A feature that these conditions all share is that the individual with the condition is at a disadvantage in dealing with some aspect of the physical or social environment. However, many conditions which place an individual at a relative disadvantage are not usually considered medical disorders, for example, short stature, tone deafness, greediness, poor sense of humor, unattractive appearance, and limited intelligence (but not mental retardation). Conditions such as these are usually regarded as the inevitable consequence of "normal variation" rather than a result of "something having gone wrong." This is the case even if medical intervention can be used to change the condition, as with plastic surgery for an unattractive nose.

The designation of a condition as a disorder on the basis of disadvantage without intrinsic distress or disability is heavily dependent on social definitions of the degree of the disadvantage, the undesirableness of the behavior, and other considerations as to the consequences of considering the condition as a medical disorder. For these reasons, all the conditions considered medical disorders on the basis of this criterion *alone* are the ones that are most apt to be a source of intense controversy, particularly those regarded as mental disorders.

The history of the classification of various sexual conditions is illustrative. For a long time masturbation was regarded as a disease (4). In part this was undoubtedly due to factual errors regarding its presumed association with other disorders. However, in large part it reflected a value judgment that the behavior was extremely undesirable, and therefore placed the afflicted individual at a serious disadvantage. There was an overt call to action and various treatment procedures were forced on the unfortunate individuals so diagnosed who were then coerced into the patient role. In time, with the realization that masturbation had no inevitable dire consequences and was common, and with a general shift in the attitude toward sexuality, masturbation *per se* was no longer viewed as a disorder.

Homosexuality was up to very recently firmly established in the psychiatric nomenclature as a medical disorder for a variety of reasons. The removal of homosexuality from the nomenclature was in part a recognition of factual errors that had been made regarding the inevitable association of homosexuality with either distress or disability in numerous areas of functioning. However, many who acknowledged these factual errors still insisted that the inability of many homosexuals to function heterosexually was a sufficient disadvantage to warrant the designation of medical disorder, regardless of whether or not the condition was egosyntonic. Many of those who opposed this view asserted that as long as an individual could function sexually in an interpersonal context, regardless of the sex of the partner, there was no disadvantage of sufficient magnitude to justify the label of medical disorder in the absence of acknowledged distress.

On the other hand, lack of orgasm in women was until recently viewed by Western society as of either no significance or desirable. Now the same condition, at least in an extreme form, is regarded by many as undesirable, evidence of an organismic dysfunction, and sufficiently disadvantageous as to justify its classification as a medical disorder. Although logically it is possible to have a disorder for which there is no treatment, the fact that a condition, such as lack of orgasm, can often be changed by a technical intervention adds weight to the logic of conceptualizing it as due to an organismic dysfunction rather than due to normal variation. Some of the current controversy about the limits of "normal" sexual response, particularly in females, has been influenced by evidence regarding which aspects of sexual response are modifiable and which are not.

The following forms of disadvantage, even when not associated with distress or disability, are now considered, in our culture, as suggestive of some type of organismic dysfunction warranting the designation of medical disorder.

The first three forms of disadvantage are applicable to nonmental medical disorders and would appear to be sufficient to explain the rationale for designating a condition as a medical disorder if it failed to meet the criteria of either distress or disability.

a. *Impaired Ability to Make Important Environmental Discriminations*

This would be the basis for classifying color blindness or lack of pain perception as medical disorders. It is of interest to note that tone deafness would also seem to qualify as a medical disorder on the basis of this criterion. However, presumably society does not regard that condition to be a serious enough disadvantage to warrant designation as a medical disorder.

b. *Lack of Ability to Reproduce*

On the basis of this criterion, sterility is viewed as a medical disorder, even when the cause is not known. Some would argue that this criterion would apply to homosexuality, whereas others would argue that in this condition there is no impairment in the reproductive function, since conception is possible without coitus.

c. *Cosmetically Unattractive Because of a Deviation in Kind, Rather than Degree, from Physical Structure*

People come in all manners of size, shape, and appearance. Quantitative variation, such as a big or small nose, even when grossly unattractive, tends not to be viewed as a disorder, even if plastic surgery is employed to improve the condition. On the other hand, some even minimally cosmetically unattractive conditions, such as a small port wine stain or fused toes (syndactyly), are regarded as medical disorders because they are qualitative deviations which suggest that some organismic function has gone wrong.

The following three forms of disadvantage are applicable to mental disorders. They have been chosen by us from a larger pool of potential criteria. They seem to adequately cover the few conditions in the standard psychiatric nomenclature which are not intrinsically associated with either distress or disability. In addition, they reflect common clinical criteria used in the evaluation of patients who may not evidence either distress or disability. Finally, they are not so broad as to bring about the inclusion of all forms of behavior or functioning which are less than optimal.

d. *Atypical and Inflexible Sexual or Other Impulse-Driven Behavior Which Often Leads to Painful Consequences*

Examples of conditions covered by this criterion include sexual sadism, kleptomania, and pathological gambling. Homosexuality frequently leads to painful consequences in environments which demand heterosexual functioning or punish homosexual behavior. In environments which support or are indifferent to such behavior, there is no necessary association with a painful outcome. On the other hand, it is hard to imagine a society which can be generally indifferent to sexual sadism, kleptomania, or pathological gambling.

e. *Impairment in the Ability to Experience Sexual Pleasure in an Interpersonal Context*

Examples of conditions covered by this criterion include anorgasmia and fetishism.

f. *Marked Impairment in the Ability to Form Relatively Lasting and Nonconflictual Interpersonal Relationships*

Examples of conditions covered by this criterion include narcissistic personality disorder and hysterical personality disorder. Admittedly, this criterion is highly dependent on cultural definitions of appropriate interpersonal relationships. Since few people have completely nonconflictual interpersonal relationships, only a marked impairment warrants an inference of an organismic dysfunction.

Criterion B. The controlling variables tend to be attributed to being largely within the organism with regard to either initiating or maintaining the condition.

As noted previously, implicit in the concept of a medical disorder is the notion that something is wrong within the organism that has either started the condition or is responsible for maintaining it. This does not mean that factors outside of the organism are of no importance. The phrase "tend to be attributed" acknowledges our lack of certainty regarding the locus of the trouble but does reflect that generally the profession assumes that the locus of the disturbance in a medical disorder is at least partly within the organism. The nature of what is wrong may be known or unknown, and may or may not be conceptualized in somatic or physiological terms. Some dysfunctions may be understandable only on the basis of psychological concepts, such as learning or conflict, and may never be reducible to biochemical or neurophysiological constructs.

Operationally, this criterion is determined by the following:

A condition is included only if it meets both of the following criteria:
1. Simple informative or standard educational procedures do not lead to a reversal of the condition.
2. Nontechnical interventions do not bring about a quick reversal of the condition.

These two criteria exclude conditions in which the organism appears to be intact but its functioning has been negatively affected by the absence of information or by unfortunate environmental contingencies.

There is no example of a nonmental medical condition in Table 1 for criterion B.1. Even where information or standard educational procedures are of value in preventing or modifying medical disorders, some environmental or behavioral change is required. For example, an elementary knowledge of nutrition can prevent or reverse vitamin deficiencies, but only by modifying the diet, not by mere knowledge alone. In contrast, some mental conditions can be reversed by information alone. Thus, anxiety regarding physical health which is relieved by negative laboratory tests is not a medical disorder, whereas the persistence of anxiety, even with the information, does suggest hypochondriasis. Similarly, illiteracy which is relieved by standard educational procedures does not suggest a medical disorder, whereas unresponsiveness to such procedures suggests either a specific reading developmental disorder or mental retardation.

The best way to explain the concept involved in criterion B.2 is an analogy with an automobile that will not start. Although in a sense something is wrong with such an automobile regardless of the cause, it is useful to distinguish between such conditions as being out of gas and having a defective carburetor. If the car is simply out of gas, no special technical knowledge or skills are required to reverse the condition. All that is needed is the nontechnical intervention of providing gas. On the other hand, repair of a defective carburetor requires a specialized knowledge of how automobiles work.

If one's foot is caught in a door causing intense pain, the condition would not be regarded as a medical disorder if the pain quickly subsided with the opening of the door. On the other hand, if the pain did persist, it would suggest that there had been an injury (medical disorder) to the foot. Similarly, if a child's inattentiveness and hyperactivity in school quickly disappear with a simple change of teachers, he would not be considered to have a mental disorder. However, if such behavior persists despite changes in school environment, and also occurs in other settings, the diagnosis of an attentional deficit disorder (DSM-III term for hyperactive syndrome) is suggested.

The distinction between a nontechnical and a technical intervention here depends on whether or not some specialized knowledge or training with regard to biological functioning is required, other than that which is part of the general knowledge of all informed members of society. Thus, it is common knowledge that water and food must be taken regularly to avoid various signs of organismic discomfort. On the other hand, the knowledge that a diabetic must take sugar to reverse a hypoglycemic crisis is regarded as specialized, and such an intervention is regarded as technical. It should be noted that a technical intervention can be made by a person who does not himself have medical training.

The operational criteria for criterion B help differentiate distress or disability that is primarily due to something wrong within the organism from that which is primarily due to noxious environmental influences. The violation of this principle results in labeling dissidents in certain countries as mentally ill on the basis of their inability to conform to the political and social norms of a particular repressive society.

In practice it is often difficult to determine whether the distress or disability associated with a noxious environment (e.g., poverty, irritable wife, lack of opportunity for job advancement, warfare) represents an expected and "normal" reaction—in which case the organism is functioning properly—or a sign of organismic dysfunction, a disorder. At times a noxious environment may overwhelm the adaptive capacity of the organism resulting in a dysfunctional state. For example, this is the conceptual basis for distinguishing between a "normal" reaction of depressed mood to a business failure and an adjustment disorder with depressed features. In practice, making such distinctions often requires knowledge of subcultural norms and the frequency of various forms of reaction to environmental contingencies.

Criterion C. Conditions are not included if the associated distress, disability, or other disadvantage is apparently the necessary price associated with attaining some positive goal.

Some human conditions associated with distress or disability are not considered medical disorders because the intrinsic negative consequences are regarded as a necessary price for some positive goal. For example, the pain and disability associated with a wanted pregnancy are regarded as the price a woman must pay in order to have a child. Simple grief upon the loss of a loved one is apparently the price that one pays for having attachments.

When individuals undergo deprivation and distress in order to obtain some understandable positive goal, we assume that the organism is working and do not infer a dysfunction. Thus, the pain associated with repeatedly exposing oneself to the criticisms of one's esteemed colleagues in an effort to define mental disorder is not, by itself, evidence of a mental disorder. Clinically, the distress is less likely to be considered as due to a mental disorder to the extent that the positive goal is understandable and in keeping with reality.

Frequently the conditions which would be excluded on the basis of criterion C have widespread subcultural supports or sanctions. For example, there are nonmedical institutionalized ways of dealing with simple grief, and the medical care given to pregnant women is understood by all as preventing possible complications of pregnancy. It is the complications of pregnancy which are considered disorders.

Criterion D. Distinctness from other conditions in one or more of the following features: clinical phenomenology, course, response to treatment, familial incidence, or etiology.

The purpose of the criterion of distinctness is to ensure that the condition is conceptualized at the syndromal or disease level of understanding rather than being a mere symptom. A symptom is a condition that may be associated with many different disorders and therefore has only limited power to predict other facts of interest. A syndrome is a collection of symptoms (or signs) that co-vary and has more power than a symptom but nevertheless may be associated with a variety of underlying pathophysiological processes. A disease, on the other hand, implies knowledge of etiology or underlying processes. As is well known, most of the mental disorders represent syndromes rather than diseases since rarely is the etiology or underlying process known.

The operations by which syndromes and diseases are distinguished from each other and from symptoms consist of examining the extent to which the external correlates of interest differ. The more they differ, the more likely it is that the conditions represent syndromes or diseases and not mere symptoms. Tuberculosis is considered a medical disorder whereas cough is merely a symptom. Similarly, panic and depressive disorder (as defined in DSM-III) are disorders at the syndromal level although mere nervousness or unhappiness is considered a symptom.

DISTINCTION BETWEEN MENTAL DISORDERS AND OTHER MEDICAL DISORDERS

Examination of the entire medical classification system reveals that no single principle accounts for the allocation of disorders to various subgroupings. Some assignments appear to be on the basis of the organ systems that are involved, for example, there are subgroupings of circulatory disorders and endocrine disorders. Other subgroupings depend on knowledge of the etiology, for example, the subgroup of infectious and parasitic diseases.

For the most part, the disorders listed in the mental disorders portion of the medical classification system are those in which the presenting symptoms or behavioral manifestations are psychological rather than physical. Psychological manifestations as used here refer to disturbances in subjective feelings (other than physical pain), ideation, reality testing, and purposeful behavior. For this reason, as noted previously, we have merely defined mental disorders as the subset of medical disorders in which the manifestations are primarily signs or symptoms of a psychological (behavioral) nature, or if physical, can be understood only using psychological concepts.

The border between neurological and mental disorders is more blurred than that between mental disorders and the other medical disorders. To a great degree, whether or not a condition is considered neurological or mental depends on whether or not the manifestations are focal and stereotyped, or generalized to involve many aspects of personality functioning. Thus, psychomotor and temporal lobe epilepsy are considered neurological disorders, even though their manifestations are purely behavioral, whereas senile dementia and mental retardation are considered mental disorders, even when the specific brain pathology is known. (On the basis of this principle it has been argued that Gilles de la Tourette's disorder would best be classified as a neurological disorder, although traditionally it has been considered a mental disorder. It will be listed in DSM-III as a mental disorder only because failure to do so would remove it entirely from the current official classification system for medical disorders.)

In a few disorders the overt manifestations are primarily physical, yet they are regarded as mental disorders because the etiology is viewed as understandable only in psychological terms. Examples are conversion disorders and some sexual dysfunctions.

GUIDELINES FOR DETERMINING WHETHER AN INDIVIDUAL HAS A DISORDER

The discussion up to now has focused on the definition and criteria for determining whether a *condition* is a medical or mental disorder. The clinical problem is different in that it focuses on the individual patient and the need to determine whether any disorder can be presumed to be present. The clinical question can be loosely phrased as "Is this person sick?"

Agreed upon clinical or laboratory criteria are available for many medical disorders. DSM-III will contain specific operational criteria for all of the conditions listed (16). If a subject meets criteria for one of the disorders, it can be assumed that the disorder is present. It should be noted that frequently for both mental and other medical disorders the criteria for making the diagnosis do not require distress, disability, or overt signs of other disadvantage. For example, a diagnosis of lung cancer can be made on the basis of X-ray findings prior to any symptomatic manifestations of the disorder. Similarly, it is possible, although unlikely, for a diagnosis of schizophrenia to be made on the basis of clinical phenomenology using the DSM-III criteria in the absence of distress, disability, or other specific forms of disadvantage.

Frequently individuals have various symptoms or signs of impaired functioning that cannot be clearly classified into a distinct disorder. If the individual does not meet the criteria for any specific disorder, a reasonable assumption can be made that some form of disorder is present if his condition meets criteria A, B, and C for a medical disorder.

An example of such a situation might be an individual who demonstrated significant signs of anxiety or depressed mood (criterion A) but failed to meet the criteria for any specific DSM-III category. Furthermore, in the clinician's judgment it was unlikely that mere information or standard educational procedures or a nontechnical environmental change would relieve the condition. Finally, the distress of the condition was not apparently the necessary price associated with attaining some positive goal (criterion C). In DSM-III, such patients would be categorized either as some residual category within a group of disorders (e.g., atypical anxiety disorder, other psychosexual disorder), or in a final residual category, other or unspecified nonpsychotic disorder.

Frequently individuals come to the attention of the mental health professions with a problem that appears to be primarily related to environmental factors so that no inference of organismic dysfunction seems warranted. If the individual is distressed, the distress does not appear to be excessive or inappropriate given the circumstances. We expect grief following the loss of a loved one, and distress associated with a marital conflict that does not appear to be secondary to significant psychopathology is generally not viewed as a disorder. These examples are perhaps analogous to the earlier example of experiencing pain while one's foot is caught in the door.

DSM-III provides a list of such conditions under the rubric of "conditions not attributable to a known mental disorder," e.g., interpersonal relationship problem, occupational problem, life circumstance problem, and simple bereavement.

APPLICABILITY OF PROPOSED CRITERIA
TO DEVELOPMENT OF DSM-III

As we have noted earlier, since almost all of the traditional psychiatric disorders are associated, in their fully developed or extreme form, with either distress or disability, the utility of the proposed definition is best demonstrated by examining its relationship to decisions made about those conditions whose inclusion or exclusion from the nomenclature is controversial.

As mentioned before, homosexuality *per se* does not meet the criteria for the specific forms of disadvantage that we have proposed and will not be included in DSM-III as such. However, in environments which demand heterosexual functioning or punish homosexual functioning, homosexuality is frequently associated with distress. Therefore, according to our previous discussion, obligatory homosexuality could be viewed as a vulnerability. We recognize that slightly different specifications for the types of disadvantage other than distress or disability would have the effect of including homosexuality as a disorder. (Some have argued that both obligate homosexuality and obligate heterosexuality are disadvantageous as compared to bisexuality!)

On the other hand, there is another condition which is characterized by homosexual orientation and dissatisfaction or distress either regarding the inability to respond heterosexually or with the homosexual impulses themselves. This condition in the extreme form in all environments is directly associated with distress. For this reason, individuals with this condition frequently wish to assume the patient role and technical interventions may be of value in modifying the condition. Therefore, this condition does meet the criteria for a medical disorder and will be called dyshomophilia in DSM-III. Some homosexual activists assert that the distress associated with this condition is merely the result of environmental attitudes and sanctions. According to this logic, the condition would then not qualify as a disorder because it would presumably be reversible by nontechnical environmental changes or the provision of information. That this is the case is by no means clear, and we believe that the more prudent approach is to recognize the condition as a disorder so as to legitimize the patient role for those individuals with the condition who desire treatment.

The problem of categorizing lack of sexual responsivity highlights the problems involved in defining the boundary of medical disorder. Certainly, lack of sexual responsiveness is not intrinsically associated with distress or disability in a wide variety of areas. On the other hand, there is a clear organismic function involved in sexual response, such that the total absence of the response in appropriate circumstances supports the inference of an organismic dysfunction which is of some disadvantage.

In the earliest discussions of the Task Force's Advisory Committee on Sexual Disorders, the majority viewed lack of sexual responsiveness by itself as not sufficient to designate a mental disorder, unless accompanied by subjective distress or dissatisfaction. This was consistent with our first attempt to define mental disorder. Part of the appeal of this approach was the wish to avoid labeling as disordered individuals who were not distressed and had no signs of generalized disability. With our more recent definition, it is clear that the extreme form of lack of sexual responsivity represents a disadvantage which in our culture is viewed as significant enough to be considered a medical disorder. It is recognized that it will not be easy to develop criteria which sharply distinguish normal variation for this function from the disorder. However, subjective distress will not be required to make the diagnosis, although its presence will undoubtedly be a factor in a clinical judgment of the saliency of the condition in terms of the need for treatment.

Our conception of medical disorder forces us to recognize that frequently the so-called sexual dysfunctions are not medical disorders but are conditions that are the result of lack of information or are highly dependent on a specific environment (e.g., sexual partner's techniques). The claim for including these conditions as disorders in such instances is obviously much weaker than when there is evidence that they are clearly due to some internalized psychological conflict.

The Ninth Edition of the *International Classification of Diseases* lists Tobacco Dependence as a medical disorder within the mental disorder section. As they define the condition, mere physiological dependence is sufficient for the diagnosis even if not accompanied by any signs or symptoms of distress. If physiological dependence on a drug were by itself sufficient to regard use of that drug as a medical disorder, then one would have to categorize almost all tobacco users as well as most regular coffee drinkers as having a mental disorder. Application of the proposed criteria for medical disorder to the problem of tobacco use has helped the Task Force define tobacco use disorder in a more restricted and, we think, useful way. Thus, the essential feature of tobacco use disorder is described in the following manner:

> Just as alcohol and some other forms of drug use are by themselves not considered a mental disorder, so the use of tobacco is considered here as a disorder only when it fulfills the following criteria: the use of the substance is directly associated with either (1) distress at the need to repeatedly take the substance, or (2) there is evidence of both a tobacco related medical disorder and physiological dependence on tobacco. Heavy use of tobacco, with or without physiological dependence on nicotine, that does not meet the above criteria, is not regarded as a mental disorder here, although such behavior clearly predisposes to the development of Tobacco Use Disorder as well as a variety of serious medical disorders which are noted below under complications.

As here defined, the justification for regarding this condition as a medical disorder is criterion A.1 (distress) or A.3.d (atypical and inflexible sexual or other impulse-driven behavior which often has painful consequences).

Applying the four criteria to the problems of personality types has led the Task Force to distinguish between personality traits and personality disorders. Personality traits are habitual and pervasive predispositions to relate to the environment in a specific style, but any disadvantage from the possession of such traits is viewed as within the normal range of expected variability. Personality disorders, on the other hand, are by definition conditions in which the personality characteristics are so inflexible and maladaptive that they result in distress, disability, or significant disadvantage, such as marked impairment in the ability to form relatively stable and nonconflictual relationships.

The classification of conditions associated with antisocial behavior is also controversial. In both DSM-I and in DSM-II a distinction was made between antisocial behavior which was a consequence of a personality disorder and antisocial behavior which was associated with membership in a subcultural group which accepts or encourages the behavior. The former was considered a mental disorder, and the latter classified in DSM-II as one of the "conditions without manifest psychiatric disorder." If one applies the criteria for a medical disorder proposed here, this distinction is maintained. DSM-III will define antisocial personality disorder in such a way that a lifelong pattern of ineffectual social and occupational adjustment is required (criterion A.2 of disability in a wide variety of areas). Antisocial behavior which has strong subcultural supports, as in group delinquent activity, or in organized crime, or in apparent response to extreme poverty, will by itself not be evidence of a mental disorder, and will be classified as either childhood or adult antisocial behavior in the category of conditions not attributable to a known mental disorder.

Some individuals may engage in antisocial behavior which meets the criteria for a medical disorder on the basis of disadvantage associated with atypical and inflexible impulse-driven behavior which often has painful consequences (criterion A.3.d). Two distinct conditions which have been identified and which will be included in DSM-III on this basis are kleptomania and pyromania. Certainly the incomprehensibility of these conditions to the untrained observer is further support for viewing these conditions as evidence of an organismic dysfunction.

Undoubtedly, a large proportion of individuals involved in criminal behavior meet the criteria for antisocial personality disorder. Unfortunately, there may be little that the mental health professions now have to offer in treating such individuals. We do not regard these two facts as good reasons for excluding antisocial personality from the mental disorders as has been suggested elsewhere (11). Criminal behavior in an antisocial personality, as well as criminal behavior associated with other mental disorders, is now, for the most part, handled by the criminal justice system. The classification of a condition as a medical disorder and the response of society to manifestations of that condition are separate issues which should not be confused. Although it is true that the "sick role" implies some exemptions from certain responsibilities, the specific exemptions given by society vary considerably from condition to condition. Thus, the common cold or a wart receives far fewer exemptions than does a myocardial infarction. Similarly, criminal behavior which is part of an episode of psychotic illness usually is viewed as exempt from legal responsibility, whereas that associated with antisocial personality disorder is not.

The principle involved in criterion D, distinctness, has led the Task Force to exclude some conditions that were in DSM-II and appear in ICD-9. For example, the psychophysiological disorders, which were by and large listed by organ systems, have been excluded as specific mental disorders. Furthermore, listing a disorder such as asthma as a psychophysiological respiratory disorder violates the principle that mental disorders are a subset of medical disorders with primarily behavioral manifestations. Asthma is first of all a nonmental medical disorder and should be coded as such. However, there will be a provision in DSM-III for noting the degree to which psychological factors are judged of importance in the etiology or maintenance of any specific nonmental medical disorder, but this coding is not a diagnosis in the sense of a specific disorder.

ANTICIPATED CRITICISMS OF THE DEFINITION AND CRITERIA

We anticipate four major criticisms of the proposed definition and criteria: it is too broad; it is too narrow; it is atheoretical; and it is not useful (and this criticism hurts the most).

There are many who agree with the Schwartz's (11) that the concept of mental disorder, particularly in this country, has become "broad, diffuse, and vague" resulting in the inclusion of "almost any type of maladaptive or socially unacceptable behavior." They argue that even the traditional categories of personality disorders, drug and alcohol abuse, and sexual deviations should be removed from the official psychiatric nomenclature. Surely, such a view is incompatible with the definition and criteria proposed here which provide a rationale for including such disorders within the broad rubric of medical disorder.

One of the reasons for their desire to limit the concept of mental disorder to the major classic disorders, such as schizophrenia and affective disorders, is to focus the psychiatric profession on caring for the seriously ill, leaving individuals with less severe problems to nonphysician caretakers. This makes as much sense to us as arguing that the milder physical disorders, like the common cold and hay fever, should be removed from the medical nomenclature so that the attention of physicians can be directed toward more serious conditions, such as tuberculosis and coronary artery disease.

Some prominent psychologists also apparently believe that the DSM-III approach to defining mental disorder is too broad. At the April 1976 St. Louis Conference on Critically Examining DSM-III in Midstream, Dr. Maurice Lorr, representing the American Psychological Association, expressed the view that mental disorders (as medical disorders) should be limited to those conditions for which a biological etiology or pathophysiology could be demonstrated. Dr. George Albee (1), Ex-President of the American Psychological Association, recently expressed his concern that DSM-III was "turning every human problem into a disease, in anticipation of the shower of health plan gold that is over the horizon."

As we have tried to make clear throughout this chapter, not all pain or distress represents evidence of a medical disorder. To remind clinicians of this elementary observation, DSM-III provides a list of problems which frequently come to the attention of psychiatrists under the rubric of "conditions not attributable to a known mental disorder." Just as it makes no sense to argue that trigeminal neuralgia is not a medical disorder because of the lack of demonstrable pathophysiology or anatomical defect, so it seems unduly limiting to require the demonstration of a biological or pathophysiological etiology for a mental disorder.

Obviously there are professional boundary problems between psychiatry and psychology, and to a lesser extent with other mental health professions such as social work, pastoral counseling, and some forms of special education. The listing of a condition as a mental disorder for us says nothing about whether it can also be appropriately conceptualized as a psychological disorder, or which profession can best study or treat it.

At the other extreme, there are those who believe that any deviation from optimal functioning is synonymous with mental disorder. For example, Waugh (19) has proposed the following: "An emotional disorder is a psychological pattern or state that to some degree handicaps the individual from utilizing his or her own abilities and capacities." As Waugh acknowledged, his definition is such that essentially no one would meet the countercriteria for "normal."

It seems to us that such a broad definition of mental disorder is virtually meaningless, particularly as a guide toward the development of a classification of mental disorders. It has no more virtue than does the World Health Organization's (3) definition of health as "a state of complete physical, mental, and social well-being and not merely the absence of disease or infirmity." This approach in psychiatry would result in a different set of conceptual problems than we have addressed in this chapter as the profession would then have to agree on what represents optimal psychological functioning. This is no easy task.

Our approach has been criticized as being atheoretical. Other authors have attempted to define medical disorder within a biological or evolutionary framework. Klein (*this volume*) has defined disease as "covert, objective, suboptimal, part dysfunction, recognizing that functions are evolved and hierarchically organized." Scadding (10) first proposed the notion that disease represented biological disadvantage but failed to indicate the exact form that the disadvantage took. Kendell (7) attempted to use Scadding's approach with the classic psychiatric disorders and interpreted biological disadvantage to mean conditions which reduce fertility or shorten life. He acknowledged that such a restrictive interpretation excluded such ordinary medical disorders as postherpetic neuralgia and psoriasis. He concluded that even with this restricted definition of medical disorder, the major psychiatric disorders, such as schizophrenia and manic-depressive psychosis, could be justified as bona fide medical disorders.

Implicit in our approach to defining disorder is the concept of disadvantage. However, it differs from that of Scadding and Kendell in that it first focuses on the obvious disadvantage of distress and disability, and then deals with more subtle forms of disadvantage. In addition, our approach makes explicit an underlying assumption that is present in all discussions of disease or disorder, i.e., the concept of organismic dysfunction. In this sense it is similar to Klein's approach but we have ignored issues of evolution and the hierarchical organization of functions.

The ultimate issue in judging the proposed definition and criteria for medical and mental disorder is simply that it is useful. As eminent a nosologist as Feinstein (6) has asserted that "the only workable definition of disease is that it represents whatever the doctors of a particular era have defined as disease." We disagree. We believe that whether we like it or not, the issue of defining the boundaries of medical and mental disorder cannot be ignored. Increasingly there is pressure for the medical profession, and psychiatry in particular, to define its area of prime responsibility. We believe that the definition and criteria proposed here can contribute to such efforts by at least focusing on some of the major issues.

We recognize that some of the component terms in the operational criteria are not without some ambiguity. For example, when does a nontechnical environmental intervention become a technical intervention? (One of our critics asked whether it was a nontechnical intervention when a grandmother suggests to a parent that the bratty child should be ignored when he is fussy, but that it is a technical intervention if the grandmother happens to have a Ph.D. in behavioral psychology.) How soon does the reversal of the condition have to be after the nontechnical intervention of criterion B.2 for the condition to be excluded as a medical disorder? Whose value system determines whether or not a goal is positive, as noted in the exclusion criteria C? Other examples could be given.

The reader will have to determine for himself whether the examples of decisions made regarding DSM-III categories which were influenced by the definition support our contention that the definition and criteria have been useful. We now see no need to apologize for the fact that there has been a back and forth interaction between the formation of the definition and criteria and decisions made about what conditions to include or exclude from DSM-III and how they are to be defined. We contend that having a proposed definition helped focus the discussion and clarify the issues with regard to specific conditions, particularly all of the conditions on the border between what is generally considered obvious medical disorder and variations in normal functioning.

In the often polemical discussion of the appropriateness of the medical model for psychiatry, clearly the absence of an agreed on definition of both medical and mental disorder has been an obstacle seeming to give support to the view that mental illness has little in common with physical illness. We believe that we have demonstrated that core definition of medical disorder is applicable to the traditional mental disorders and that for those few medical and mental disorders which require additional justification, the same concept, disadvantage, is applicable to both.

CONCLUSIONS

For hundreds of years the medical profession has managed without a set of criteria for defining which conditions are to be considered medical disorders. There are those who argue that any attempt to provide such a definition, even with the recognition that it is tentative, is doomed to failure and will cause more problems than it will solve. We disagree. We have proposed a set of criteria for defining medical disorder which takes into account the complexities of the problem and is remarkably concordant in its classification of conditions which have traditionally been considered medical disorders, including the mental disorders. The principles involved in this definition have been useful in determining which conditions should be listed as mental disorders in DSM-III and in defining their boundaries. Finally, the successful application of the criteria for medical disorder to that subset termed mental disorders demonstrates the appropriateness of the medical model as applied to mental disorders.

ACKNOWLEDGMENTS

The authors gratefully acknowledge the assistance of the other members of the Task Force on Nomenclature and Statistics, in particular, Drs. Donald Klein and Rachel Gittelman-Klein. However, the views expressed here are the responsibility of the authors alone.

REFERENCES

1. Albee, G. W. (1977): Letter to the editor. *A.P.A. Monitor*, Vol. 8, February issue.
2. Ausubel, D. P. (1971): Personality disorder is disease. *Am. Psychol.*, 16:59–74.
3. Callahan, D. (1973): The WHO definition of "health." *Hastings Cent. Stud.*, 3:77–88.

4. Engelhardt, H. Tristram, Jr. (1974): The disease of masturbation: Values and the concept of disease. *Bull. Hist. Med.,* 48:234–248.
5. Feinstein, A. R. (1967): *Clinical Judgment.* Williams & Wilkins, Baltimore.
6. Feinstein, A. (1977): A critical overview of diagnosis in psychiatry. In: *Psychiatric Diagnosis.* Brunner Mazel, Larchmont, New York.
7. Kendell, R. E. (1975): The concept of disease and its implications for psychiatry. *Br. J. Psychiatry,* 127:305–315.
8. Moore, M. (1977): Legal conceptions of mental illness. In: *Philosophy and Medicine, Vol. 5.* Reidel, Netherlands.
9. Parsons, T. (1951): *The Social System.* The Free Press, Glencoe, Ill.
10. Scadding, J. G. (1967): Diagnosis: The clinician and the computer. *Lancet,* 2:877–882.
11. Schwartz, R. A., and Schwartz, I. K. (1976): Are personality disorders diseases? *Dis. Nerv. Syst.* 37:11, 613–617.
12. Sedgwick, P. (1973): Illness—mental and otherwise. *Hastings Cent. Stud.,* 3:19–58.
13. Siegler, M., and Osmond, H. (1974): *Models of Madness, Models of Medicine.* Macmillan, New York.
14. Spitzer, R. L. (1976): Further thoughts on pseudoscience in science and psychiatric diagnosis: A critique of D. L. Rosenhan's "Sane in insane places" and the "Contextual nature of psychiatric diagnosis." *Arch. Gen. Psychiatry,* 33:459–470.
15. Spitzer, R. L., and Endicott, J. (1976): Proposed definition of medical and mental disorder for DSM-III. Presented at the Annual Meeting of the American Psychiatric Association, Miami, Florida.
16. Spitzer, R. L., Endicott, J., and Robins, E. (1975): Clinical criteria for psychiatric diagnosis and DSM-III. *Am. J. Psychiatry,* 132:1187–1192.
17. Spitzer, R. L., and Wilson, P. T. (1975): Nosology and the official psychiatric nomenclature. In: *Comprehensive Textbook of Psychiatry,* edited by A. M. Freedman, H. I. Kaplan, and B. J. Sadock, pp. 826–845. Williams & Wilkins, Baltimore.
18. Stoller, R. J., et al. (1973): A symposium: Should homosexuality be in the APA nomenclature? *Am. J. Psychiatry,* 130:1207–1216.
19. Waugh, R. L. (1975): Letter to the editor. *Psychiatric News,* December 17.

Critical Issues in Psychiatric Diagnosis,
edited by Robert L. Spitzer and Donald F. Klein.
Raven Press, New York © 1978.

A Proposed Definition of Mental Illness

Donald F. Klein

*New York State Psychiatric Institute and Columbia University College of
Physicians and Surgeons, New York, New York 10032*

PROBLEM

The recent debate within the American Psychiatric Association whether homosexuality should be included in the *Diagnostic and Statistical Manual of Mental Disorders* is a salutory event. It indicates a growing awareness that labeling some behavioral pattern as a mental disorder has important personal and social consequences. Psychiatric diagnostic concepts should pass the harsh tests of substantive content, logical consistency, and practical relevance. This chapter's purpose is to sharply focus the issues, so that debate will not bog down in imprecise terminology and unspoken assumptions, varying interpretations of the evidence, or differing goals. Before proceeding to the statement of explicit criteria, we must clarify problems in terminology and classificatory goals.

Strikingly there is no explicit statement within the *Diagnostic and Statistical Manual of Mental Disorders* that defines the sort of condition categorizable within this document. Such a logical lapse is not restricted to psychiatry, however, since the *International Classification of Diseases* also lacks such a statement. It seems plain that these compendia are actually compilations of the sorts of things that physicians treat; a circular classificatory principle but a useful historical cue. Our definitions of illness are derived from medical practice.

Linguistic terms such as illness, disease, dysfunction, and deviance are produced by cultural history. Each term embodies the perceptions and preconceptions of a particular historical period. It is hardly surprising that beliefs developed 2,000 or even 200 years ago required modification. However, as our understanding progresses, there are various degrees of linguistic and conceptual lag. A historical approach to terms, concepts, and social practices clarifies the logical, substantive, and social issues.

Also, since these concepts justify various social practices, their revision may imply changes in rules prescribing how groups of people should do things (roles). Since such roles are often heavily invested in, an apparently academic semantic discussion of unusual heat may indicate the existence of opposing social interests, as well as different concepts of human functioning. A review of role theory with special reference to illness is necessary.

EXEMPT ROLES

A socially defined role entails a system of rights and duties. It defines the expectations regarding the action of others toward you and vice versa. Actions toward an individual can be in terms of the specific individual or as the representative of an institution. Further, the action may come from an individual acting as such or as an institutional representative.

Role relationships can be *fair,* implying equal exchange, or exploitative. Equal exchange is often defined monetarily but not necessarily.

Exploitative relationships are unstable unless masked as fair relationships, or stabilized by force, or involve specifically *exempt* roles.

In exempt roles the individual receives more than he gives manifestly, but exploitation is either denied or justified on the following grounds:

1. Exploitation is temporary and represents an investment to be repaid, often with interest. This is usually contractual.
2. Exploitation is temporary, regarded as a favor, and incurs an obligation for similar reciprocal exploitation—usually not contractual but enforced by shame mechanisms.
3. Exploitation is charitable—repayment is not necessary or required. This may be motivated by altruism or implied psychic returns such as self-approval and heavenly approval, or relief of the pain induced by empathy or sympathy.

A ratified false claim to an exempt role allows exploitative parasitism. This is widely resented because it deprives others of goods and diminishes their self-esteem thus making them feel deprived, helpless, and foolish. Therefore, claims to exempt roles are carefully scrutinized.

Examples of Exempt Roles

Self-Ascribed Exempt Roles

One cannot claim an exempt role except by asserting involuntary occupation of the role, e.g., "I can't help it, I'm not responsible."

Voluntary behavior is defined here as behavior whose performance is relatively easily modifiable through the procedures of instruction or reward and punishment, is expressed externally through the striate musculature during consciousness, and post-infancy is directable by self-instruction. Voluntary behavior is particularly evident under conditions of purposive goal pursuit. The term "voluntary" does not imply a specific faculty, the will, nor does it imply free will.

This is a crude definition of a crucial concept. Research into the characteristics and prerequisites of voluntary behavior is required. It is likely that there exist degrees of voluntariness dependent on the intactness of higher cortical functions, at least.

For a self-ascribed exempt role to become operational, others must ratify the claim. Examples of self-ascribed exempt roles are the beggar who appeals to charitable motivation, the borrower who appeals to economic investment, and the ill who appeal to psychic return and prevention of future losses.

In each case the role, if legitimate, is involuntary to some degree. Evidence of involuntariness serves a useful persuasive role; eliciting ratification. With beggars it becomes crucial to be obviously and hideously afflicted. The borrower is best received when his indigent state is due to exigencies beyond his control rather than self-indulgence. The ill person is most easily declared exempt if he has not predisposed himself toward illness—by pursuing private voluntary goals, e.g., overindulgence.

A particularly poignant aspect of exemption relates to criminal guilt. The standard is that a criminal action must be voluntary. It is generally conceded that illness, e.g., febrile delirium, is a defense against criminal responsibility although there is considerable argument concerning the details. If it can be claimed that voluntariness is impaired by illness, a strong exemption defense is possible. The theme of evidence for involuntariness will return in the definition of illness.

Assigned Exempt Roles

An exempt role may be declared by solicitation and affirmation or simply by assignment by others. Independent assignment by others may be reaffirmed, ignored, or resisted by the subject.

A specific controversial category of the other-ascribed exempt role is the dependent role where the individual does not have the full capacity for self-care. Care is then provided by others for the individual's own good; if necessary, over his objections.

This is a dangerous situation requiring careful scrutiny, since the assertion of protectorship may mask exploitative intent just as does the fallacious self-ascription of an exempt role.

Examples of assigned developmental exempt roles are preadult and senescent status. Assigned exempt roles also occur when there is impairment of ability to initiate a request for exempt status, as in unconsciousness, idiocy, or mental illness with impairment of insight and judgment.

If social needs are declared superior to individual rights, despite objections of the individual, there may be a judicial declaration of dependent status, as with the leper or typhoid carrier, or some psychotics.

A further danger is that social deviants who are not actually criminal or ill may have their civil liberties abrogated by being assigned to a dependent role, e.g., mentally ill, thus masking a repressive act as medical care. Such repression is possible only when the legislature, judiciary, press, and medical profession have accepted servile roles.

Unfortunately, concern for this risk may lead to an overreaction which prevents those with impaired insight and judgment from being assigned dependent status, and thus receiving needed care, unless they are immediately dangerous.

INVOLUNTARY SUFFERING, ILLNESS, AND EXEMPTION

Suffering is a perennial human problem. Certain forms of suffering appear part of anyone's lot, given certain life contingencies, e.g., hunger and thirst upon food and water deprivation, cold during the winter. These sufferings are predictable even with a low level of technology. They are related to universal biological needs and vulnerabilities in interaction with environmental stresses and deprivations.

Such easily recognizable, regularly occurring, predictable, potentially universal sufferings have led to individual, familial, and social practices designed to ameliorate or prevent them. Society's common working institutions, e.g., hunting, gathering, agriculture, herding, and construction, are remedies for distress of this nature. If this sort of suffering is unavoidable, self-application for exempt status income is common; usually to relatives or friends, more recently to the state. A positive response is contingent on the degree of involuntariness. Conversely, refusal often is justified by attribution of voluntariness: "He's just lazy."

Other contingent sufferings occur irregularly due to trauma, e.g., broken limbs or lacerations. Another body of social practice developed concerning such afflictions, the ancestor of traumatic surgery and nursing. Individuals suffering from disabling trauma generally request and receive exempt status. If the trauma interferes with brain function, e.g., concussion, delirium, unconsciousness, or amnesia, dependent status may be imposed. The involuntary affliction basis for exemption is evident.

Other irregularly occurring sufferings are due to psychological rather than physical trauma, induced by personal losses and deprivation. Here, too, society has developed a number of comforting practices, e.g., religious counsel and psychotherapy, to lessen the degree or shorten the period of suffering.

Grieving individuals are regularly granted moderate, transient exemptions, e.g., paid absence from work, neglecting household duties. Again, the emotional state is clearly involuntary and partially incapacitating. If prolonged, grief needs ratification as an illness (depression), or will lead to the withdrawal of exemptions on the basis that, "they're just feeling sorry for themselves," which implies willfullness.

All the above plights have an evident causation. In contrast, it was undoubtedly known from prehistoric days that individuals would begin to feel badly, suffering from pain, dizziness, malaise, etc., for no apparent reason. Further, these episodes of inexplicable discomfort were often accompanied by manifest bodily changes, e.g., rash or wasting, and behavioral changes and incapacities, e.g., cough, anorexia, or delirium.

This led to the social definition of the "patient" (Latin *pati;* I suffer), and the compensatory medical institution centered on the physician developed. Illness, like starvation, trauma, and bereavement, was an involuntary affliction, i.e., inflicted on the organism rather than self-inflicted, and justified a particular exempt role: the sick role.

THE SICK ROLE

Parsons (8) describes various aspects of the sick role. The sick person has involuntarily impaired functions. Consequently, it is only reasonable to exempt him from normal responsibilities, since such impairment cannot respond to voluntary effort. He cannot help being ill and cannot get well by an active decision. He wants to get well as soon as possible and will seek and employ appropriate help, usually a physician.

The sick person is expected to reduce being a social burden by those means under his control, e.g., seeking appropriate medical help. The expectation of help-seeking presumes that a sick person is able to recognize that something is wrong and what to do about it, demonstrating insight and judgment. When he does not, it is most frequently attributed to cognitive inability to evaluate his condition correctly, justifying a dependent sick role. If the inability to assess one's impaired condition correctly is attributed to other sources, e.g., an attempt to preserve self-esteem or a defensive maneuver such as denial, there is room for debate whether to assign a dependent sick role.

To recapitulate, illness was defined, prescientifically, as an inexplicable involuntary impairment or suffering that could not be attributed to understandable antecedents, i.e., need deprivation or physical or mental trauma, and implied that something had gone wrong. It was often accompanied by manifest bodily changes, but not necessarily. The attribution of illness entitles the patient to occupy a specific exempt status—the sick role.

IS THE SICK ROLE AN ARBITRARY SOCIAL LABEL?: DEFINITION OF ILLNESS

Sedgwick (10) states that the term "illness' is irreducibly evaluative. There is no mental or physical illness in nature; there is simply a variety of things happening to a variety of organisms. The human evaluation of certain conditions as being deviant and undesirable leads to their segregation as states of illness. This point of view is plausible but suffers from both overinclusiveness and a failure to understand the systematic implications of modern biology.

As indicated above, not all deviant, undesirable states are called illness, but rather only prescientifically obscure involuntary conditions implying that something has gone wrong, that result in suffering or incapacity. For instance, poverty-engendered theft, although both deviant and undesirable, is not called illness. The necessary crucial inference is that something has gone wrong, not simply that something is undesirable.

The historical social term "illness" can now be recognized as a hybrid concept, with two necessary components; something has gone wrong involuntarily, and the results are sufficiently major to justify the sick, exempt role by a particular society. The latter component is plainly a variable related to historical stage and cultural traditions. However, with increased biological understanding, determinable impairments of evolved functions provide a material, objective basis to the determination that something has gone wrong. To develop this necessary idea requires some extended discussion.

CLASSIFICATION AND CAUSATION OF ILLNESS

In early society, medical practices were necessarily primitive, and usually nonspecific, considering the lack of comprehension of pathogenic processes. They were primarily derived, on the one hand, from religious and demonological concepts, and on the other from environmental and culinary manipulation.

Great clinicians, such as Hippocrates and Sydenham, observed certain regularities about patients. Initially, illnesses were usually labeled in terms of single, discrete clinical manifestations. Therefore, diagnostic terminology initially contained monosymptomatically defined conditions such as fever, rash, or asthma.

Sydenham developed two taxonomic concepts of great utility: syndrome and course. In a syndrome several clinical manifestations coexist frequently and, therefore, deserve segregation as a single descriptive entity. With regard to course, an illness is described not only according to immediate manifestations but with regard to the evolving clinical history. This concept is particularly trenchant in psychiatry. On a cross-sectional basis many behavioral patterns may appear simply normal variations, but from the point of view of life history a peculiar inflexibility and repetitiveness can be noted that raises the question of illness.

Using these concepts, Sydenham separated the clustered temporal pattern of gout (acute inflammatory joint exacerbations with complete remissions) from rheumatism (chronic inflammations with intercurrent deficits). The resemblance of Sydenham's work to Kraepelin's distinction between manic-depressive and schizophrenic illness is unmistakable.

Once phenomenological regularities were classified, the search for causation became possible. Given historical ignorance, the various etiologic nosologies propounded were understandably crude.

Since much suffering was acute and self-limiting, a hypothesis developed that it was due to a temporary invasion by invisible external agents. Although elaborated into demonological possession theory, the basic inference of external invasion was a good one, later validated by the discovery of bacteria and viruses.

Noteworthy as a precursor of later theories of dynamic harmony was the belief that the healthy organism contained a certain balance of humors; illness was best understood as a chaotic disharmony due to relative humoral imbalances. It is generally characteristic of prescientific explanation that a wide variety of phenomena are explained by appeals to single causes or the balance of contending forces. The attempt to stipulate causation is often contested on the basis that things are simply chaotic. Sydenham (3) repudiated the general supposition "that diseases are no more than the confused and irregular operations of disordered and debilitated nature, and consequently that it is a fruitless labor to endeavor to give a just description of them." Unfortunately, speculative hypotheses and philosophical systems did much to cloud the perception of regular patterns; what is now called the natural history of disease.

The basic problem was, to use engineering talk, of analyzing the human "black box." One could not look within the body and empirically analyze the underlying process. Therefore, early medicine was stuck with pure descriptive nosology and speculative causation. However, with the development of the microscope, chemistry, and autopsy began the empirical study of the processes underlying illness.

During the nineteenth century an enormous wave of new knowledge indicated that clinically discrete syndromes were frequently associated with specific morphological or physiological deviances. Further, with the germ theory of disease, and knowledge of cellular function, biological defenses, and immunity, relatively complete explanations of certain illnesses developed that stipulated both necessary and sufficient causal networks.

General medicine has undergone a historical evolution. Its field of relevant practice is now socially defined as the treatment of illness by affecting underlying pathogenic processes, empirically if necessary, but preferably based on rational understanding.

Because of this evolution there is now some question as to the appropriate limits of medical practice. Previously the doctor treated any help-seeking or dependent, obscurely suffering, or incapacitated person. Since the most rational medicine is based on understanding and ameliorating underlying pathogenic processes, treating suffering without understanding causation is often considered second-grade symptomatic intervention at best or quackery at worst. Therefore, there is considerable pressure for practitioners to assert a scientific understanding of the pathogenesis of illness. In general, the self-serving testimony of interested parties requires meticulous scrutiny.

Once it was possible to objectively detect covert disease, the concept of illness expanded with tremendous public health impact. It appeared evident that manifest clinical illness was simply a late stage of progressive subclinical process. If chronic hyperglycemia and glycosuria were demonstrated in an asymptomatic person, he was still considered to have diabetes.

It is conceptually helpful to distinguish between clinical manifestations and underlying processes, and to develop appropriate labels. Feinstein (4), for instance, suggests the straightforward model that the *host* acquires a *disease* and manifests an *illness*. Historically, from unclassified observations and airy speculation, we have progressed to discovering "illness" (clinical nosology) through classifying "disease" (morbid anatomy) to understanding "disease process" (etiology and pathophysiology). I shall adopt the term "disease" to refer to covert pathogenic processes, recognizing that many consider the terms "illness" and "disease" as synonyms. Disease is covert dysfunction. With scientific advance covert dysfunctions, even psychological ones, have become more and more accessible.

However, not all manifest dysfunctions will receive the social appellation of illness and thereby justify the sick role. Only dysfunctions of sufficient magnitude so as to incite social concern and a tolerance for exemption have been referred to as illnesses in the past.

This is plainly a social evaluation and indicates what is right about Sedgwick's (10) critique. Referring to a person as ill is a social evaluation but not a simply arbitrary one. To support this label requires evidence allowing a reasonable, necessary inference of an underlying dysfunction. The class of dysfunctions is inclusive of the class of illnesses.

Also, whereas the term "illness" was socially applied in previous years only to cases of manifest severe disability, three trends have resulted in the term "illness" being applied more widely. First, with rising affluence minor indispositions become socially acceptable as warranting an exempt role. In line with this, personal testimony that one is incapacitated is more often accepted at face value. Finally, since illness has been shown to be a late stage of subclinical process, by extension the term "illness" has been applied to those who show no manifest dysfunction at all, but are potentially ill. Nonetheless, despite this broadening of the range of applicability of the term "illness," all legitimate usages imply actual dysfunction.

Unfortunately, psychiatry is still largely in the seventeenth century, diagnosing black boxes by syndromal and course analysis and treating them with empirical, often poorly validated, procedures. Since many suffering people who seem ill have no demonstrable morbid anatomy or physiological dysfunction, we are still participating in the debate between specific organic causation versus various functional disharmonies (e.g., intrapsychic conflict, aversive conditioning) versus a role playing model.

FUNCTIONAL ILLNESS, DISEASE, ABNORMALITY, AND THE DEFINITION OF DYSFUNCTION

Illness was originally indicated by inexplicable suffering or incapacitation. Many suffering people were found to be diseased, i.e., manifesting specific structural or physiological abnormalities. However, one could persistently panic and have insomnia after a severe fright, thereby manifesting illness, without apparent physiological cause, as in traumatic neurosis. Further, one could incapacitate and induce manifest chronic distress in animals by confronting them with situations of insoluble conflict. The illness seems the outcome of requiring the experimental animal to cope in a situation that exceeds their coping. These experimental interventions produce no physical trauma and no apparent immediate physiological damage, yet the psychological mechanisms are impaired. Such illness is clearly an involuntary affliction. Thus arose the concept of functional illness, that is, psychological impairment, often resulting in maladaptation, without physiological or structural pathology.

Could one be diseased without being ill? Obviously one could detect a covert lung carcinoma by X-ray, prior to any clinical manifestations. Such a person was diseased even if not ill. However, the historical reason that carcinoma was defined as a disease was that it was often found in ill people. Further, its growth pattern was such that it was readily comprehensible that it would eventually produce suffering. Subclinical disease was originally defined by the predictable appearance of an associated illness.

The question arises: can one define disease in a fashion conceptually independent of illness? Is there a positive, scientifically definable criterion for pathogenic process or disease? Can one distinguish an abnormal disease state from simple biological variation without using illness as a necessary criterion? Unless we can do this we will not be able to meet Sedgwick's criticism that all illness and disease categories fundamentally represent nothing but arbitrary social evaluation. How do we know that something has gone wrong?

There are two usual definitions of abnormality. The common statistical definition of abnormality simply means unusual. Something is abnormal if it is rare. There is no necessary implication that something has gone wrong since there is biological variability among people, and someone is bound to be at an extreme!

Nonetheless, there is a strong presumption that something has gone wrong if something is sufficiently unusual. If a patient has a hemoglobin count of 5 g/100 ml, any doctor would be certain that this does not represent simply a normal biological variation. Something has gone wrong with the usual hemoglobin regulatory mechanism, e.g., dietary peculiarity, hemolytic disease, or covert bleeding. Therefore, infrequency is a useful indicator that something may have gone wrong, but it is not essential or sufficient.

If we do not equate infrequency with dysfunction, we need another basis to infer abnormality: deviation from a specific standard. This conception of abnormality is particularly useful when you wish to refer to a common condition as being nonetheless pathological, e.g., the ubiquitous dental caries. Plainly, dental caries are frequently associated with a specific illness—toothache. But can we define caries as due to a disease without referring to the associated illness?

By extension, the same question arises about every discernible variation in physiological or psychosocial functioning. If we do not refer to an associated illness, what justifies considering any particular variation as disease? Can we arrive at a standard that is not simply an expression of personal preference, but is given to us by the biology of the situation? I propose that evolutionary theory allows us to infer such a standard—suboptimal functioning—and further helps us to objectively specify the optimum. This often allows us to state that something is biologically wrong, not simply that it is rare or objectionable.

EVOLUTION AND DISEASE

Our current scientific beliefs concerning evolution (in brief, oversimplified form) involve the following factually supported hypotheses:

    I. The basis of life is a self-duplicating molecular structure.

    II. These self-duplicating structures develop variations (mutations), some of which are also self-duplicating.

    III. These variations interact with the environment.

    IV. Certain heritable variations result in maximizing self-duplication and, therefore, become more common. Other variations result in less self-duplication and, therefore, tend to become extinct. This process is known as natural selection.

    V. Since the rate of self-duplication is a function of environmental circumstances, species develop a variety of ancillary biological equipment and practices, through variation and selection, fulfilling specific adaptive functions. Those equipments that foster survival for a period of effective self-duplication tend to be retained and form the basis for successive genetic modifications to the degree that they are hereditary.

    VI. These equipments allow many ancillary adaptive functions. To list a few we have:

    A. Energy gathering
      1. Photosynthesis
      2. Predation
        a. Herbivore
        b. Carnivore
    B. Information gathering
      1. Hearing
      2. Sight
      3. Touch, etc.
    C. Homeostatic preservation of the internal milieu
    D. Patterns of differentiation and development

E. Psychological functions
   1. Perception
   2. Learning
   3. Thinking
   4. Memory
   5. Emotion
   6. Motivation, etc.
F. Goal-directed behavior
   1. Appetitive
   2. Consummatory
   3. Avoidant
   4. Agonistic, etc.

This list could be indefinitely extended, but the point should be clear that each species has developed, through evolution, a complicated webwork of interacting adaptive, regulatory, and behavioral processes. Many of these processes are self-regulatory. Through the intricate processes of negative feedback and error comparison, these processes act as if they had goals or even a hierarchy of goals. This makes the detection of functional goals simpler, since they appear as invariants despite environmental perturbations.

VII. Since the organism must survive to allow reproduction, most adaptive mechanisms serve an overall organismal goal of survival and minimization of biological disadvantage, in addition to their specific functions.

The biologist studying life processes makes hypotheses as to the functional goals of the various bodily systems. These hypotheses are just like any other hypotheses; they integrate what is known and allow the development of new knowledge. They can be disproven if their implications are false.

For instance, it seems evident that among the functions of the digestive tract are processing and absorption of nutrients and discarding of wastes. If peristalsis stops, as in intestinal atony, these functions cannot be carried out. It is certainly no arbitrary statement on my part, reflecting social or individual values, if I state that lack of peristalsis is a dysfunctional state—a suboptimal deviation from evolutionarily determined process and the result of disease. Sedgwick's critique ignores the possibility of objectively determining correct biological function. No one will deny that this is difficult in practice. Sedgwick, however, has implied that this cannot be accomplished, even in principle, and this is plainly false. As Aubrey Lewis (7) states, "the concept of disease, then—and of health—has physiological and psychological components, but no essential social ones."

It is my contention that all such suboptimal part dysfunctions may be considered diseases of the specific function in question, without any reference at all to the question of whether there is an associated illness. Obviously any serious dysfunction, interfering with a major regulatory process, is likely to cause suffering or incapacitation and, therefore, a recognizable illness. However, manifest illness is not necessary to define suboptimization.

With growing biological knowledge, we will be able to make more and more exact statements concerning optimum part and integrative functioning from an engineering point of view. When an engineer studies a thermostat's structure, he should be able to state its degree of responsiveness and efficiency and whether certain structural or wiring patterns will interfere with its functioning. Such patterns would be definable as defects even without actually putting the thermostat to an operating test. Our grasp of our own biological engineering (physiology) is still primitive. Therefore, we usually investigate disease processes only after dysfunction has been made manifest by illness.

Yet another complication must be raised here. Optimum functioning can be defined only with regard to specified environments. It seems evident that certain physiological functions are optimum and adaptive to the Arctic but would be suboptimum and maladaptive for the tropics, e.g., spheroidal versus elongated body. The need to relate the assessment of optimum physiological functioning to specific environments makes for great complexities but still does not relegate the notion of optimum to the arbitrary category of pure idiosyncratic evaluation.

Also, the idea of dysfunction must be related to the organism's compensatory hierarchical organization. Function A may be impaired and function B may pick up the load so that some superordinate function C is maintained unimpaired. Under these circumstances function A is diseased, whereas function B is not, and, therefore, function C is not. Function B may well have changed, but insofar as it is one of B's functions to compensate for dysfunction in A, there has been no suboptimization of function B. In this particular case there would be dysfunction at one level but no dysfunction at a superordinate level—one example of disease without illness.

Since "illness" implies that something has gone wrong, all illnesses are secondary to disease, that is, suboptimal functions. However, we can have functional impairment at all levels of integration including psychological functions. It is true that inferences are more difficult in functional illnesses, because of our ignorance. Therefore, the evidence for mental illness needs careful review.

EVIDENCE OF MENTAL ILLNESS

What evidence provides strong support for the allegation of mental illness? By mental illness we mean a subset of all illnesses that presents evidence in the cognitive, behavioral, affective, or motivational aspects of organismal functioning. Attribution of such illness often entitles the patient to the exempt status of the sick role. Clear evidence of involuntary impairment is the crucial issue since this has the dual role of implying an underlying dysfunction and eliciting social concern.

We have the following types of contributory evidence:

1. There is clear-cut evidence of physical disease that regularly leads to the behavioral syndrome displayed, e.g., syphilis and general paresis, senile brain deterioration and confusion.
2. The behavioral syndrome is clearly associated with a necessary specific genetic predisposition.
3. The syndrome has a regular physiological abnormality antecedent to the behavioral syndrome.
4. The syndrome is regularly associated with premature death.
5. There is a manifest impairment of a definable psychological function.

Aubrey Lewis (7) has put this succinctly:

Besides subjective feelings and degree of total efficiency, the criterion of health is adequate performance of functions, physiological and psychological. So far as we cannot designate formal, major functions of the human organism and lack means for judging whether they work efficiently, we are handicapped in recognizing health and illness in a reliable and valid way. The physiological functions can be thus designated and judged far more satisfactorily than the psychological. We can, therefore, usually tell whether an individual is physically healthy, but we cannot tell with the same confidence and consensus of many observers, whether he is mentally healthy.

In the extreme this is simple. If an adult does not remember what he had for breakfast he has a memory defect. One can develop a roster of all psychological part functions, e.g., memory, anticipation, and deductive thinking, and with sufficient normative study develop procedures for grossly defining rare defect states, to be followed by engineering process analyses.

Other evolved capacities can be stipulated at a more molar level. The hedonic organization of human behavior is well known. Evolutionary theory indicates that the utility of the pain mechanism derives from the fact that it is regularly aroused by dangerous situations. Usually traumatic pain incites the individual to either leave the situation or decrease the danger (flight or fight). Pain or suffering, intrinsic to illness, is good evidence that a derangement has occurred since usually no external adaptive purpose is served.

Pleasure is almost always related to situations that foster either individual survival or reproduction. Therefore, hedonic organization has a key reality evaluative, behavior organizing function. In addition, the primary pleasure-pain axis is related to a variety of positive and negative affective behavioral steering states.

Plainly, if the hedonic affective steering system itself is not performing well, then the individual is ill, as in the case of those who suffer from depression where there is no actual loss, fear where there is no danger, or elation where there is no reward. This concept subsumes intrinsic distress as an illness criterion.

Humans also have developed a remarkable anticipatory mechanism that produces behavioral steering affects such as anxiety and hope. The occurrence of such affects out of proportion to perceived positive or negative future states, or, conversely, the absence of such affect when a person should be able to clearly anticipate such eventualities, speaks for a disorder of the anticipatory mechanism.

If none of the above holds, we are less certain, but logical inference is still possible.

PUTATIVE DISORDERS

For both ego-syntonic and ego-dystonic putative disorders the following criteria suggest that some function has been impaired and that the condition is not better considered as malingering, unhappiness, ideological conviction, personal preference, or normal inflexible variation.

The general positive indications of dysfunction are listed below:

1. Syndromal clarity.
2. Normalization of syndrome by pharmacological or physical interventions.
3. Endogenous course.
4. If precipitated, resembles states with endogenous course.
5. Resists self-instruction.
6. Resists negative consequences and cannot be markedly modified by positive rewards.

Indications of Dysfunction Specially Relevant to Ego-Dystonic Putative Disorders

If one convincingly presents disability or distress, without the likelihood of a fallacious purposive claim, illness is generally confirmed, especially if any of the stronger indications, such as syndromal clarity, are present. Useful evidence that makes malingering or unhappiness unlikely includes:

1. Benefits of sick role far exceeded by distresses entailed.
2. No evident gains such as defense against criminal charges, prosecution of personal injury claims, or excuse from arduous or hazardous life circumstances.
3. Willing cooperation with examination and treatment.

4. Distress intrinsic to condition rather than secondary unhappy reaction to misfit with environment.
5. No lying, inconsistency, or exaggeration with regard to functional loss.
6. History of competent social performance (the converse does not hold).

All of these indications weigh against the conclusion that the disorder is feigned.

Indications of Dysfunction Specially Relevant to Ego-Syntonic Putative Disorders

Possible ego-syntonic disorders are obviously not malingering since there is no attempt to achieve the sick role; rather, the reverse.

Nonetheless, there may be good reason for considering someone ill despite his protestations. The psychotically intoxicated LSD user who insists he has X-ray vision and isn't that grand offers one example. Difficulties arise where cause is not obvious and gross disorganization or incapacity is not apparent. Useful indications are:

1. Syndrome strongly resembles syndromes where either spontaneously or with medical treatment the patients change their opinions concerning formerly ego-syntonic wishes or belief (e.g., suicidal wish in depression or delusions in schizophrenia) in a direction consonant with normal adaptation.
2. Patient unable to persistently modify behavior to demonstrate that it is under voluntary control.
3. Behavior not due to special ideological stand, supported by subcultural values.
4. Behavior is incomprehensibly out of proportion to ideology of upbringing or even in direct opposition to it, persisting despite severe sanctions.
5. Patient's actions do not promote desires we find intelligible in the light of rational beliefs. This is not a sufficient indicator of illness as it raises thorny problems of social deviance.
6. Behavior markedly inflexible. This is also not a sufficient indication of illness, but does incite suspicion.

Being left-handed is an ego-syntonic involuntary inflexibility, usually due to a normal variation in cerebral dominance. The usual debate will be over the likely normality of the cause, i.e., biological variation or diseased left cerebral hemisphere. It is hard to believe that the inflexible attitudes of the transsexual are due to a normal biological variation. Further, if the behavior regularly incurs severe negative consequences, the question arises why it continues to be ego-syntonic.

Humans are capable of an almost species-specific flexibility in goal pursuit as well as the capacity to shift from subgoal to subgoal in the pursuit of overall goals. The lack of such flexibility is viewed by me as possible evidence of psychological dysfunction. This is not an intrinsically social criterion of illness, although inflexibility may be made most apparent by fluctuating social circumstance.

Inflexibility can most easily be ascertained when a behavioral pattern (that may have once been adaptive) is maintained under circumstances where it incurs suffering. This may meet the primary criterion of involuntary impairment since simple voluntary self-instruction does not work.

The problem is that we do not know the boundaries of our species' flexibility, except by unsystematic consensus. When we are confronted by involuntary inflexibility, combined with the common experience that similarly aged and trained people can be flexible in such circumstances, the belief that such inflexibility indicates that something has gone wrong receives support. An even more problematic situation occurs when a behavior can be considered inflexible, but due to a good ecological fit, suffering and failure do not occur.

Another problem is that moderate inflexibility may be a matter of early training or overtraining. Therefore, atypical inflexibility that is out of proportion to training is probably a more refined criterion of psychological dysfunction than unqualified inflexibility. However, conflict of opinion is certainly possible concerning the degree of disproportion.

Are "bad habits" to be considered as possible disorders because of their inflexibility? The term "habit" refers to a relatively simple acquired act which by repeated performance and reinforcement has become prepotent. Nonreinforcement of operant acts usually leads to extinction. Learning theorists hold that if it appears that a behavior should extinguish, but it persists, either there is covert reinforcement or something is wrong with the extinction procedure or mechanism. Further, behavior is molded by both positive and negative consequences of the act. Habitual behavior regularly associated with negative consequences tends to disappear. In humans such extinction seems supplemented by self-instruction.

It is not clear that most socially identified bad habits are necessarily manifested of inflexibility. Many are simple tension release devices without marked aversive consequences. For instance, the person who publicly picks his nose has immediate tension relief and very slight, if any, social negative feedback. No serious attempt is usually made to either self-instruct in opposition to such behavior or to develop systematic aversive consequences for the continuation of this behavior. Plainly, such "bad habits" cannot *a priori* be considered as evidence of inflexibility, but may be simple deviant behavior.

However, some bad habits are reputed to abnormally resist change. If true, they seem not to obey the same laws of acquisition and extinction as ordinary habits. The social learning theorists have not dealt critically with this question. If one must postulate some peculiarity, e.g., Eysenck's lack of reactive inhibition, to account for a habit's inextinguishability, then this behavior is due not to ordinary learning but to extraordinary learning.

Other conditions, such as compulsive smoking, are sometimes loosely considered bad habits. The appetitive pattern of keen immediate pleasure followed by cognitively vague future negative effects is apparent, which is not a part of ordinary habit formation. The possibility of pharmacological withdrawal producing aversive steering affects further complicates matters by raising the issue of a special class of addictive behavior. The frequent marked inflexibility of this behavior is evident, but stopping is no problem; staying stopped is the difficulty.

Significantly, what may be the most successful form of treatment does not consist of the usual habit breaking techniques, i.e., extinction with non-reward and/or coupling with aversive conditioning, but rather in the expansion of the impact of the anticipatory mechanism via forceful instruction or hypnosis to the effect that the person is clearly damaging himself and is self-responsible.

Human behavior is often the result of a conflict between the anticipation or experience of immediate pleasures and the anticipation of future losses, or, psychoanalytically, between the pleasure and reality principles. Reinforcement of the vividness of negative anticipations creates an inhibition of immediate pleasure seeking behavior, and even the loss of conscious pleasurable anticipation. This educative procedure apparently breaks through the defensive denial and minimization that prevents the adequate anticipatory aversive affect (anxiety) necessary for overcoming pleasurable anticipation and consequent self-damaging activity.

This formulation seems as persuasive as the simple learning formulation but accounts for certain phenomena better. For instance, smoking has declined more among doctors than among other comparably well-educated professionals as a response to the now well-publicized dangers. An obvious guess would be that their exposure to illness and better understanding of pathogenesis make their anticipatory imagery more vivid, anxiety producing, and, therefore, more behavior molding. It is not likely that doctors are particularly gifted in modifying habits in general.

Another type of change-refractory habit occurs when one has learned to avoid upon receipt of a signal of an aversive stimulus, e.g., the trained dog who gets off a potentially electrified grid when warned by a bell signal. This behavior does not extinguish; the dog can never learn if the shock is turned off since he is no longer on the grid. Ignorance maintains the behavior. This bears some resemblance to traumatically induced phobias and lends some rationale to an empirically effective treatment: forced *in vivo* extinction.

However, humans with traumatic phobias claim to know that their fears are unfounded but cannot bring themselves into the feared situation, experiencing strong negative affects when they make the attempt. Self-instruction has become ineffective in the face of the affective state. The unrealistic affective state implies an overactive anticipatory mechanism that effectively prevents experiential extinction.

Therefore, I suggest that habits that are atypically change-refractory, even though they incur negative consequences, do imply an involuntary inflexibility in the unlearning mechanism that qualifies for the term "dysfunction." The anticipatory anxiety mechanism may be at fault, by ineffective underactivity with regard to pleasurable but self-damaging habits and by overactivity with regard to avoidant habits. No claim is made that this necessarily arises from underlying physiological abnormality, although this is possible. On the other hand, developmental experience may modify anticipatory capacity; a researchable question.

I propose that marked inflexibility be considered a possible indication of human mental dysfunction but recognize operational measurement difficulties. However, if a person evidences an earnest attempt to change a certain behavior or goal and is unable to do so, then there is a case for inflexibility and involuntary impairment, if such behavioral change is commonly attained.

A recurrent problem is whether illness should be attributed to ego-syntonic deviant patterns that are characterized only by inflexibility, obligate behavior, and minority aspirations. A prime case is obligate homosexuality. It is possible that such behavior is secondary to impaired psychosexual functions, and many claim that this is the case. The evidence is not overwhelming, however. Since the mental illness label still has power as a stigma, we should be as conservative as possible and not attribute illness to purely inflexible behavior without decisive evidence of impairment.

If an obligate homosexual becomes unhappy with his lot, tries to perform heterosexually and cannot, he thereby demonstrates operationally an intrinsic involuntary incapacity sufficient to elicit social concern, should be considered ill, and is entitled to the sick role. The happy homosexual may be suspected of underlying disease, but currently the issue is moot.

SOCIAL DEVIANCE AND ILLNESS

Until recently behavioral deviants were considered either physically ill, ignorant, bad, stupid, or insane. Physical illness as an involuntary incapacitation justified related social deviance by subsuming it under the sick role. Therefore, no behavior-correcting action was called for nor would it be effective.

Ignorance could be modified by education. Badness could be deterred by punishment or modified by reward of alternative behaviors. These methods were on the whole quite successful in producing desired behavior or removing undesired actions.

On occasion, however, some deviant people did not respond as expected. Some had great difficulty in learning, although they seemed responsive to reward and punishment. These people had impaired educability; thus developed the concepts of stupidity, degrees of intelligence, and mental defectiveness.

Confusingly, some bad people seemed intelligent enough but their transgressions did not respond to punishment. Such incorrigible deviants were of two types. One group seemed to be pursuing understandable, although socially undesirable goals, such as theft or rape, presumably as voluntary acts. When they broke laws they were classified as criminals. If they did not respond to punishment, they were labeled incorrigible criminals.

Another group of social deviants also seemed incorrigible, but their goals and actions were incomprehensible. Such people were considered, in common parlance, irrational, crazy, or, legalistically, insane. Many but not all appeared to be suffering or involuntarily incapacitated, so that the legitimacy of considering them ill engendered much debate. Further, they were often not help-seeking, which made treatment impossible unless it was stipulated that "insight" was impaired and the gravity of the situation required assignment to a dependent role.

The entire group of incorrigible social deviants, the mentally defective, the criminal, and the insane were often exposed to successively severer forms of punishment in the dim hope that this usually effective mode of social shaping would finally work. The failure of punishment led to exclusion from society in the form of vagabondage, jails, asylums, exile, starvation, execution, etc. Theories of theological retribution for sinfulness were useful in easing this process of social exclusion.

Those with chronic medical illnesses, especially when reduced to a socially parasitic role, often underwent similar processes of stigmatization and social rejection. This indicates that the exemptions of the sick role are a grudging concession by society, justified by the hope of remission. Under conditions of relative economic scarcity, parasitism is resented; it is expected that everyone pulls his own weight. Therefore, societal acceptance of the sick role becomes strained by chronicity, and there is a distinct tendency to withdraw support. This may account for the peculiar situation whereby the allocation of resources for the treatment of acute illness far outweighs those devoted to the much more important problem of the treatment of chronic illness.

With the recognition that illness was often the manifestation of a demonstrable underlying disease, and that not all diseases caused manifest suffering, the question was then raised whether the various incorrigible deviant behavioral syndromes were not secondary to incapacities deriving from covert diseases, and that they were erroneously conceived as simple voluntary behavior. The lack of help-seeking behavior was explained as a lack of "insight"—the ability to recognize one's illness. Failure to seek help is comprehensible as another incapacity, analogous to unconsciousness and delirium.

Understandably, the hypothesis of underlying disease was often most staunchly defended by humanitarians who wished to extend the sick role to defectives, criminals, and the insane and treat them with the same consideration given the medically ill. It is a mistake, however, as Begelman (2) has indicated, to assert that mental illness was simply a metaphorical extension of the notion of physical illness. It was instead a contrademonological hypothesis asserting that mental illnesses belong within the same naturalistic framework of understanding as physical illnesses. This assertion is substantive and not metaphorical.

Ironically, changes in social attitudes have, for some socially deviant groups, converted this previously liberal humanitarian stand into what some believe to be a hampering, stigmatizing one. For instance, obligate homosexuality has long been recognized as a social deviation. It has been stigmatized as bad or even criminal in many societies. The categorization of homosexuality as due to underlying disease and, therefore, an illness, rather than a type of incorrigible criminality, was viewed by many liberal people as a distinct social advance. As an illegal act, punishment, obloquy, and social extrusion were indicated. As an illness, medical study, therapy, and social pity were engendered even though suffering and help seeking were not intrinsic parts of the syndrome.

Recently, due to a marked moral shift, sexual acts between consenting adults are more generally considered a private affair. Therefore, homosexuality has been effectively decriminalized in many jurisdictions. However, homosexuals are still confronted with social rejection. They have a fair claim that the stigma of mental disease is used as a discriminatory economic device by those who would like to see previous criminal sanctions maintained. Since the belief that homosexuality was regularly associated with other symptomatic or reprehensible behavioral deviations (neurosis, antisocial character disorder, criminality, etc.) has either not been supported or found explicable on the basis of learned reactions to a punitive society, it is not surprising that some homosexuals have pressed for removal of the socially approved stigmatizing label—mental disorder. The nub of their argument is that their behavior is simply voluntary rather than the result of an incapacity, or if involuntary it is on a par with involuntary heterosexuality. Therefore, they reject the sick role.

Parallel developments led to the application of the underlying disease concept to the insane and, more abortively, to the chronically criminal. This was a distinct social advance and resulted in marked humanitarian ameliorations as in the scientific and administrative work of Pinel. The mental disease concept was understood by many in the nineteenth century to mean the mentally ill had organic brain disease that had not, as yet, been discovered, e.g., general paresis.

This concept was challenged, more recently, by those who aver that since no brain pathology has been found in most mental disorders, the peculiar behaviors were simply learned maladaptive procedures; no more evidence of an underlying disease than a bad habit. Other attacks on an organic disease model were stimulated by psychoanalytic theory which provided an explanation, convincing to many, deriving both symptomatic distress and abnormal behavior from intrapsychic conflicts and unconscious motivation. Further, animal experiments produced both behavior disorder and manifest distress by simply manipulating life experience.

This too was seen by many liberal humanitarian people as an optimistic conceptual advance since it held out the hope that proper specialized reeducation, e.g., psychoanalysis or deconditioning, could allow the patient to cast aside his maladaptive processes and be once again, simply, a fellow human being.

One problem with applying the illness label to social deviants is that it is a mixed blessing. The sick role has two advantages and one disadvantage. It legitimizes an otherwise exploitative relationship by sanctioning unreturned support for the patient. It prevents blame for parasitism of either the civil or criminal sort, and thus prevents civil or criminal retaliatory action, i.e., shaming, suit, or state punishment.

Its defect is that it exposes an otherwise independent adult to assignment to a dependent role, providing him with a protector who, while attempting to foster the best interests of the dependent will, if necessary, overrides objections.

Obviously, the parent does this for the child who goes to school or else. Few would object to the treatment of the unconscious adult, where illness has grossly impaired the ability to care for self, although unsolicited care may be considered an invasion of privacy. However, the issue gets progressively more controversial with the delirious alcoholic, the dangerous paranoid, the suicidal depressive, the feckless manic, the exploitative psychopath, those with obligate deviant sexual object choices, the deviant ideologue, such as the racist or anarchist, and the rigid personality.

Libertarians assail the potential for the abrogation of civil liberties in assignment to the dependent role. Authoritarians assail the acceptance of dependent behavior, e.g., the family chronically on relief, and the consequent prevention of criminal sanctions.

Some civil libertarians view the state as so malevolent as to claim that the potential for deprivation of civil liberties through assignment to a dependent role is so great that this mechanism should never be used. Even if the person is ill, the social dangers of abrogation of freedom outweigh any conceivable personal benefits.

This clearly is a debatable social judgment. If our state were of this monolithic repressive nature, the Watergate and CIA investigations, etc., would have been impossible; on the other hand, the abuses did occur. The libertarian stand points to a real danger, but concentrates its fire on an unimportant symbolic area. Does anyone believe that if commitment were outlawed the FBI would be better controlled?

Authoritarians, on the other hand, claiming that mental illness is a myth, condemn assaultive paranoids to jail and suicidal depressives to death. I believe that their real covert agenda is the promulgation of a heartless individualism whose target is not the malingerer or the criminal disguised as mentally ill, but the poor, disadvantaged, and socially deprived.

The havoc wrought by the suicidal depressive, belligerent paranoid, etc., is persuasive to me that enforcement of the dependent role requires strict safeguards rather than a blanket prohibition. What should be the prerequisite for assignment of the dependent role, which may include involuntary hospitalization or treatment? The basic prerequisite is a diagnosable illness. Usually the issue will not arise except in the case of mental illness. However, it should be noted that society has forced the dependent role on physically diseased people who were not manifestly ill, but either endangered society or refused to care for themselves, e.g., lepers and typhoid carriers.

Diagnosis of illness is not sufficient but is essential. According to the criteria offered in this chapter, mental illness will not be diagnosed unless the evidence is compelling. In addition, for ascription of the dependent role there has to be social danger or a disruption of functioning so grave that the patient: (a) is unable to appreciate his urgent need for care and treatment; (b) is unable to function effectively in self-care; or (c) endangers himself or others.

It is ironic that just at the point where committed psychotic patients may receive effective medical treatment, there is an attempt to abolish the commitment process or to so limit the grounds for commitment as to make the process meaningless, e.g., by limiting the criteria to manifest immediate danger.

UNHAPPINESS AND ILLNESS

What about unhappiness over involuntary limitations that may be biological variants rather than functional impairments? Unhappiness is egodystonic; if it stems from a bad fit between a limitation and society, the person is truly afflicted. A person with large buttocks may meet with social rejection in the United States, but not in some African tribes. Such problems are not usually considered illness because there is no conviction that some psychobiological process has gone wrong.

It is illogical to extend the sick role to involuntary limitations, e.g., uglinesses that are not necessarily associated with incapacitation but can be associated with secondary unhappiness. It would be best not to blur the defining line between illness and limitations.

This does not deprive us of social procedures to deal with those whose involuntary limitations might be ameliorated. If they have sufficient resources, no social action is required. But if they request subsidization by the community to relieve their unhappiness, then they are in priority conflicts with other unhappy people, e.g., the unemployed, and social policy is required.

Cosmetic surgery for the burned, for instance, follows in an attempt to repair the effects of the primary trauma, whereas cosmetic surgery for the receding chin does not. Social policy decisions are necessary and should not be avoided by syncretically amalgamating limitations with illnesses in order to justify social support of amelioration.

DEFINITION REVIEW

Having developed the necessary conceptual background and terminology, we will now critically review some alternative definitions.

Ausubel (1) in an article succinctly entitled "Personality Disorder is Disease," defines disease as "including any marked deviation, physical, mental, or behavioral, from normally desirable standards of structural and functional integrity."

This definition is unsatisfactory since "normal desirability" may well be defined differently by different social groups. If one wishes to stipulate an ideal standard of normality it should be as unequivocal and ideology resistant as possible. Further, it is not clear if this definition implies dysfunction in an evolutionary context.

Scadding (9) states, "a disease is the sum of the abnormal phenomena displayed by a group of living organisms in association with a specific common characteristic or set of characteristics by which they differ from the norm for their species in such a way as to place them at a biological disadvantage."

This embodies two key concepts. Although divergence from the species norm as a criterion of abnormality is a handy practical indication of probable dysfunction, statistical abnormality does not qualify as a logical necessity.

"Biological disadvantage" does seem crucial, however. In my terms, biological disadvantage is the probable end result of uncompensated dysfunction. Therefore, Scadding's definition of disease is narrower than mine and actually refers to one subset of the possible outcomes of diseased functions. However, biological disadvantage is a less equivocal and ideology-ridden concept than deviation from normally desirable standards, and can be a most useful indicator of probable dysfunction when this cannot be directly demonstrated.

Kendell (5) has recently applied Scadding's criteria to mental illness with the result that the field of mental illness has been constricted considerably. Many patients with manifest dysfunction, e.g., anxiety states, are placed at no substantial biological disadvantage and would be excluded.

Interestingly, Kendell interprets biological disadvantage to include reduced fertility, arguing that this is justified by an evolutionary framework since differential fertility determines which species and genotypes flourish. On these grounds homosexuality could be considered a biological disadvantage and therefore a disease. Unfortunately, this argument would also apply to rational contraception.

The flaw in this argument is that the evolutionary mechanisms that engender fertility cannot depend on cognitive understanding of the process of conception. Therefore, the incentives for fertilization are distinctly noncognitive: the mechanisms of sexual attraction and excitation. If such mechanisms are still active but rational contraception takes place, there has been no dysfunction but only increased planfulness. This sort of reduced fertility may have implications (positive and negative) for species survival, but hardly implies individual dysfunction. The fact that the usual mechanisms of heterosexual attraction do seem to have gone astray in obligate homosexuals does raise the question of an underlying disorder and is discussed elsewhere in this chapter.

Spitzer (11) attempts to develop a useful definition of mental illness when disease cannot be demonstrated. He defines mental disorder (illness) as:

I. The manifestations of the condition are primarily psychological and involve alternations in behavior. However, it includes conditions which are manifested by somatic changes (e.g., psychophysiologic reactions) if an understanding of the etiology and course of the condition is largely dependent on the use of psychological concepts, such as personality, motivation, and conflict.

II. The condition in its full-blown state is regularly and intrinsically associated with either:
  (a) subjective distress, or
  (b) generalized impairment in social effectiveness or functioning, or
  (c) voluntary behavior that the subject wishes he could stop because it is regularly associated with physical disability or illness.

Spitzer first reflects the classic etymological root of illness by insisting on intrinsic suffering or subjective distress as a key criterion of illness. This would avoid applying the illness label to socially deviant behaviors that do not result in subjective distress, e.g., belonging to a cult or having unusual hobbies, or to secondary unhappiness.

However, if Spitzer asserted that subjective distress was a necessary component, many involuntary conditions historically considered psychiatric illness, e.g., euphoric mania, would be excluded. To deal with this, Spitzer expands the definition to include "generalized impairment in social effectiveness or functioning." Although not stipulated, it is likely that the "impairment" is in pursuit of the patient's goals and therefore involuntary, rather than simply being a deviant social goal.

Spitzer's third alternative criterion of illness consists of "voluntary behavior that the subject wishes he could stop because it is regularly associated with physical disability or illness." However, how voluntary is behavior one cannot control? Spitzer's definition of illness gains coherence from its implicit substrate—involuntary dysfunction.

Aubrey Lewis (7) in his remarkable critique, "Health as a Social Concept," offers three criteria for mental illness:

1. The patient feels ill—a subjective datum.
2. He has disordered function of some part of him—an objective datum.
3. He has symptoms which conform to a recognizable clinical pattern—a typological datum.

Lewis specifically states, "though our estimate of the efficiency with which functions work must take account of the social environment which supplies stimuli and satisfies needs, criteria of health are not primarily social. It is misconceived to equate ill health with social deviation or maladjustment." Lewis states,

> "there were, however, always physicians who regarded . . . (insanity) . . . as forms of ill health. Why do they do so? What principles led them to bring insanity and physical disease under one heading, while leaving crime, for example, apart? The common feature was, surely, the evident disturbance of part-functions as well as of general efficiency. In physical disease this needs no demonstration; in mental disorders it is shown by the occurrence of, say, disturbed thinking as in delusions, or disturbed perceptions as in hallucinations, or disturbed emotional states, as in anxiety neurosis or melancholia. Deviant, maladaptive non-conformist behavior is pathological if it is accompanied by manifest disturbance of some such function. . . . If non-conformity can be detected only in total behavior, while all the particular psychological functions seem unimpaired, health should be presumed, not illness.

As Lewis points out, a crucial difficulty arises with psychopathic personality, and the general category of personality disorder. He offers the definition:

> . . . a person although not insane, psychoneurotic or mentally defective, who is persistently unable to adapt to social requirements on account of quantitative peculiarities of impulse, temperament and character. . . . Unless the category of personality disorder is further defined and shown to be categorized by specific abnormality of psychological functions, it will not be possible to consider those who fall within it to be unhealthy, however deviant their social behavior.

An alternative possibility is to recognize that we are still in a primitive state in the detection of disturbances of psychological functions. Perhaps just as "biological disadvantage" can be a useful presumptive indicator of "physiological dysfunction," marked inflexibility under circumstances where flexibility is generally possible may be a behavioral nonsocial index that is a possible indicator of "psychological dysfunction," applicable to the personality disorders.

Comparison with Spitzer and Lewis

Spitzer, like Lewis, feels that intrinsic subjective distress is sufficient for diagnosis of mental illness. "Intrinsic," however, is not well defined. It should be clear that intrinsic refers to the organism's condition and not to interaction of the organism and a specified environment. My definition emphasizes subjective distress that does not reflect actual deleterious influences (realistic distress) but is due to the dysfunction of hedonic aberration. Therefore, although unrealistic elation fits my definition of illness, it is ignored by Spitzer and Lewis.

Distress experienced by some patients can readily be understood as due to an accurate perception of their punitive environment or their life failures. For instance, the distress level of many homosexuals falls abruptly upon entering specialized social enclaves, clearly indicating the extrinsic social basis of their distress.

Another difference lies in Spitzer's specification of generalized impairment in social effectiveness or functioning as a key criterion. It is true that the more generalized the social deficit, the more likely it is that major atypical inflexibility and involuntary impairment exist; however, part-function deficit is also clear evidence of illness. Specific idiosyncratic minor defects in social effectiveness may be considered illness. A patient afraid of snakes may manage his life very well; he merely refuses to go to the snake house at the zoo. Nonetheless, psychiatry considers this evidence of phobic illness. Therefore, generalized impairment in social effectiveness seems an excessive requirement; the criterion of involuntary impairment is overriding. A propensity for unrealistic affective response to specific triggers speaks for an involuntary functional impairment. Spitzer's emphasis on widespread impairment is useful, however, considering that not all dysfunctions are socially considered illnesses. The more widespread the dysfunction, the more likely it is that it will not be considered simply a quirk.

Spitzer's third criterion, "voluntary behavior that the subject wishes he could stop because it is regularly associated with physical disability or illness," is also simply subsumable under the concept of involuntariness. This particular criterion has value as an operational way of specifying beyond doubt that both goal pursuit inflexibility and involuntary impairment are occurring since the person is unable to change his own behavior in the face of very marked incentives.

Personality disorders cannot be defined as illnesses simply on the basis of personality traits, e.g., dependency or suspiciousness. Spitzer and I agree that given current knowledge such traits must cause the person manifest difficulties to operationally warrant consideration as a disorder; otherwise they are simply personality descriptors. The criterion that the traits engender manifest difficulty fulfills the usual dual role, that of implying underlying dysfunction and engendering social concern sufficient to warrant the illness exemption.

Also, the notion of inflexibility points to the cardinal feature of the personality disorder, i.e., that the maladaptive traits are maladaptive precisely because they are inflexible. Depending on circumstances it may very well pay a person to be dependent or suspicious. Given environmental fluctuation, however, if his adaptive repertoire is fixed he cannot help but get into difficulties.

However, if no specific functional impairment is discernible, defining personality traits within mental illness is unwarranted. Only if manifest incapacity occurs does categorization as ill seem justified.

Historically, the case of chronic criminality has been debated primarily because it appears to be voluntary behavior. Also, Aubrey Lewis did not consider psychopathic personality as an illness since no defect of part-function was apparent to him.

The belief that psychopathic personality is an illness stems largely from the fact that despite reward, punishment, self-instruction, and good intentions—the central characteristics of voluntary behavior—such personalities are continually in trouble.

Is it possible that their behavior is actually partially involuntary; that they lack the internal mechanisms that allow for voluntary self-control? In this context voluntary self-control is not an ethereal psychic phenomenon but a psychobiological decision process dependent on adequate cognitive anticipatory mechanisms which develop steering affects (anxiety, embarrassment, disgust, hope, etc.).

I believe that a strong case can be made for considering psychopathic personality a mental illness on the basis of atypical inflexibility and probably part-function defect, i.e., the relative impairment of aversive steering affects. Chronic criminality attributable to psychopathic personality (as well as psychosis, etc.) should be subsumed under mental illness.

However, in contrast, some chronic criminals are in a life situation where chronic criminality actually provides greater payoff than the noncriminal life. In this latter case a diagnosis of mental disorder would be incorrect.

One difficulty with adjudging various patterns of sexuality as due to dysfunction is that sexual goal seeking or avoidance behavior is voluntary. Chastity can be voluntary, although some have considered it the most peculiar perversion.

Consider the happy, exclusive, obligate boot fetishist. Certainly most psychiatrists would consider this *prima facie* evidence of mental illness, but on what grounds? He is not suffering, or a social failure. His inflexibility has not resulted in intrinsic suffering; his appetitive actions appear voluntary.

Plainly the presumption is that so outré an object choice must reflect an involuntary impairment. Total sexual abstention may be voluntary, but boot fetishism is hard to understand except as an internalized *faute de mieux* adjustment, i.e., secondary to involuntary impairment of interpersonal sexuality or inflexible positive fixation. Should we consider it an illness then?

Personally I would defer resolution of the question of the well-functioning person with obligate deviant sexual object choice since we are just developing a scientific understanding of this area. However, I would consider manifestly ill those with deviant object choices who show clear-cut incapacity by earnestly trying to change their adaptation without success; or who persist in sexual behavior that is likely to result in marked social sanctions, e.g., pedophilia or exhibitionism. It is hard to consider such behavior as entirely voluntary, and therefore, impairment is inferred.

The differences in criteria are particularly sharp with regard to sexual difficulties. Using Spitzer's definition, obligate homosexuality does not qualify as a mental disorder. There is no intrinsic subjective distress, no generalized impairment in social effectiveness, no voluntary behavior that they wish they could stop because it is associated with physical disability or illness.

To deal with the fact that homosexuals may apply for psychiatric help because of distress, Spitzer has recommended that the term "sexual object choice disorder with distress regarding homosexual arousal" be used. The important issue is that the term "disorder" applies to the distress and not to the homosexuality. Since these patients have subjective distress, they may seem to qualify as mentally ill by Spitzer's definition.

However, Spitzer is inconsistent as shown by his stipulation that it is not enough for somebody to have subjective distress to be considered mentally ill; he must have a condition where mental distress is intrinsic. However, the mental distress of the homosexual patient can readily be attributed to his interaction with a punitive environment engendering realistic unhappiness.

Exactly the same logic applies to other sexual difficulties. For instance, it has been suggested that there be a category entitled "sexual object choice disorders with distress regarding non-human objects, i.e., zoophilia, fetishism, transvestism." Again the distress is comprehensible, not evidence of a disorder.

However, in voluntary patients we usually have marked inflexibility and refractoriness to self-instruction, operationally defined by the fact that in spite of distress and effort, the patient has been unable to change his behavior and has sought help. Therefore, it is not distress over homosexuality but involuntary heterosexual incapacity that indicates a disorder. It would be gratuitous to label a homosexual as mentally ill unless he himself professed that he was trying to change his behavior and was unable to do so despite severe subjective distress.

Plainly, the whole field of ego-syntonic behavioral inflexibility is the most problematic area. Our problem is to walk the fine line between classifying deviant behavior as ill simply because it is deviant and classifying deviant behavior as well simply because it is ego-syntonic. Detailed analyses of part-function impairment and the nature of involuntary behavior may prove the way out of this dilemma.

IDEOLOGICAL PROBLEMS

I have stipulated certain function norms which derive from our current grasp of human evolutionary development.

Recently, a number of evolutionary behavioral norms have been promulgated, e.g., territoriality, that have not received widespread scholarly acceptance although they have made for much popular discussion. There is a marked problem in that different social interests may attempt to legitimatize their methods and goals by ascribing them biological status. In the nineteenth century the sociopolitical movement described as "social Darwinism" insisted that competitiveness was a law of nature, thus supporting a free enterprise capitalist ideology.

Similarly, some have insisted that evolutionary theory demonstrated that social adaptability was an organismal necessity; therefore, social reformers and revolutionaries demonstrated defect by their lack of adaptability. This stand ignores the human capacity for planfully changing the environment. Interestingly, Lenin (6) in *"Left Wing" Communism; An Infantile Disorder* inveighed against those revolutionaries who lacked flexibility in the pursuit of revolutionary goals, considering them to have an infantile disorder; that is, an illness.

Because ideological apologetics present serious problems for objective science, we should lean over backward to be meticulously critical of supposedly scientific conclusions that clearly support one of a set of contending social interests. I believe that the principles stipulated above are reasonably ideology-free and current but unlikely to be final. As our grasp of evolutionary development deepens, more precise and detailed norms will be possible, thus modifying our specific criteria for dysfunction; the necessary precondition for the illness label.

SUMMARY

The definition of mental illness presents thorny semantic and social issues. Social process has required the development of a variety of approved parasitic roles, here termed exempt, of which the sick and dependent roles are examples. The attribution of illness both legitimatizes the sick role and is a defense against criminal prosecution, so that the definition of illness has marked social impact.

Prescientifically, illness was defined as an involuntary impairment or suffering that could not be attributed to understandable antecedents and implied that something had gone wrong of sufficient magnitude to warrant social exemption, in the form of the sick role. Modern science has developed the concept of objective underlying disease processes, demonstrating that the inference that something has gone wrong is not simply arbitrary. Disease is defined here as covert, objective, suboptimal part dysfunction, recognizing that functions are evolved and hierarchically organized. It is argued that disease is not simply an arbitrary social evaluation but is derivable from the concept of optimal biological functioning, within an evolutionary context. Illness is always secondary to disease, but also requires a social judgment that there is sufficient incapacity to warrant the assignment of the exempt sick role.

Mental illness is the subset of all illness that presents evidence in the cognitive, behavioral, affective, and motivational aspects of organismal functioning. It must be believed that something has gone wrong to attribute illness. For functional disorders, involuntary impairment is a key inference, supported by a range of evidence including lack of response to self-instruction, evidence of intrinsic suffering, clear incapacity, the likely production of overriding negative consequences, etc.

Inflexibility as a relatively species-specific incapacity that raises the question of dysfunction is discussed. Difficulties in the thoughtful application of these criteria are reviewed. Categorization is usually clear, but there are gray areas where the evidence is not conclusive.

Ego-syntonic inflexible behavior without undesirable effects, and personal limitations that incur negative social reactions and cause unhappiness pose many problems. Such conditions should not be considered illnesses given current knowledge. If it can be demonstrated that the limitation is actually due to an incapacity, then the illness label could be justified given sufficient historically determined social concern.

ACKNOWLEDGMENTS

This chapter has benefited from many discussions with Jean Endicott, Rachel Gittelman-Klein, and Robert L. Spitzer. The conclusions are the author's responsibility despite good advice. Phyllis Skomorowsky provided valuable editorial assistance.

REFERENCES

1. Ausubel, D. P. (1971): Personality disorder is disease. *Am. Psychol.*, 16:59–74.
2. Begelman, D. A. (1971): Misnaming, metaphors, the medical model, and some muddles. *Psychiatry*, 34:38–58.
3. Faber, K. (1923): *Nosography in Modern Internal Medicine*. Paul B. Hoeber, New York.

4. Feinstein, A. R. (1967): *Clinical Judgment.* Williams & Wilkins, Baltimore.
5. Kendell, R. E. (1975): The concept of disease and its implications for psychiatry. *Br. J. Psychiatry,* 127:305–315.
6. Lenin, V. I. (1921): *"Left Wing" Communism; An Infantile Disorder.* Marxian Educational Society, Detroit.
7. Lewis, A. (1967): *The State of Psychiatry.* Science House, New York.
8. Parsons, T. (1951): *The Social System.* The Free Press, Glencoe, Ill.
9. Scadding, J. G. (1967): Diagnosis: The clinician and the computer. *Lancet,* 2:877–882.
10. Sedgwick, P. (1973): Illness—mental and otherwise. *Hastings Cent. Stud.,* 3:19–58.
11. Spitzer, R. L., and Wilson, P. T. (1975): Nosology and the official psychiatric nomenclature. In: *Comprehensive Textbook of Psychiatry,* edited by A. M. Freedman, H. I. Kaplan, and B. J. Sadock, pp. 826–845. Williams & Wilkins, Baltimore.

Critical Issues in Psychiatric Diagnosis,
edited by Robert L. Spitzer and Donald F. Klein.
Raven Press, New York © 1978.

A Behavioral Analysis of Diagnosis

Kurt Salzinger

*Polytechnic Institute of New York, New York State Psychiatric Institute,
New York, New York 10032*

To the writing of diagnosis there is no end; nor is it easy to locate that far away point in time when a human being first caught some others in a category, first damned them to a diagnosis which formed a sturdier prison than one constructed of more solid matter.

Why do we continue to talk about diagnosis as if it were the weather? To be sure, over the years we have learned a little about diagnosis. As with forecasts of the weather, we have become accustomed to inaccuracy. As with the experiments in weather modification, we have learned to seed the clouds of observations in order to sometimes precipitate a sprinkling of information —not enough to make a tree of knowledge grow, but occasionally, enough to revive a wilting plant of psychiatric anecdotes. I dare say that our discussants will not be moved by the drifts of snow produced by our papers on diagnosis to admit that "the winter of our discontent" has changed to "glorious summer." Yet would I rather melt one snowflake than curse the low reliability of diagnosis. Herewith, then, my prescription for the problem.

THE RELIABILITY PROBLEM

Let us begin with that concept of reliability which students of psychopathology have so readily, and greedily, made their own. Even Rosenhan (6), who was able to incur the righteous wrath, not only of the psychiatric, but of the psychological establishment (see the *Journal of Abnormal Psychology,* Vol. 84, No. 5), responded to his critics, not with a bang, asking for another kind of system of classifying humanity in trouble, but with a whimper, begging for a higher reliability score. "Would you believe 81% of the variance to be assigned to agreement?" pleaded Rosenhan (6). "No," remonstrated the fierce stepmother, Spitzer (18), "that's unrealistic. Even true Mother Medicine won't do that for her offspring." (These quotations have benefited from poetic license.) And thus we are counseled to be content in the thought that psychiatric diagnosis is no worse than other medical diagnoses.

Yet the problem of diagnosis lies not in the reliability coefficients—high or low, for those are but poor indicators of the basic measurement problem that needs to be addressed. Substituting a kappa whose variance can be obtained without squaring for a product-moment correlation coefficient whose variance can be obtained only through self-multiplication to tell us about true subject variation is too much like increasing the light in one room when you know the coin you lost is in another.

Where does the problem of reliability reside? Of course, ultimately in the validation of the diagnosis—the homogeneity of the members of the group designated by the diagnostic category with respect to the origin and course of the disorder, and its response to treatment. But wait; before we get to that part, we must first struggle with how we arrive at the diagnosis: how we obtain information; how much we view the potential patient as informant; how much as subject whose behavior is to be observed, and when to view the person as informant and subject at the same time; how much we and the context in which we examine the person affect what the patient says and does, and how much we (influenced by our reinforcement history) and the context in which we examine the person affect what we say and do; how we select the information that we obtain—through planned or unplanned but still systematic observations, proddings, and reinforcements, biased memories, premeditated record keeping, theoretically determined analysis, and synthesis of the information we have deemed relevant to our purpose—all of which we have endowed with the sacrament of the official DSM-II and soon with its reincarnation in the form of DSM-III.

AGREEMENT AMONG OBSERVERS VERSUS AGREEMENT AMONG INTERVIEWERS

And after we have done all that, i.e., examined the behaviors and their interactions and made our procedures and assumptions explicit so that others may do the same, then we must first grapple with the problem of the meaning of reliability—such simple questions as the reliability of raters observing the same interview versus reliability of two different interviewers conducting independent interviews of the same person. It has become the fashion of late, because of the "Drang nach Reliability," to measure that reliability which will fare best rather than the one we need to know. It is interesting, but insufficient, to discover that several observers can sometimes agree in their diagnosis when that diagnosis is based on observing the same interview. Why is such reliability not impressive? The answer lies in the fact that a substantial part of the variation of diagnoses is due to interviewers (20), who differ not only in the material they evoke from the potential patient but also in the extent to which they follow up what the patient says or does as a function of their differing interpretations and the manner in which they synthesize the often conflicting pieces of information they obtain. Thus the observers who look at a canned interview are truly presented with processed food—information already partially digested. Some investigators feel that the structured interviews, which sometimes guide the course of the questions to be asked, reduce the degrees of freedom the interviewer has in what leads to follow-up, but since they are interviews rather than questionnaires, the interviewer still can "manage" the outcome of the interview. The artifact in interrater agreement for canned interviews consists of the series of clues that the interviewer inevitably supplies in how he/she follows up various statements made by the patients, thus producing agreement among raters, not because of consistent patient observation, but because of consistent interviewer observation.

What is interesting is that despite the artifacts conducive to inflationary agreement among observers, even these conditions do not inevitably produce the desirably high reliability. Langer and Abelson (2) found a significant amount of disagreement among raters observing the same canned interview as a function of whether they were told that they were observing a patient or an employment interview, and whether their theoretical background was behavioral or psychodynamic—even though the person interviewed was, in fact, *not* a patient. It is worthwhile noting that clinicians of behavioral persuasion were not influenced by the extraneous information that this was a patient, i.e., they were influenced by the behavior of the person they observed; the psychodynamically oriented clinicians, on the other hand, saw the person as significantly more maladjusted when called a patient than when the same person was called a prospective employee.

IS A RELIABILITY INDEX ENOUGH?

We must remember that the reliability score is merely an index; viewed separate and apart from the behavior involved in arriving at the labels we call diagnosis, the indices provide no information of interest. Psychologists have for a long time demonstrated agreement in labeling, as in the area of the psychology of stereotypes. The pattern (syndrome?) of characteristics that have consistently been assigned to such unknown groups as the Turks has long ago achieved a consistency to marvel at. Were we to use agreement as an index of this "diagnostic" procedure, we would draw all sorts of incorrect conclusions. When an example of this kind is given, it is the fashion to point out that the measurement of the validity of the judgment would show the stereotype to be the slander that it is.

Unfortunately, the validity test is not as useful as it may seem at first thought. First, the validation of diagnostic "findings" is even more difficult to achieve than the validation of such stereotypic judgments as "cruelty" in Turks, but secondly and more importantly, the basic problem with the stereotypic patterns of characteristics, the "syndromes" assigned to Turks, vis-à-vis reliability, is not that they are false, invalid descriptions of people—which they are—but rather that they were arrived at on the basis of a procedure we would not accept as potentially providing us with insights into the behavior of the people being judged. The point is not to increase the reliability, but to make an explicit, well-planned, judicious choice of the conditions under which the diagnostic judgment is made. When the measurements performed are operationalized, then the reliability coefficient will be meaningful.

THE EFFECT OF THE ENVIRONMENT— CONDITIONS OF OBSERVATION

I believe that there is a more productive way of viewing the problem of reliability of diagnosis than the mechanical method applied so far. It requires an extension of the concept of reliability, which brings me back to the title of my chapter—a behavioral analysis of diagnosis. Please note that I am making no judgment here about the medical model's validity in classifying psychiatric patients. I have done that elsewhere (e.g., 10). I wish to discuss here only the general interview method one ought to use to arrive at a diagnosis. Two general assumptions that I make are, I believe, universally acceptable at all levels of observation: first, the phenomena we observe are influenced by the fact that we observe them, and, second, they are *differentially* influenced by different conditions of observation. Physicians have not only become aware of the possibility of artifacts in blood pressure and heart rate measurements due to their subjects' running around the block; they have more recently begun to take advantage of the effects of running by taking measurements after the patient was rested as compared to measurements after the patient has run on a treadmill. We also have more subtle ways of modifying heart rate and blood pressure and a large variety of other bodily functions by means of conditioning (3). No behavior occurs in a vacuum. Not only is behavior affected by the environment in which it occurs; behavior is shaped by that environment. Most important of all, we must remember that behavior of individuals who act peculiarly, as do our patients (never mind ourselves), is still affected by the environment. Therefore, we do not have the option in any diagnostic examination, to pay attention to the so-called biological factors alone. We cannot get at them at all without paying attention to the environment.

The idea of a behavioral analysis of diagnosis is then simply an extension of this generally acceptable idea that if we are to improve our techniques of obtaining information, no matter for what purpose, we ought to have a systematic way of going about it. Certainly, the idea that we ought to determine the effects of the interviewer on the verbal behavior of the patient who is being interviewed has been around for a long time. The fact that psychologists have continued to spend any time at all examining the procedural monster of the interview is almost entirely, it seems to me, to be laid at the feet of Joseph Zubin (22), who long ago systematized what is going on in the interview and who inspired the more recent work both in structuring what is being discussed (19) and in determining how the interviewer may, by subtle means (which sometimes are so subtle that they are unknown even to the interviewer), influence the outcome of an interview (7,8,13–17).

A BEHAVIORAL ANALYSIS OF DIAGNOSIS

Let us look now at what the behavioral analysis proposes. The central concept is the reinforcement contingency $(9):S^D \ldots R \to S^R$. S^D is the discriminative stimulus, that is, the occasion on which a response is emitted and reinforced. The occasion refers to the entire context of stimuli surrounding the behavior and reinforcement and includes such factors as the room and the general physical environment in which the interview is conducted; the sex of the interviewer; his/her attire; the interviewer's behavior, both verbal and nonverbal; the place from which the individual being interviewed just came; noises occurring in the course of the interview; the questions—their order, repetitiousness, and emotional quality; the consequences of what the patient says—both immediate, in the form of verbal and nonverbal reinforcers, and remote consequences whose likely occurrence is signaled by the interviewer's behavior or about which the patient has already correctly or incorrectly been informed.

R stands for the response of the patient and is defined by its membership in a class of responses (12) which have been shown to vary together as a function of some empirical variable. R refers to verbal as well as nonverbal responses, that is, to such behavior as the patient's grimaces, head shaking, smiling, crying, as well as the content of what he/she actually says and to whom the conversation is directed.

S^R is the reinforcing stimulus, by which is meant the consequence of the response, or, completely empirically, what happens after the patient has emitted a response. There are positive and negative reinforcers, that is, those that increase the rate of the responses that produce them, and those that increase the rate of the responses that avoid or eliminate them, respectively.

We must note that by negative reinforcer, we do not mean a punishing stimulus which is contingent on the occurrence of a response; rather, we mean a contingency that allows a response to avoid or escape an aversive event. Punishing stimuli also occur in interviews, but their effect, interestingly enough, has not been studied. Such stimuli would merely suppress the behavior they followed (the exception being the case of traumatic punishment, which is not what we are talking about here).

Before giving examples of the kinds of events and interactions that behavior analysis explains, I should point out that the concept of reinforcement contingency can also be used to explain the behavior of the interviewer. The events that constitute discriminative stimuli for the interviewer are, like the patient's discriminative stimuli, the physical environment and other conditions surrounding the interview, including what just happened in the last interview or whatever else preceded the interview in question. Presumably the most important S^D's for the interviewer are the behavior and appearance of the patient, in conjunction with the interviewer's reinforcement history, which has trained him or her to pay attention to particular behaviors in conducting the interview. Thus the patient, like the interviewer, is engaged in a conditioning experiment. The patient provides the S^D's and the S^R's for the interviewer's behavior just as surely as the reverse is true.

The Patient as Subject

In a series of studies (13–17), we were able to show quite clearly that a response class described by a concept such as shallowness of affect (which we defined operationally to be measured by the number of self-referred affect statements such as "I like," "I hate," "I am angry," "I am sad," "I am happy") does vary systematically with the conditions of reinforcement currently operative, that is, the number of reinforcers delivered, the nature of the period immediately preceding the reinforcement condition, and the amount of conditioning preceding it during a previous session. Thus what the interviewer did during the interview that used a standard series of questions but systematically varied the presence and number of reinforcers determined a great deal of the content of what the schizophrenic patient or the normal individual said, the only difference between normals and patients arising in the extinction condition. There the schizophrenic patient emitted a smaller number of affect statements than the normal, that is, the normal carried over the effect of the reinforcement for a longer period of time than did the schizophrenic. Now, that by itself is an important finding, not only as I have shown with respect to a theory of schizophrenia, which I have summarized under the concept of immediacy [according to which the stimuli most immediate in the environment of the schizophrenic control behavior (11)], but also respect to the differential influencibility associated with the kind of diagnosis the individual gets in the first place. Life is very complicated, and what the individual brings to the situation in which his/her behavior is measured, and that situation itself do not interact in a simple way. As far as I know, no structured interview to date has paid any attention to the manner in which the interviewer reinforces the patient, and, given that situation, I can only assume that the reliability obtained under such conditions cannot be free of artifact.

The Interviewer as Subject

Before developing the significance of the effect of the interviewer on the patient, let me throw in the patient-as-reinforcer complication. Not only does the interviewer reinforce the patient, but the patient also reinforces the interviewer. That wise Columbia University student who drew the cartoon showing the subject (a rat, in that case) reinforcing the experimenter put his finger on a universal truth relating to any kind of behavioral interaction— there is mutual reinforcement. Two experiments demonstrate the reality of the interviewer modification by the interviewee. Rosenfeld and Baer (4) set up an experiment in such a way that the interviewer was instructed to rein- force the interviewee whenever the latter rubbed his chin. The chin rubs, however, were made contingent on the interviewer's emission of the verbal responses "yeah" or "mm-hm." The interviewer's verbal behavior varied with the contingency, and the interviewer showed no awareness of being re- inforced. The other experiment was also done by Rosenfeld and Baer (5). In this case, the "interviewer" was instructed to condition fluent speech by de- livering points to the interviewee. In fact, however, the interviewee's fluencies and disfluencies were contingent on the interviewer's emission of such verbal behavior as "next word" or "O.K." Again the experimenters showed the expected changes and the subjects (the interviewers) showed no awareness of having had their behavior manipulated.

These studies have two implications: The first is that the behavior of an interviewer is susceptible to influence, apparently even when that person's behavior is somewhat programmed, as it was in the two experiments de- scribed. How much more susceptible is the behavior of the interviewer whose verbal behavior is *not* programmed! But secondly, the fact that even so simple and straightforward a manipulation as was described above was not detected makes it clear that we cannot trust the report of the interviewer as to what happens during the interview.

Some Implications of the Behavior Theory Model

What are the implications of these examples of bidirectional influence? The first is that the behavior of the interlocutors in an interview situation varies in a lawful, predictable way. The second is that the individuals par- ticipating may not know of the influences involved. Suggestive as was the study by Ward et al. (20), simply asking two interviewers to discuss their reasons (guesses) about why they arrived at different diagnoses is not a foolproof way to find out the source of their disagreement. Nevertheless, the fact of the matter is that patients do seem to tell some interviewers one thing and others another. The reinforcement-contingency analysis provides a tool for the isolation of the variables that might be responsible for those differ- ences. We cannot simply continue to blame that vague but all-purpose waste- basket category of personality to explain the differences in the type of information that different people evoke from patients; we must refer the dif- ferences in the kinds of material evoked to some nameable variables. Person- ality, as Zubin (21) long ago told us, is a shrinking universe. It retains within its borders all of our ignorance, occasionally transferring those items to other areas which we have come to understand. Thus, what we cannot explain in terms of behavior theory or biochemistry, social norms or neurology, we sequester from investigation and condemn to the personality category.

But what can we do with the first implication, namely, that the behavioral interaction between people during the interview is lawful? The lawfulness suggests, to return to the medical example of monitoring potential heart attack victims, that we too study our patients under varying conditions. Note that all this means that we must study which variables affect what the patients tell us and what the content of their responses is. Some of the necessary research has already been done. I submit that on the basis of the literature of psycholinguistics and the operant conditioning of verbal behavior, we can make good guesses on setting up the proper research to improve how we arrive at our diagnoses.

The most important fact in an interview is that two people continue to converse with one another. When one interlocutor ceases to speak altogether, then, that rare exception of the psychoanalytic session notwithstanding, the conversation ceases altogether; even in the psychoanalytic interview, where only one person speaks, we are told the therapist often fills the patient's pauses with "mm-hm's's." It follows that the interviewer should be fully aware of when he/she uses the unobtrusive reinforcers that seem so natural. Interviewers may tell us the reinforcers are being used merely to keep things natural and the talk flowing. But we have already shown that one can reinforce either speech in general, or affect in particular (17), depending on which of these two classes the reinforcer is contingent on. Thus it is not too hard to imagine that the diagnostician who is collecting, say, according to the latest DSM operational criteria for a depressive episode, the necessary four out of the eight from which the diagnostician may sample, and has already found three, might be under some pressure to obtain the fourth. The interviewer who questions the patient about recurrent thoughts of death, suicide, or any suicidal behavior might well ask more pointed questions (use stronger S^D's) and reinforce even closer approximations to the desired answer.

We must add to this picture the findings by Chapman and Chapman (1). The vaunted advantage of diagnosis produced by being able to take advantage of the clustering of symptoms and signs might simply reflect an illusory kind of clustering brought about by theories that are taught and accepted, so that even when symptoms do not co-occur, they are perceived or remembered to have occurred together. The criteria are still vague to some extent and they probably will continue to be. So much the more reason for specifying the conditions under which the patient makes particular statements. We can view the recurring thoughts about suicidal behavior in terms of the reinforcement contingency model. What are the conditions, that is, the reinforcement contingencies, under which a person will admit to having suicidal thoughts, or will admit that they are recurring? Obviously, different ethnic groups or people of differing religious backgrounds might well have been differentially reinforced for talking about such things, never mind for thinking about such things. Clearly, patients' reinforcement history should be taken into account when determining what to make of their statements in response to interviewer questions (which can be variously phrased—sympathetically, belligerently, inquisitively, etc.), e.g., whether they have been thinking of committing suicide.

We can view the variety of conditions conducive to evoking such information from the point of view of artifacts or errors that we shall never be able to get rid of. On the other hand, we can also view the varying S^D's and reinforcement conditions as exactly the kinds of variables that will aid us in gauging the strength of the various behaviors we are seeking to monitor. Thus we can, for example, see how long it takes, in the course of an interview, for a patient to tell us about suicidal ideation without ever being asked about it, and then see how direct the question must be in order to evoke that response. We can then compare the kind of S^D necessary to evoke that class of information from the patient to the kind of S^D necessary to evoke equally intimate details, for example, of the patient's sexual experiences. Thus it would be possible by proper systematization to include in each interview the proper comparative measures of response strength that would provide us with the quantitative measures that we have so long lacked vis-à-vis the diagnostic procedure in psychiatry.

BEHAVIOR ANALYSIS AND RELIABILITY

How does this approach relate to reliability of diagnosis? Rather than seeking duplication of symptoms as derived by one interviewer or another, we must look for replications of the *relationships* between our examination procedure and the responses from the patients. In addition, we must seek the lawful relationships between the variables acting on the patients and their resultant behaviors outside the interview situation. By these criteria, the reliability of diagnosis would depend not on the amount of overlap in the responses evoked by two different interviewers, but rather on their agreement on the functional relationships between the stimuli each used and the responses each obtained from the same patient.

PRIVATE EVENTS AS DISCRIMINATIVE STIMULI

We have not yet discussed the problem of the patient's verbal behavior. A good deal of it is assumed to reflect such private events as feeling sad, happy, or angry. Unfortunately, the learning of verbal responses to discriminative stimuli that are private events does not take place with the same uniformity and accuracy as does the learning of verbal responses controlled by external events. Psychotherapy often turns out to be a matter of teaching patients how to describe their emotions or private events in terms that society considers appropriate. That learning, in turn, allows the patients to make the appropriate responses to the external stimuli that evoke these private events in them. Unlike the clinical psychologist and psychiatrist, the general practitioner has the advantage of being able to resort to a number of tests that do not depend on the patient's verbal responses; this is also true of the dentist who can take X-rays of the teeth or simply observe the patient while probing a certain area to determine whether the patient is in pain. In psychopathology, we must simultaneously plumb the depths of something called a thought disorder, and rely on that thought disordered person as an informant. Without physical tests to aid us, we must program most carefully the stimuli we apply to the patients we interview, for clearly those stimuli, which constitute the reinforcement contingency, ought to serve as the context for the patients' responses, not as the sole stimuli determining them.

No matter how carefully we conduct the interview, however, if the problem of private events inheres in the patients' not having been conditioned to respond to their private events in a manner explicable to the diagnostician, then we cannot escape the task of training the interviewee, our informant, to emit known verbal responses under the control of private events. Behavior therapists do that kind of thing when they first train the patients to observe the conditions under which and how frequently they emit disturbing behaviors. It is often the experience of behavior therapists that the behaviors the patients complain about do not take the shape that the patients first say they do. Thus, behavior originally described as ubiquitous occurs only at selected times and places, and sometimes other behaviors not initially described by the patients turn out to be crucial to them after a period of self-observation. Although it is more difficult to train patients to respond to their private events than to public ones, it can be done. What is more important than the question of whether it can be done or not is that unless it can, no purpose is served in having interviewers pursue their patients' private events if their verbal responses do not reflect them.

WHERE DOES RADICAL BEHAVIOR THEORY LEAD US WITH RESPECT TO DIAGNOSIS?

It provides us with a systematic way of viewing the relative evocability of various classes of verbal and nonverbal behaviors. Although it is not possible to gauge the probability of each class of behavior that might be asked for in a diagnostic interview, it does make available the methods that could be applied to those pieces of information that are crucial for the diagnosis. The determination of the presence of suicidal thoughts is obviously more important than other information the interviewer might obtain. Behaviors like that can be gauged with respect to their strength by determining the kinds of S^D's that evoke them.

Behavioral Analysis and the Diagnostician's Judgment

Behavior theory has another use with respect to the diagnostic process, and we have already alluded to it above. The diagnostician, like the patient, is also controlled by S^D's and S^R's. It is therefore critical that the diagnostic manual be prepared in such a way that global judgments not precede the gathering of information, that the diagnostician not be inspired to prove that a given individual belongs to a particular category, but rather that the information be collected in such a way that the diagnostic category grows out of the cumulative collection of data. The order of questions which is typically guided by a hypothesis, in order to complete the interview as fast as possible, might well not be the ideal way to go from facts to synthesis of facts. It might be more helpful to program questions in an order that deliberately makes it difficult to reach a conclusion without being able to review the responses, combine and evaluate them, and determine the conditions under which they were emitted.

I realize that I have suggested a number of problems and that my solutions have not been spelled out, nor have they been time-saving devices. The point is that all questions are not easily answerable and the quick answers are not always the correct ones, even if they have been used for a long time and even if we all feel comfortable continuing to believe in them.

One final demurrer: I have been speaking about the medical model-diagnosis interview throughout. That is not to be taken as evidence that I have shifted my position to believe that this is the best model on the basis of which to obtain information relevant to psychopathology. On the other hand, whether you believe in the pure medical model or in a more behavioristic formulation of psychopathology, the problems of obtaining the relevant information are the same and the importance of the variables of the interviewer and the environment are not surmountable by fleeing into biochemical hypotheses, since the conduct of the interview is a behavioral affair. So if you are content to use the medical model, if you are impressed by accumulating evidence that biochemistry will supply us with answers regarding psychopathology, then you still ought to make use of the appropriate field of science to shed light on the diagnostic interview, and that is radical behavior theory.

ACKNOWLEDGMENTS

The writing of this chapter was supported in part by NIMH Grant MH 22890, Behavior Modification: Evaluating Effects on Patients. As usual, the author has profited from R. S. Feldman's careful editing.

REFERENCES

1. Chapman, L. J., and Chapman, J. (1969): Illusory correlation as an obstacle to the use of valid psychodiagnostic signs. *J. Abnorm. Psychol.*, 74:271–280.
2. Langer, E. J., and Abelson, R. P. (1974): A patient by any other name . . . : Clinical group differences in labeling bias. *J. Consult. Clin. Psychol.*, 42:4–9.
3. Miller, N. E. (1973): Autonomic learning: Clinical and physiological implications. In: *Psychopathology*, edited by M. Hammer, K. Salzinger, and S. Sutton, pp. 127–146. John Wiley & Sons, New York.
4. Rosenfeld, H. M., and Baer, D. M. (1969): Unnoticed verbal conditioning of an aware experimenter by a more aware subject: The double-agent effect. *Psychol. Rev.*, 76:425–432.
5. Rosenfeld, H. M., and Baer, D. M. (1970): Unbiased and unnoticed verbal conditioning: The double-agent robot procedure. *J. Exp. Anal. Behav.*, 14:99–107.
6. Rosenhan, D. L. (1975): The contextual nature of psychiatric diagnosis. *J. Abnorm. Psychol.*, 84:462–474.
7. Salzinger, K. (1959): The experimental analysis of the interview. In: *Experimental Abnormal Psychology*, edited by J. Zubin. Columbia University Press, New York.
8. Salzinger, K. (1969): The place of operant conditioning of verbal behavior in psychotherapy. In: *Behavior Therapy: Appraisal and Status*, edited by C. Franks, pp. 375–395. McGraw-Hill, New York.
9. Salzinger, K. (1969): *Psychology: The Science of Behavior*. Springer, New York.
10. Salzinger, K. (1970): Diagnosis: Who needs it? *J. Clin. Iss. Psychol.*, 1:25–27.
11. Salzinger, K. (1973): *Schizophrenia: Behavioral Aspects*. John Wiley & Sons, New York.
12. Salzinger, K. (1967): The problem of response class in verbal behavior. In: *Research in Verbal Behavior and Some Neurophysiological Implications*, edited by K. Salzinger and S. Salzinger, pp. 35–54. Academic Press, New York.
13. Salzinger, K., and Pisoni, S. (1958): Reinforcement of affect responses of schizophrenics during the clinical interview. *J. Abnorm. Soc. Psychol.*, 57:84–90.
14. Salzinger, K., and Pisoni, S. (1960): Reinforcement of verbal affect responses of normal subjects during the interview. *J. Abnorm. Soc. Psychol.*, 60:127–130.
15. Salzinger, K., and Pisoni, S. (1961): Some parameters of the conditioning of verbal affect responses in schizophrenic subjects. *J. Abnorm. Soc. Psychol.*, 63:511–516.
16. Salzinger, K., and Portnoy, S. (1964): Verbal conditioning in interviews: Application to chronic schizophrenics and relationship to prognosis for acute schizophrenics. *J. Psychiatr. Res.*, 2:1–9.
17. Salzinger, K., Portnoy, S., and Feldman, R. S. (1964): Experimental manipulation of continuous speech in schizophrenic patients. *J. Abnorm. Soc. Psychol.*, 68:508–516.
18. Spitzer, R. L. (1976): More on pseudoscience in science and the case for psychiatric diagnosis. *Arch. Gen. Psychiatry*, 33:459–470.
19. Spitzer, R. L., and Endicott, J. (1973): The value of the interview for the evaluation of psychopathology. In: *Psychopathology*, edited by M. Hammer, K. Salzinger, and S. Sutton, pp. 397–408. John Wiley & Sons, New York.
20. Ward, C. H., Beck, A. T., Mendelson, M., Mock, J. E., and Erbaugh, J. K. (1962): The psychiatric nomenclature. *Arch. Gen. Psychiatry*, 7:198–205.
21. Zubin, J. (1954): The measurement of personality. *J. Counsel. Clin. Psychol.*, 1:159–164.
22. Zubin, J. (Ed.) (1959): *Experimental Abnormal Psychology*. Columbia University Press, New York.

Critical Issues in Psychiatric Diagnosis,
edited by Robert L. Spitzer and Donald F. Klein.
Raven Press, New York © 1978.

Discussion of the Spitzer-Endicott and Klein Proposed Definitions of Mental Disorder (Illness)

Michael S. Moore

Harvard University, Cambridge, Massachusetts 02138

I shall discuss here only the chapters of Drs. Spitzer and Endicott, and Dr. Klein, both of which deal with a single question: how should 'mental illness' be defined?

There are two very general ways of proceeding when one defines a phrase such as 'mental disorder'. (I shall use 'mental disorder' as a synonym for 'mental illness' as used by Dr. Klein.) The first is an analysis of what the phrase means as it is used in a body of discourse. One proceeds by analyzing the various ways in which a phrase is employed, either in the general population or within some subgroup, and one attempts to isolate the criteria *implicit* in such ordinary usage as the meaning of the term. Robinson (9) has called these "lexical" definitions, and I shall follow his usage.

The second mode of definition proceeds by disregarding the ways in which a phrase is actually used in a body of discourse, and focuses on how it ought to be used. One defines a phrase, in other words, by making a proposal as to what it ought to mean to people. Let us call these "stipulative" definitions, because in making them one stipulates (as opposed to discovers) the criteria that are henceforth to govern the use of a term.

Although I don't think ultimately either Dr. Klein or Drs. Spitzer and Endicott wish to claim complete freedom from giving us an analysis of how 'mental disorder' is used, nonetheless I take it that the prima facie nature of their proposals is just that: *proposals* as to how one ought in the future to use the phrase 'mental disorder'. Because these are seemingly stipulative definitions, their accuracy is not in issue, for they are not purported descriptions of how we in fact use the phrase. In criticizing, one thus first faces the task of articulating the criterion by virtue of which we judge a stipulative definition as good or bad. Drs. Spitzer and Endicott in their chapter correctly point out the general nature of this criterion: stipulative definitions are either more or less useful, and are to be judged accordingly.

One may at this point legitimately ask, useful for what? What one needs, in other words, is a clear idea of what such definitions seek to accomplish before one can even begin to criticize them. Hence, I shall first proceed by seeking the purpose(s) behind proposing definitions such as these. Only then will I discuss the definitions themselves.

WHY DEFINE 'MENTAL DISORDER'?

Because of the close tie of these chapters to the forthcoming third edition of the *Diagnostic and Statistical Manual,* two questions need to be distinguished here: the first is, what purposes are served by classifying mental disorders into the various categories of schizophrenia, etc.? The second is, what purposes are served by going further and attempting to define mental disorder in general (as opposed to defining schizophrenia, antisocial personality, etc.)?

Drs. Spitzer and Endicott seem to conflate these two distinct concerns when they tell us that their proposed definition of the general phrase 'mental disorder' "helps clarify the goals of medical classification," and then go on to rely on "the purposes of a classification of medical disorders" as if it were the purpose of the general definition. Dr. Salzinger's critique of Drs. Spitzer and Endicott blurs this distinction as well; he assumes that if he demolishes the categories of psychiatric diagnosis, he has undermined the general definitional efforts of Drs. Spitzer and Endicott. The truth of the matter is that the general definition efforts of Dr. Klein and Drs. Spitzer and Endicott can be neither justified nor refuted by either relying on or disparaging the purposes served by DSM-III or like classificatory efforts in psychiatry.

There are doubtlessly a number of legitimate reasons why doctors generally, and psychiatrists in particular, seek to classify disorders. The scientific and therapeutic concerns of medicine have for centuries dictated that symptoms which recur together, develop in an established course, etc., be provisionally linked as separate disorders. Such inductive procedures would seem to be a necessary first step in seeking the sorts of causal accounts themselves necessary to discover and justify effective therapies.

Those sorts of reasons, however, do not justify going beyond the stage of classification, and attempting the different task undertaken by Drs. Spitzer and Endicott, and Dr. Klein, namely, to say what the general phrase 'mental disorder' should mean. There must be purposes other than those behind the classificatory scheme of DSM-III itself that justify this more general definitional effort.

Both of these chapters suggest a number of such purposes. Although not perhaps organized quite in the way their authors suggest, there are I think three separate purposes to be served in defining 'mental disorder'. The first I shall call a jurisdictional purpose: a definition of 'mental disorder' should mark clearly the sphere of proper concern—the jurisdiction—of psychiatry. To serve this purpose, a definition of 'mental disorder' should include only those conditions which are properly the subject matter of treatment by psychiatrists.

The second purpose, explicit in the Spitzer-Endicott chapter, is probably the one which in fact has motivated both chapters' definitional efforts. That I shall call the "hard cases" purpose of giving the definition. It was a "hard case" such as homosexuality that has most recently generated the discussion about what is a mental disorder. Such hard cases can be resolved, or even intelligently debated, only if one has clearly in mind what it is one is claiming when one claims that, e.g., homosexuality is or is not a mental disorder. Hence, the hard cases purpose: a definition of 'mental disorder' should allow one to resolve cases (or at least know what we are arguing about if we cannot resolve them) when we are unsure of whether to classify a condition as a mental disorder or not.

The third purpose behind these definitional efforts is what I shall call the legitimization purpose served by the definition. The purpose of defining 'mental disorder', on this rationale, is to legitimate psychiatry as a genuine branch of medicine. A definition of 'mental disorder' serves this purpose only if it shows mental disorder to be a species of the genus, medical disorder.

Before one critiques the proposed definitions in light of these purposes, one first must ask whether these are legitimate purposes for defining 'mental disorder'. Would any definition that satisfied them be useful? Can any definition in fact accomplish these three items? Let me reexamine them one by one.

Jurisdictional Purpose

One very important caveat needs to be stressed here: no definition of 'mental disorder' can or should have as its purpose the staking out of a claim to *exclusive* jurisdiction by psychiatry over the conditions so labeled. At several points Drs. Spitzer and Endicott seem to suggest such a purpose. They urge that their definition "helps delineate the areas of responsibility of the medical system from that of other social systems which also have as their purpose improving or otherwise changing human functioning, such as the educational or criminal justice systems." Elsewhere they urge that use of 'mental disorder' is a "call to action" on the part of society, in the sense that those to whom the label is truly applied may claim exemption from moral and legal responsibility or other social duties, and in the sense that its true application would justify third-party payments for medical care.

Dr. Klein is even more forceful in his urging that doctors define 'mental disorder' in order to determine when a person may legitimately be exempted from his social responsibilities: "the attribution of illness," he states, "both legitimizes the sick role and is a defense against criminal prosecution, so that the definition of illness has marked social impact." One purpose of the definition of such a view would be to separate the jurisdiction of medicine—the sick who are treatable—from that of the criminal law—the bad who are punishable.

These claims of definitional purpose are not consistent with the disclaimer later in the Spitzer-Endicott chapter that "The classification of a condition as a medical disorder and the response of society to manifestations of that condition are separate issues which should not be confused." I simply wish to emphasize the latter disclaimer to the exclusion of any implication from the former statements. As I have argued elsewhere (7), no definition of mental disorder for the psychiatric profession can or should be controlling of other disciplines' definitions of the phrase. The law, for example, in defining 'mental disorder' in the many legal contexts in which the phrase appears, must govern its definitions by its own purposes. Thus, if alcoholism or drug addiction is defined by doctors as a mental disorder, that should not control whether such a condition cannot constitutionally be made the subject of criminal sanctions. Nor can inclusion of, e.g., antisocial personality as a disorder be relevant to determining whether such condition should constitute an excuse from punishment.

The matter of third-party payment is a bit more complicated. In the first instance, of course, the separation made above holds: the purposes behind whatever insurance or other compensation scheme that may be set up should govern the definition of 'mental disorder' (or like phrase) appearing in the laws or contracts creating such schemes. There thus should be no automatic transposition of the concept of mental disorder of psychiatrists, to such compensation contexts. On the other hand, one might argue that such compensation schemes might have as their purpose the compensation of those conditions properly treatable by doctors—i.e., those conditions labeled 'mental disorder' by definitions such as those proposed. Whether such compensation schemes should adopt such psychiatric definition is I think an open question. It would seem to depend in part on how much attention is paid to the idea stressed more by Dr. Klein than by Drs. Spitzer and Endicott —the idea of voluntariness. If one of the purposes of a definition of 'mental disorder' is to make it attractive to those who will define the phrase for compensation purposes, then it would seem some attention would have to be paid to limit mental disorders to conditions that are involuntary; for compensation systems generally exist to compensate misfortune, not self-improvement schemes.

Finally, with regard to any claim of exclusive jurisdiction, neither Dr. Spitzer nor Dr. Endicott would wish to claim that categorizing a condition as a mental disorder under their definitions could or should preclude different conceptualizations of the same condition by other disciplines, notably psychology.

Having taken such effort to say what I take it this jurisdictional purpose should not be, let me now say what I think it should be. The other "calls to action" mentioned by Drs. Spitzer and Endicott are those to the medical profession and to the person with the condition—to treat, and to seek treatment, respectively. The definition is intended as a "trigger for treatment," that is, to state the general conditions under which treatment by a psychiatrist is appropriate (again with the caveat that this does not preclude other modes of treatment by other professions from also being appropriate). One may state this rationale more precisely as follows: 'mental disorder' is defined in such a way that if one has a mental disorder, that is sufficient to justify treatment.

I am unclear whether Drs. Spitzer and Endicott wish to say that their definition of mental disorder is intended also to state a necessary condition justifying treatment. That is, should people seek treatment from and be treated by psychiatrists if they do not have a mental disorder as defined? If one of the purposes of the definition is to mark out the area of therapeutic concern of psychiatrists in a systematic way, presumably 'mental disorder' should be defined so that it is a necessary as well as a sufficient condition of treatment. (My only hesitation in saying that Drs. Spitzer and Endicott do in fact attempt this stems from their criterion C, which excludes as medical disorders some things doctors properly treat, e.g., pregnancy; yet I am unable to find any mental condition similarly excluded, so perhaps 'mental disorder' and 'treated by psychiatrists' are intended to be extensional equivalents, even if 'medical disorder' and 'treated by doctors' are not.)

Having said all of this, it is still not clear why a general definition of 'mental disorder' is necessary, above and beyond an elucidation of the categories of mental disorders in DSM-III. For one could define the jurisdiction of psychiatry simply by pointing to DSM-III and saying, "psychiatrists treat whatever conditions are listed therein as mental disorders." Indeed, Busse (3) once pointed out that is in fact how many psychiatrists do define the domain of their concern.

I find myself out of sympathy with the latter mode of proceeding. Surely it is a legitimate enterprise to attempt to discover what all such conditions have in common that make psychiatrists think of them as mental disorders. It may be that there is no unity to the various conditions we are prepared to say are mental disorders; perhaps psychiatrists treat so many different conditions that nothing of interest can be said about them in general. That would not show psychiatry to be without a jurisdiction; it would have as many jurisdictions as there were different mental disorders. But it surely would be troubling to think that one's profession deals with a large number of different things which have nothing in common with each other, other than the juxtaposition of their names in a manual issued by the professional association.

The "Hard Cases" Purpose

This purpose behind the definitions of Drs. Klein and Spitzer-Endicott is comparatively straightforward and unproblematic. One does need to know what one is arguing about (what are the characteristics of a mental disorder) before one can even intelligently disagree about whether homosexuality is or is not a mental disorder. It might be thought that one can argue by analogy in such cases, e.g., "homosexuality is like sterility because both render one unable to reproduce." And, indeed, one can meaningfully debate borderline cases in such ways; only, when one does so, one does unsystematically what Drs. Spitzer, Endicott, and Klein attempt to do systematically, namely, articulate the criteria by virtue of which such analogies hold.

The Legitimization Purpose

It is no secret that the medical approach to the treatment of mental disorders has been under severe attack from numerous directions in the last two decades. Can a definition of 'mental disorder' serve as an argument against this attack?

It may sound odd to think of a definition as constituting an argument at all. If Drs. Spitzer, Endicott, and Klein were merely stipulating a meaning to 'mental disorder' to serve the first two purposes, then such a definition would not be itself an argument. Yet in fact both chapters do engage in analysis, not stipulation, in their attempt to give a (lexical) definition of 'medical disorder'. The strategy is a familiar one in the literature: one first analyzes what 'medical disorder' means in physical medicine, and then stipulates that the only conditions properly thought of as mental disorders are those that are medical disorders of a mental sort. If successful, one does show that 'mental disorder' as defined is a species of the genus, medical disorder; one has thereby legitimated the medical approach to mental disorders, because by definition the only conditions properly so called are medical matters.[1]

It is worth stressing that this purpose requires an accurate analysis of the general criteria that doctors implicitly use to decide what is and what is not a medical disorder. One necessarily gives up Humpty Dumpty's freedom to make a word mean what one pleases, for this part of the definition is not free from factual inquiry. A successful definition of 'medical disorder' will classify as such all and only those conditions doctors agree are medical disorders. It is thus a legitimate form of objection to this part of the definition to argue by counterexample: if the criteria suggested include conditions most doctors do not regard as medical disorders, or if the criteria suggested exclude conditions most doctors do regard as medical disorders, the criteria are wrong. 'Wrong' in the sense that the definition cannot then serve the third, legitimizing purpose.

THE SPITZER-ENDICOTT DEFINITION OF 'MENTAL DISORDER'

Drs. Spitzer and Endicott follow the classic, Aristotelean (1) pattern of definition in which a word or phrase is defined in two steps. One first shows

---

[1] If one actually wishes to complete the argument, one further step remains: one must show that the conditions psychiatrists treat, as listed in DSM-III, in fact fit the general definition of 'mental disorders' stipulated in these chapters.

the larger class of things to which the item to be defined belongs, here, medical disorders; one then states the principle that differentiates the item to be defined within that larger class, for Drs. Spitzer and Endicott, psychological symptoms or comprehension only in psychological terms.

Since Drs. Spitzer and Endicott spend little time on the second step, I will as well. It is worth noting in passing that there are some issues lurking here: should one classify as mental disorders those with mental causes, or those with mental symptoms? It is a common assumption that the difference between physical and mental illness lies in the species of causality involved. Although I think Drs. Spitzer and Endicott are right in classifying by symptoms and not by causes, it is a position that requires argument.

Secondly, it is unclear why 'psychological' is parenthetically equated with 'behavioral'. Some symptoms of mental disorder are straightforwardly behavioral (e.g., in antisocial personality), but others, as in paranoia, are behavioral only if behaviorism is a correct translation of the mental states involved. There is good reason to believe that behaviorism is not an adequate translation of mental terms such as 'belief' or 'hallucination' necessary to describe paranoia; in any case, it would seem unnecessary for psychiatrists to take a position on this general problem in the philosophy of the mind.

Turning to the main point of Dr. Spitzer's and Dr. Endicott's definition (that which defines the class of medical disorders), this definition comes in three parts: (a) organismic dysfunction that causes (b) negative consequences, which in turn give rise to (c) a call to action on the part of patients, doctors, and society. This nominally three-tiered structure obscures, I think, the true nature of the definition, and is in any event unnecessarily complicated.

Taking the third part first, the various calls to action: there are two questions one should distinguish in order to see that none of the discussion of "calls to action" is properly part of the definition of 'medical disorder'. First, is it true that if and only if there are the calls to action Spitzer and Endicott describe, there is a medical disorder? Second, even if it is true, is the fact that there is such equivalence any reason to suppose that part of the meaning of 'medical disorder' is that calls to action exist?

The first question I have already discussed in the section on the jurisdictional purpose to the definition. To repeat what was argued for there: it is not true that if doctors treat a condition as a medical disorder, then such condition exempts one from responsibility, entitles one to third-party payment, etc. There may in some of the cases doctors treat be such a "call to action" on the part of society to react to the patient in certain ways, but whether there is will be determined by purposes other than those justifying medical classification.

Secondly, even if it were true that society, e.g., exempted persons from certain responsibilities if and only if they had a medical disorder as defined by doctors, surely such exemption is not part of anyone's meaning of 'medical disorder'. To say otherwise is to confuse mere equivalence (A is true if and only if B is true) with "meaning the same as." Consider the *Oxford English Dictionary's* former definition of 'gold' as "the world's most precious metal." Suppose that these expressions are equivalent, that is, whenever 'gold' is used, "the world's most precious metal" could be substituted without change of the truth value of the expressions in which they occur. Such equivalence does not show 'gold' to mean the world's most precious metal. To say that 'gold' does mean this reduces the statement that gold is the world's most precious metal to an analytical truth; when in fact a rise in the price of silver could make it false. 'Gold' does not mean "the world's most precious metal," even if it is a contingent truth about gold that it is presently the world's most precious metal.

As a second example, consider the following definition of 'death' (a condition doctors, lawyers, and philosophers are currently much concerned to define): " 'Death' means to be buried by a mortician." Suppose it were true in our society that all and only dead people are buried by morticians (i.e., 'dead' and 'buried by morticians' are extensionally equivalent expressions). Even so, the definition misses entirely the meaning of 'death'; otherwise, the idea of being *buried alive* could not constitute the plot of a chilling horror story but only a conceptual impossibility imagined by someone who did not know the meaning of the word 'death'.

In short, the calls to action are not part of the meaning of 'medical disorder'. They may be consequences of having a medical disorder (although one of them, the call to society, I have argued is not even that); they may be one of the purposes of giving the definition, as I have argued the triggering of treatment rationale is; but they are not themselves part of the meaning of 'medical disorder' as doctors or anyone else employs the phrase.

The first and second parts of the definition collapse into one basic requirement, I think, for "organismic dysfunction" carries no weight in the definition that I can ascertain beyond the negative consequences it engenders. It suggests, perhaps, something wrong about the organism; but what that more specifically means is that one of the negative consequences—distress, disability, or disadvantage—has come about. Accordingly, the heart of the definition turns on these three negative consequences.

These three are proposed as the positive conditions which govern the proper use of 'medical disorder'. All of the other criteria—B, C, and D—are limitations posited to exclude counterexamples. The necessity of positing such limiting criteria stems in part from the breadth of the positive criteria, and from the fact that they are disjunctive, that is, any one being satisfied is sufficient to label someone as having a medical disorder.

Coming then to the heart of the matter, the "three D's" of distress, disability, and disadvantage: the first two, distress and disability, I shall not discuss directly; they (along with death, which Drs. Spitzer and Endicott include under disability) are the traditional criteria mentioned in the literature for having a medical disorder. The third, disadvantage, is, as Drs. Spitzer and Endicott recognize, much more problematical. 'Disadvantage' as used by Spitzer and Endicott is far removed from its usage in the literature [e.g., Kendell (5) and Scadding (11)] as a traditional criterion of illness or disease, where it refers to the ability to function effectively, to survive, or to reproduce. The most critical difference from this traditional usage is Drs. Spitzer and Endicott's willingness to allow the adverse reaction of society to count as placing the individual at a disadvantage. Sexual sadism, kleptomania, and pathological gambling are said to disadvantage the individual because such activities lead to painful consequences, namely, the police pick you up. If one were to keep extending such examples, one would include all seriously immoral or illegal activity as "leading to painful consequences in all cultures and thus a disadvantage," and thus all dispositions to such activity as medical disorders.

Drs. Spitzer and Endicott exclude masturbation and homosexuality from this criterion only by virtue of the fact that some societies do not punish such activities. If it were hard to imagine a society which could be indifferent to such activities, presumably they too would be included as medical disorders.

Surely Drs. Spitzer and Endicott do not want to say this. One does not want to give up the line between medical judgment and moral evaluation this easily (I will discuss when I get to Dr. Klein's chapter the comparatively anemic sense in which all medical judgments are normative). It strikes me that we might well wish to consider some forms of theft, sexual brutality, or gambling as forms of medical disorder, but not because well-ordered societies necessarily attach painful consequences to these activities. After all, all well-ordered societies attach such painful consequences to many forms of these activities which no one would want to consider as disorders, e.g., organized car theft. Surely it is something else about kleptomania, sexual sadism, or pathological gambling that inclines us to regarding them as disorders, something other than the fact that no society can tolerate such activities.

The "something else" which suggests itself is to be found in the compulsive and irrational nature of the activities. It would seem that, e.g., kleptomaniacs might be regarded as having a mental disorder because they do not know why they steal what they do, and they find it difficult if not impossible to stop. The difference between a kleptomaniac and a habitual thief would seem to lie, as Max Friedman (4) once suggested, in these two dimensions, lack of rational motive and compulsion. If so, kleptomania could seemingly be regarded as a disorder under the first two criteria, distress and disability, for one who is irrational and compelled is necessarily one who is impaired from acting in ways in which both he and society would wish him to act. That would seem to qualify as a disablement (the second criterion), usually leading to distress (the first).

One would doubtlessly wish to do further analysis in order to make out the last thesis. One might want to modify the range of activities required to be impaired before one is said to have a disorder, to accommodate these cases of compulsion. One would also want to be clear on the distinction between compulsion and mere causation, so that one is not led to the error of thinking that because one is merely caused to act in certain ways one is therefore impaired in the relevant sense from acting otherwise. Still, this approach seems more promising than does the open invitation Spitzer and Endicott's notion of 'disadvantage' gives to all who wish to argue that psychiatry is covert moral philosophy, thinly disguised as science.

The last two subcategories of disadvantage are "marked impairment in the ability to form relatively lasting and nonconflictual interpersonal relationships" and "impairment of the ability to experience sexual pleasure in an interpersonal context." These are expressly included by Spitzer and Endicott as disadvantages, not disabilities, because of their normative nature. I will not deal with them until I discuss Dr. Klein's chapter, which raises the normative issue explicitly. To anticipate the results of that discussion: in a nonharmful sense, all medical classification is normative; that includes what we call 'disability' no less than the things Spitzer-Endicott call 'disadvantage'; thus, these items, if they are to be disorders at all, should be handled as disabling conditions under the second criterion. If they cannot be fit there, perhaps one should simply recognize that psychiatrists, like all doctors, treat conditions that are not disorders.

I will be as brief as possible with the three limiting conditions. Taking them in reverse order: criterion D, distinctness, is added because of the background of Spitzer and Endicott's definitional efforts. Their general definition of 'mental disorder' was generated by the classification problems of DSM-III. Hence, a criterion such as D is necessary to build into the definition of 'mental disorder' the classic attributes of any such medical classification, in terms of syndrome, course, etc. One should note that such a criterion is unnecessary if the question were not "what is a mental disorder?" but were, "Is this patient disordered (sick, ill)?" For a patient could be disordered (sick, ill) by suffering the negative consequences of organismic dysfunction, yet not fit any category of disorders established by DSM-III. Drs. Spitzer and Endicott recognize this; DSM-III will classify such cases in residual categories. It is probably nit picking, but if distinctness is retained as a criterion of 'mental disorder', such residual categories are not, as far as we know, disorders, for by definition there is no clinical distinctness in terms of syndrome, course, etc.

Two things are disturbing about criterion C. One is that it seems essentially *ad hoc* posited to avoid specific counterexamples. This is really no more than an aesthetic objection, but its force derives from the following *reductio:* imagine a definition of 'medical disorder' in terms of some very general positive criterion—e.g., "disorder is any state of the organism"—and hundreds of negative criteria, each posited to take care of foreseen counterexamples. Although such a definition might well fit the conditions doctors treat as medical disorders, and thus satisfy some of the purposes of the definition, one would doubtlessly seek a simpler definition, that is, a definition with more precise positive criteria and correspondingly fewer negative ones. (In addition, it would be a much less satisfying demonstration of the unity of psychiatric interest—the jurisdictional purpose of the definition—if all one did was make clear what psychiatrists do not treat.)

Apart from its aesthetics, one may also question this criterion's correctness. To begin with, it may be true to regard the distress and disability of pregnancy as the price women have to pay to bear children. "He who wills the end necessarily wills the means." But does one really want to say the same of grief, namely, that it is "the price that one pays for having attachments?" Kierkegaard, the Danish philosopher, once thought something like this about deep emotional attachments. Being in love, he wrote, was like being suspended over ten thousand fathoms, because of the risk one exposed oneself to that the loved one would leave or die.

The difference in the two cases is that one hardly regards grief as the necessary price of emotional attachments to others, as one regards pain and disability as the necessary price of pregnancy and childbirth. One hopes and probably believes otherwise when one forms personal attachments; one may have to pay the price, but certainly did not expect to pay it. Hence, the acceptance of the pain of childbirth, and the contrasting nonacceptance of the gratuitousness in the death of a loved one.

In any case, even if grief could be analogized to childbirth in the way Drs. Spitzer and Endicott suggest, surely the criterion as stated is too broad. It would seemingly exclude all medical disorders known to be caused by activities we think to be desirable. Thus, the necessary prices associated with (the positive goods of) mining and smoking are, respectively, black lung disease and lung cancer; by virtue of criterion C, these are not medical disorders.

Such cases would suggest to Dr. Klein, I would suspect from reading his chapter, that the exclusionary condition be framed in terms of voluntariness —pregnancy and grief are voluntarily incurred as known concomitants of certain activities, and therefore are not disorders. Yet this is surely much too strong. A disorder voluntarily incurred is still a disorder. One has lung cancer whether due to smog or cigarette smoking.

The first part of criterion B ("the controlling variables tend to be attributed to being largely within the organism") introduces explicitly what was implicit in the idea of "organismic dysfunction," namely, that the cause of the condition be internal. With regard to physically caused disorders, this requirement is unproblematic, for we know what it means to say that a virus or a chemical imbalance is in the body. Once one recognizes that "some dysfunctions may be understandable only on the basis of psychological terms," however, one has all the problems surrounding the location of mind in assigning sense to the phrase, "within the organism." One is reminded of Gilbert Ryle's (10) intentionally paradoxical remark that if one must think of minds (and all of their furniture that might serve as psychological causes) as being somewhere, they are "in" the external world.

Understandably enough, Drs. Spitzer and Endicott seek to avoid this problem by giving an "operational definition" of criterion B in terms of what types of interventions reverse the condition: if "simple informative or standard educational procedures" or "non-technical interventions" reverse the condition, then it is not thought to be "within the organism," that is, the condition is not a medical disorder. In light of the difficulties alluded to earlier that are involved when one attempts to define a thing by focusing on contingent connections it may have with other things, be they consequences or methods of correction, it is preferable to regard criterion B as consisting of its operational part only.

Even so, this second part raises potentially serious problems. For the ideas of "simple informative or standard educational procedures" and "non-technical interventions" come perilously close to meaning no more than "non-medical procedures." One of the purposes of the definition is to define psychiatry's (and medicine's) jurisdiction. That cannot be accomplished if one defines the conditions medicine treats (disorders) in terms which beg the question, namely, terms dependent for their meaning on a prior understanding of what is and what is not medical. The reduction such definition leads to is that medical disorders are the conditions doctors treat, a useless statement that Spitzer and Endicott rightly reject as not accomplishing the jurisdictional purpose of the definition.

In closing my remarks on the Spitzer-Endicott chapter, let me turn to the criticisms they anticipated (but which I have not made). These are the criticisms that the definition of mental disorder is either too broad or too narrow. Most of the motive for making these criticisms, it seems to me, evaporates if one accepts the limited purposes outlined earlier for giving the definition. As long as one realizes that neither DSM-III nor this definition of 'mental disorder' drawn from it is determinative of social issues, such as moral or legal accountability, third-party payments, or different forms of treatment, and that the only thing at issue is an in-house specification of the (nonexclusive) jurisdiction of psychiatry, then much of the fury surrounding such matters will doubtlessly abate. That does not, of course, mean that there is not room to criticize on grounds of breadth or narrowness. Only that what is at stake is not a large social issue but a matter of stipulating a meaning to 'mental disorder' consistent with the conditions psychiatrists in fact treat. For the kinds of legal, moral, or other social issues often *thought* to turn on definitions of this kind by psychiatrists, the Spitzer-Endicott definition of 'mental disorder' and DSM-III on which it is based are probably much too broad.

DR. KLEIN'S PROPOSED DEFINITION OF 'MENTAL ILLNESS'

Like the Spitzer-Endicott chapter, Dr. Klein regards mental illness as a species of the general class of illnesses, differentiated by "evidence in the cognitive, behavioral, affective, or motivational aspects of organismal functioning." Also like Drs. Spitzer and Endicott, Dr. Klein devotes almost all of his attention to defining the general class to which mental illness belongs (illness) and pays relatively little attention to the principle of differentiation.

In his discussion of the concept of illness, I am unclear as the precise role Dr. Klein assigns to the "sick role." To the extent that the exemptions society usually grants to those who are sick are meant as criteria of 'illness', Dr. Klein makes the same error as Drs. Spitzer and Endicott with regard to confusing equivalence with identity of meaning. To the extent these exemptions are meant to constitute the purpose of defining 'mental illness', for reasons earlier mentioned I don't think any definition useful to psychiatrists can *ipso facto* be transferred to other social settings.

Most of Dr. Klein's chapter deals with a definition of 'mental illness' in terms other than its supposed social consequences. Although there is an unfortunate lack of clarity about the difference between "evidence," "indicators," and criteria in the balance of Dr. Klein's chapter, his central analysis of the criterion of illness is plain enough; we are ill only if we are diseased, and we are diseased only if we have suboptimal, part dysfunction. The crucial notion in terms of which we are to understand both illness and disease is, for Dr. Klein (and ultimately for Drs. Spitzer and Endicott as well via the idea of disability), the notion of function. Since in this I think Dr. Klein is ultimately correct, and because it focuses the normative issue on which Dr. Klein is I think incorrect, I will direct my comments on his chapter to explicating the notion of function and its relation to (mental) illness.

The Logic of Functional Analysis

A familiar use of 'function' is one such as: "The function of the heartbeat is to circulate the blood." This could be paraphrased without change of meaning to: "The heartbeat serves the purpose of circulating the blood," or to: "The heart beats in order to circulate the blood." The elements most commonly found in the unpacking of such statements are four: a system (S) is tacitly assumed; an end-state (ES) of the system is also tacitly assumed; an identifiable part of the system or a process (P) occurring within the system (which is the item for which an explanation is sought) is expressly mentioned; and effect (E) of the process or part (that is also a state of the system) is expressly mentioned.

In such an explanation the information content is that the existence or activity of the part or process P is a contingently *necessary condition* to the occurrence of the effect E; the tacit assumptions further assert that E is itself a contingently necessary condition to the maintenance of the system as a whole in some general end-state. Thus, "the function of the heartbeat is to circulate the blood" implies the existence of a system (the human body), labels an identifiable part (the heart) or process (the heart's beating), and specifies an immediate effect of that process, namely, a state of the system in which the blood circulates. The function assigned to the heart is the effect named in the statement (the circulation of blood), and the information content is that in certain living systems with which we are familiar (namely, vertebrates), the heart's beating is a necessary condition for the circulation of blood. This effect (the circulation of blood) is of interest to us only because it itself is in turn a necessary condition for the survival of such organisms. Hence, the ultimate empirical content of such a functional statement will be that the beating of the heart is a necessary condition for the survival of the organism.

It is important to stress that P is a necessary condition to E (and to ES) only relative to some system. Hearts are not logically necessary for blood to circulate in all living systems; some other mode of circulation is certainly logically possible. Hearts are necessary only for the survival of those living systems we classify as vertebrates. Since the class of vertebrates is not defined as "creatures with a heart," the asserted connection between having a heart and being a live vertebrate is a genuinely empirical claim. If there were no way to specify for what system S P is a necessary condition for E, then the quoted statement would be either meaningless or false.

It is equally important to stress that it is only relative to some ES in S that a function may be assigned. Absent the end-state of health of the human body, one would be free to pick any consequent E of the heart's beating (e.g., the noise it makes in the chest cavity) to call its function; for freed of the requirement that E itself causally contribute to the maintenance of some general ES, one consequence of the heartbeat is as good as another to be emphasized as *the* function of the heart.

Thus, although the statement with which we began did not expressly mention either a system or an end-state, both must be tacitly assumed if sense is to be made of such statements. In fact, of course, the contexts in which such statements are made will often expressly provide definitions of S and of ES.

What such explanations tell us is that there is a causal connection between the part or process to which a function is attributed, and the existence of the end-state. In vertebrates, the heart must beat in order for blood to circulate. This is a genuinely empirical claim that may be expressed equivalently in nonfunctional language as, "the blood circulates (in vertebrates) *only if* the heart beats." In our symbolization: for all systems, E only if P.

Thus, functional explanations involve causal laws, but "in reverse": rather than explaining the heart's beating by reference to its *causes,* a functional explanation explains it by reference to one of its *effects* (the circulation of blood). The relationship of cause and effect is asserted in such explanations, but we are told what has been *caused by* the part or process about which we are curious, not what *causes it* to be or do what it does.

It has struck many people as decidedly peculiar that an *effect* of an event should be cited to explain it; it sounds much like the Aristotelean notion of a Final Cause, where some end causally determines the events that are its means. Yet nothing of the sort need be asserted in one's use of 'purpose' in the sense of function. In the first place, much of the use of functional statements such as that about heartbeats is not explanatory of the heartbeat at all; the attribution of functions in such statements is often merely a description of the heart or heartbeat that emphasizes certain of its features. Secondly, where function is used in an explanation, the effect (e.g., the circulation of blood) that is called the function does not play the role of a cause of the item to be explained, the heartbeat. Each of these two legitimate uses of 'function' merits some discussion.

Where scientists share a common concern for a particular system and the maintenance of some particular end-state in the system, the attribution of functions is a useful descriptive task. Thus, in physical medicine one is concerned with the human body; and there is widespread agreement among doctors on the desirability of maintaining that system in the particular end-state we call health. In such circumstances it is useful for medical texts to attribute functions to organs and other physical structures, or to their activities. Formulating medical information in this way serves to emphasize the causal contribution each such organ or process makes to the maintenance of an end-state that it is the business of doctors to preserve. It is a way of referencing a great deal of information in such a way that one knows immediately the contribution of each part of the system to the end-state desired for that system.

To be sure, the referencing of a good deal of causal information in this way, so as to emphasize just those features relevant to a particular undertaking, does not lead to full-fledged explanations of why, for example, a heart beats. Functional statements in such situations are simply a mode of organizing information about parts of a system and their relationship to each other around a central concern. One can see this by schematizing functional statements such as the one quoted, as: for all S, ES only if P. From such a premise nothing can be deduced about any particular individual's heart beating or not. Yet such a premise does tell us that, if in general we are interested in maintaining S in state ES, we must make certain P occurs. If we wish to keep patients alive, we must keep their hearts beating.

Beyond the organizational benefits of attributing functions, one may use such attributions as part of a genuine explanation of the event in question. To do this one must add the premise that the system in question will tend (within certain boundary conditions here ignored) to return to some particular end-state. The structure of the argument is then:

1. The heart's beating (P) is a necessary condition for health (ES) in vertebrates (S) [ES only if P for all S]; *and* 2. The body will maintain itself in a state of health [for all S, ES]. From these premises the conclusion, P, follows by the rules of elementary logic. Thus, for systems which do in fact tend to return to some end-state despite varying conditions in the environment, it is a legitimate form of explanation of a part or process to cite its function in the maintenance of some larger system. It is a matter for empirical discovery to what extent such self-regulating systems are to be found in nature or in human artifacts, such as homing devices on missiles, thermostats for furnaces, etc.; where there are such regularities, the attribution of functions and explanations in terms of them are appropriate.

Physical medicine is an obvious example that fits both of these requirements. It is concerned with a well-defined system in which numerous homeostatic balances are maintained (e.g., body temperature); and the maintenance of a particular state of that system is one about which doctors are much concerned. The latter is a sufficient ground for attributing functions to parts and processes in the body; the former allows one, in addition, to use that attribution of function as part of a genuinely empirical explanation of why we should expect to find that part or process occurring in some particular vertebrate's body.

The suspicions functional explanations engender outside of physical medicine or biology are largely due to the fact that functions are assigned in situations that do not meet either of the two criteria just discussed. Rather, some effect of a social practice or habit is singled out as *the* function of the practice in question, and treated as an explanation of such practice, without: (a) any reason being given as to why we should be concerned about the particular end-state of the system relative to which the function is assigned; or (2) any reason being given to believe that the system in fact tends to achieve the end-state relative to which the function is assigned. We may be told, for example, that the function of a ceremonial rain dance among certain tribes is to reinforce group solidarity. Although the reinforcement of group solidarity may be an effect of the practice in question, so are a lot of other things—tired feet, satisfaction at the completion of exercise, relaxation of group anxieties, etc. Absent a precise stipulation of an end-state about which we are most concerned to maintain in such systems (societies), or which is in fact maintained in such systems, there is little to be gained by selecting this one effect of the action in question over a host of others for the emphasis as "the function." It is about as useful as saying that the function of the heart is to produce sounds in the chest cavity. Functions can be assigned only relative to end-states, and are usefully assigned only when such end-states are a matter of great interest to us to preserve, or are preserved irrespective of our interests in nature.

Suboptimal Part Dysfunction and Value Judgments

With this analysis of function in mind, let me apply it to two problems raised by Dr. Klein's definition: the sense in which mental illness can be said to be "part dysfunction"; and the sense in which all judgments of illness are normative because they rely on the notion of functional impairment.

It should by now be apparent where Dr. Klein's definition of disease is most comfortable, namely, with those impairments of the function assigned to various parts of the human body. For here a clear distinction can be maintained between Klein's idea of "part-function" and the kind of function social scientists frequently ascribe to total behavior ("his reading Shakespeare served the function of making him a better politician"). Less clear is how the distinction between part function and functions served by total behavior can survive when we move to examples of mental illness. For the distinction between the functions assigned by biologists and those assigned by social scientists seems to lie in the object to which the function is assigned; in the biological case, to parts of bodies; in the social science case, only to total behavior.

The problem of placing mental or "functional" illnesses on the "part function" side of such a distinction is that there is no part of the body to which to assign the functions impaired (memory, perception, will, emotion, etc.). The only unproblematic objects around are persons *in toto* and their behavior. One of course might say that it is to the "mind" or parts thereof to which mental functions are ascribed. But what is that? One of the most persuasive philosophical analyses of mind is that it just *is* an aggregation of functions, that, e.g., the will is not some object which has as its function the execution of actions, but rather it just is the function persons perform when they act [Putnam (8)]. Similarly (and I take it this is consistent with current interpretations of the structural aspect of psychoanalytic theory), the ego is not an object to which the function of conflict resolution is assigned; conflict resolution is one of the functions people perform that is named by the word 'ego'. If this reduction (of minds in general and mental faculties and other parts of mind in particular) to functional states is correct, then the distinction sought by Dr. Klein (and Aubrey Lewis, on whom he relies here) has to be cast in other ways.

The way which suggests itself (because I, like Dr. Klein, believe that there is a difference between the functional explanations of social science and those of psychiatry) is to be found in the functional interpretation of mind itself. The words naming mental faculties are crude beginnings of a functional subdivision of the mind—in order, e.g., to raise a spoonful of cherries to one's mouth, one must *perceive* the bowl in front of one, *remember* that these are cherries, *reason* that lifting the spoon will lead to cherries in the mouth, *will* the movement, etc. Beyond these crude functional subdivisions of the ancient faculty psychology, one may continue to subdivide each of these mental performances into smaller functional steps. Workers in the field of artificial intelligence work up such functional subdivisions into very fine detail indeed.

The notion of functional impairment Dr. Klein seeks, I think, lies in the impairment of a person's abilities to perform these (functionally defined) subroutines and thus to perform normally in daily behavior. The functional impairment lies "behind" the behavior, not in the sense that some part of the person is not functional, but in the sense that the normal (functional) states which are necessary to produce rational, intelligent behavior do not exist, and because of this dysfunction the behavior itself is not normal. Such an account demands no entities beyond whole persons, their behavior, and the states defined by that person's functional organization.

These functionally defined steps need not be discrete acts, even mental acts, we perform in order to exhibit normal, gross behavior. When one begins functional divisions of intelligent routines, very quickly one leaves acts one does for functional stages that had to have been passed through. Thus, functionalists about mind such as Dennett (4) speak of the "subpersonal" level at which such steps are taken—subpersonal because such functionally distinguished steps are not acts persons perform at all. It is here, I think, that Dr. Klein's "part dysfunction" (and Drs. Spitzer and Endicott's "organismic dysfunction" "within the organism") is to be found.

Dr. Klein's second main concern is related to his first, but is distinct; it is whether medical judgments about health and illness or disease are in some pejorative sense normative. The sense in which all judgments of illness are normative is suggested by Dr. Klein's fear that they are *arbitrary,* meaning, I should think, that they are guided by values that vary with a culture rather than by factual criteria which do not. If 'illness' or 'disease' simply meant "deviation from average physical structure," then by our ideas of illness or disease there would be no normative element in our judgments. But as Dr. Klein recognizes, structural deviation is neither necessary nor sufficient; it can indicate disease only if it indicates *functional* impairment (hence the importance of structure/function correlations in medicine).

Because function is simply a consequence of process, as earlier discussed, and because there are many consequences of any process, some judgment is necessary as to *which* consequence gets labeled "the function," e.g., of the heart's beating. That question, I should think, is guided by the *factual* question of whether the consequence (E) itself contributes to health (ES). But in what factual criterion are judgments of health fixed?

Dr. Klein's answer is that we need not ask what values inform our judgment of what is or is not healthy. Rather, evolution has made us creatures with "natural functions," that is, has endowed us with numerous homeostatic mechanisms which guide our bodily processes in such a way that certain activities tend to produce certain goals despite varying conditions. It is these goals (the immediate effects) which he believes to be discoverable and which tell us, e.g., what the function of a heart is without recourse to some ultimate end-state of health. His argument is remarkably similar to a philosophical analysis by Christopher Boorse (2) who argues that our "species-specific" functional organization provides an objective basis for medicine.

The problem with such a view is twofold. In the first place, even if this made physical medicine nonnormative, it might well not do the same for psychiatry. (Indeed, this is precisely where this kind of analysis leads Boorse.) For although there are homeostatic mechanisms in the body which might allow one to pick out one consequence of an activity as its function, there are no unproblematic homeostatic mechanisms "in the mind." There are, to be sure, psychiatrists such as Karl Menninger (6) who have purported to have discovered an analogous principle of homeostasis around which mental functions may be organized; yet such a discovery is at best a useful heuristic posit, not the kind of empirical discovery Dr. Klein would need to make out his thesis about mental functions.

Secondly, even if one could make out the analogy, I do not think the discovery of such self-regulating mechanisms is the whole story about function assignment, even to body parts. Imagine a people who did not value bodily vitality as we do, who were perhaps of an ascetic streak, who did not, accordingly, care about capacities to engage in physical exercise at all. They would have a different concept of health than we do. Because of this, they would conceptualize the functional organization of a person differently than we do, because it would be important to them to preserve *their* sense of health, not ours. This would be true even if their judgments of health were dysfunctional vis-à-vis the end-state of survival, toward which many of our homeostatic mechanisms are directed. Thus the evolutionarily-generated functional organization on which Dr. Klein relies is no guarantee that medicine is nonnormative in its judgments of illness. All medicine, with its functional organization of persons, reflects our society's judgments of well-being, and is in that sense normative.

That of course need not mean that medicine is therefore arbitrary or nonscientific. If society is arbitrary (depending on one's view of ethics) in what it likes, that hardly makes science so in trying to find ways of achieving the object of such desires, namely, health.

CONCLUSION

Having taken this much time to say what is wrong with these definitions, let me close by saying what I think is right about both of them, namely, their focus on functional impairment as the central notion of any idea of disorder, disease, or illness. Making that general notion sufficiently precise to be useful is no easy task; it is a task worth doing, however, and these chapters are serious efforts in that direction.

REFERENCES

1. Aristotle (1960): *Topics, Book VI.* Harvard University Press, Cambridge, Mass.
2. Boorse, C. (1975): On the distinction between disease and illness. *Philos. Publ. Affairs,* 5:49–68.
3. Busse, E. W. (1972): The Presidential Address: There are decisions to be made. *Am. J. Psychiatry,* 129:1–9.
4. Dennett, D. C. (1969): *Content and Consciousness,* Humanities Press, New York.
5. Kendell, R. E. (1975): The concept of disease and its implications for psychiatry. *Br. J. Psychiatry,* 127:305–315.
6. Menninger, K. (1963): *The Vital Balance.* Viking Press, New York.
7. Moore, M. S. (1977): Legal conceptions of mental illness. In: *Philosophy and Medicine, Vol. 5.* Reidel, Netherlands *(in press).*
8. Putnam, H. (1975): *Mind, Language and Reality,* Chapters 14–22. Cambridge University Press, Cambridge.
9. Robinson, R. (1950): *Definition.* Clarendon Press, Oxford.
10. Ryle, G. (1949): *The Concept of Mind.* Hutchinson and Co., London.
11. Scadding, J. G. (1967): Diagnosis: The clinician and the computer. *Lancet,* 2:877–882.

Discussion: Definition and Labeling of Mental Illness

Dr. Jane Murphy: I would like to respond to Dr. Farber's comment about the role of social conditioning and reinforcement in the production of personality traits. His view is very similar to that of anthropologists who composed the "culture and personality" school of thought before and in the aftermath of the Second World War. The idea in these early studies was that by growing up in a given culture with its special cues, symbols, and guidelines for behavior, individuals developed personality traits which matched the cultural blueprint. Furthermore, different cultural blueprints were thought to produce different personality traits.

Some of the soundest anthropological work on this topic is the recent studies by John and Beatrice Whiting (2) and by William Caudill (1). These investigations concern children and infants in a variety of different cultural settings. Their findings are much more complex than the earlier views of cultural conditioning. They point to certain aspects of personality being malleable to cultural influence and other aspects not.

If the major psychiatric disorders were the same as personality traits, and if the role of social conditioning were as strong as Dr. Farber suggests, we would by now have discovered groups of people in which psychiatric disorders were nonexistent. When one thinks of the large number of "cultural experiments," so to speak, whereby an infant is reared to adulthood—when one considers, for example, the multitude of cultural variations inherent in patterns of communication, punishment, reward, standard-setting, and many other patterns characterizing the interactions of parents and children in different cultures—surely some of these variations would have produced a formula which would have prevented psychiatric disorders if such disorders were strongly under the influence of social conditioning.

Dr. Klein: I will try to be brief, with regard to the comments made by Drs. Farber and Moore.

Dr. Farber says we have to pay attention to human needs and values in the definition of illness, and I thought I agreed with him about that.

My point was that you have disease, an objectifiable aspect of part dysfunction, and you have the social evaluation of the disease-produced distress or disability, that may or may not result in the application of the illness label. I think there are rather few societies in which a broken leg would not be considered a disorder.

As for Dr. Moore, I think he accused me of academic imperialism. The idea was that we psychiatrists are trying to legislate for the lawyers, the third party payment people etc., and I say, why let them legislate for us? (Laughter)

I think it is an obligation on the part of the psychiatric profession to try to come up with definitions that will tell the ill from the bad, for instance.

It is quite true that my definition does not preclude other people's definitions. No definition precludes any definition, unfortunately for my definition. Definitions are simply stipulations about the use of words.

The question is if there is some valid, cutting relationship that one definition leads to, that another definition does not. We will find out about that in the future.

Dr. Guze: Committed to the importance of diagnosis, as I am, I find myself a little distressed by the discussion, because it suggests that we might be drifting into a new kind of scholasticism.

To prevent this from happening we should recognize that the concept of disease (or disorder), as many have already said but not, I think, adequately emphasized is a convention, and that, quite aside from psychiatric conditions, no definition of disease is entirely satisfactory for general medicine.

The notion of disease (or illness) requires tolerance of fuzzy boundaries. And to the degree that we try to deny that fuzziness and make it sharp, we risk stultifying scholasticism.

If we are trying to pursue the medical model in psychiatry, we should consider what this model means in medical areas where there is less controversy about its appropriateness.

To apply the medical model to psychiatric disorders means to use the ideas and approaches that medical practitioners use when they deal with general medical conditions.

It is likely that we will never achieve consensus about the definition of illness, whether medical or psychiatric, but we might accomplish more if we concentrate on the definitions of individual disorders.

I am much less concerned about whether or not we can agree on the boundaries of psychiatry than I am about whether we can agree on the boundaries of mania or obsessional neurosis, for example.

Preoccupation with the definition of disease leads to a kind of armchair philosophy, and psychiatry surely has had more than enough of that.

Preoccupation with individual disorders leads to research and data, and psychiatry certainly needs a lot more of that. (Applause)

Dr. Freyhan: Since our topic deals with the question of the diagnosis of mental disorders, the question arises whether Dr. Salzinger's paper puts too much emphasis on the structured interview, the problems of reliability in evaluating the interview, and other secondary matters pertaining to the interview.

Many of you may know that Eugen Bleuler made it a rule in his clinic in Zurich that every psychiatric resident during his training time had to succeed in converting a mute catatonic patient into one who responded to questions and talked, if briefly. Brill, the pioneer American psychoanalyst, who trained in Bleuler's Clinic, described how he spent an entire Sunday afternoon, not too happily, with a catatonic patient before he succeeded in establishing verbal communication.

After World War II the sodium amytal interview was widely used for the same purpose: to facilitate verbal communication with mute-depressed or catatonic patients. In some instances this method has a "normalizing" effect, meaning that the patient verbalizes in a seemingly rational manner. In the case of catatonics, however, the verbalizations, not surprisingly, mostly consist of bizarre delusions. Most importantly, it is common with sodium amytal interviews that repeated interviews result in very dissimilar verbal and behavioral responses. Only the sum total of interviews, rarely one single interview, provides a profile of the psychopathology.

It seems to me then that we should not put too much faith in the diagnostic value of the structured interview. It has its merits. But what we need in addition is clinical observation and a whole series of interviews in order to obtain a longitudinal view for the purpose of comprehensive diagnosis.

Dr. Salzinger: I agree with Dr. Freyhan's call for the longitudinal approach; it makes sense and behavior therapists have used it, based directly on Skinner's approach to animals which followed them up for very long periods of time. Skinner and Lindsley also worked, in the fifties, following up chronic patients for many years.

In addition, I quite agree that a single interview is not sufficient, and I agree that we must observe behavior other than verbal behavior. I think that is exactly what behavior therapy is all about.

REFERENCES

1. Caudill, W. (1972): Tiny dramas: Vocal communication between mother and infant in Japanese and American families. In: *Transcultural Research in Mental Health,* edited by W. P. Lebra. University of Hawaii Press, Honolulu.
2. Whiting, J. W. M., and Whiting, B. B. (1975): *Children of Six Cultures: A Psycho-Cultural Analysis.* Harvard University Press, Cambridge, Mass.

Critical Issues in Psychiatric Diagnosis,
edited by Robert L. Spitzer and Donald F. Klein.
Raven Press, New York © 1978.

Delusional Disorder (Paranoia)[1]

George Winokur

Department of Psychiatry, University of Iowa College of Medicine, Iowa City, Iowa 52242

In practice, psychiatrists occasionally examine a patient who has nothing but delusions. Such patients have no marked depressive symptomatology although they may be unhappy. They are not euphoric although they may be grandiose as a natural response to the delusion. They are neither blunted nor inappropriate in affect. Their mind is clear. They do not have sensorium difficulties. They are not incoherent. What they have is simply a delusion, nothing more, nothing less. Such patients are not common, but they are seen both in the hospital and in the clinic. This syndrome may be called "delusional disorder." A number of synonyms have been used to name delusional disorder, including paranoia vera, paranoid state, delusional monomania, delusional insanity, and conjugal paranoia. In the French literature, delusional disorders are called *delires chroniques paranoiaques* (2). Such a syndrome has systematized delusions with ideas of persecution. There are no hallucinations. The patients "are clear, coherent, often plausible and sometimes convincing." Another group which appears similar is *délires chroniques passionnels et de revendication.* These two syndromes are to be differentiated from *psychose hallucinatoire chronique,* which is characterized by a systematized delusion and hallucinations. Also, the French separate such syndromes from chronic schizophrenia because of the lack of discordance and dissociation in them. They separate them from the paraphrenias because in the paraphrenias the delusions are absolutely incredible. Thus, as a clear and unequivocal definition, the French concept of *délires chroniques paranoiaques* is quite similar to the diagnosis of delusional disorder.

Kraepelin (5) wrote that patients with paranoia remain permanently sensible, clear, and reasonable. He did not believe genuine hallucinations occurred but did remark that occasionally patients tell of isolated or fairly frequent visual hallucinations. There is no problem in memory or retention. The patients have many delusions of reference. There is no clear mood disorder. The delusions are frequently part of an extensive system. Except for the presence of hallucinations, Kraepelin's concept of paranoia is similar to what is called delusional disorder in this chapter.

It is useless to continue to explore the fine points of differentiation between various delusional illnesses. It becomes mostly a semantic, philosophic,

---

[1] Presidential address.

epistemological experience with a Thomistic quality. To continue it is tantamount to attempting to untie the Gordian knot. Better to take the clinical observations and attempt to investigate them in a systematic fashion.

METHODOLOGY

A search was made through the computerized records of the Psychiatric Hospital of the University of Iowa for the entire length of the hospital's existence (1920 to 1975). During these 50 years, 21,000 patients had been admitted.

The computer produced 93 admissions with diagnoses that included the term "paranoia." That term was the basis for the search. Seven charts could not be found. Eight patients had had more than one admission. Seventy-eight charts were transmitted to the investigator.

Each chart was then perused and only ones that met the following criteria were accepted:

1. All patients had to exhibit an unequivocal delusion.
2. Such a delusion or delusions could have been present for any length of time.
3. The delusions had to be related to events that were possible, however implausible.
4. There were a number of exclusion critiera:
   a. the presence or suggestion of the presence of any hallucination at any time;
   b. bizarre or fantastic delusions at any time;
   c. evidence of organic brain syndrome;
   d. illness beginning after the age of 60;
   e. meeting clear criteria for depression or mania (4);
   f. inappropriateness or marked flattening of affect (frozen face).

The 78 charts were reviewed and because of the very rigid exclusion criteria the majority were rejected. Twenty-nine patients were accepted and in each case the chart was examined for data concerning the age of onset, psychiatric history, types of symptoms, personality background, family history, and follow-up.

RESULTS

Frequency

Assuming that all 93 admissions which contained diagnosis of paranoia were acceptable, the frequency of the illness in 21,000 admissions would be $0.4 \pm 0.04\%$. Between two standard errors of the proportion, we would consider the frequency between 0.3% and 0.5% of the hospital population. In fact, as only 29 patients were accepted for the study, it is highly likely that the frequency in the hospital admissions is closer to 0.1%. Because such patients have no obvious symptoms besides delusions which clearly make them look different from the population, it is impossible to estimate the frequency in the population.

Achté in Finland (*personal communication,* 1976) describes paranoia in the following way: "The most essential characteristic in paranoia is delusions which are, in general, restricted to one specific area in a patient's life. Outside of this area he functions in a normal way." He has presented material on the incidence of admissions in 1960. Sixteen patients per 100,000 (0.02%) admitted for the first time in the city of Helsinki were given the diagnosis of paranoia (9).

We may conclude that delusional disorder of paranoia is a relatively uncommon illness for a psychiatrist to see. It does exist, nevertheless. One must ultimately decide whether it is related to other diseases such as schizophrenia or affective disorder or whether it is in fact an autonomous illness.

Intelligence

As a resident in psychiatry, I was taught that patients with paranoia are uncommonly intelligent. Of the 29 patients who are included in the present

TABLE 1. *IQ in patients with delusional disorder*

IQ	No. of patients	Proportion of total group (%)
60–69	1	5
70–79	4	19
80–89	6	29
90–99	2	10
100–109	3	14
110–119	3	14
120–129	2	10
Total	21	101

study, 21 had had intelligence tests. In 11 cases, the Stanford revision of the Binet-Simon was used. In four cases, Wechsler adult intelligence scale was used. And, in the remainder of the cases, there was no specific note as to the type of test. Table 1 gives the IQ findings in the 21 patients. There is no evidence for any superior intelligence in this group. In fact, over half of the patients scored under 90 IQ.

Sex Ratio

Kraepelin (5) remarked that males predominated over females in paranoia, 70:30%. Of the 29 patients, 20 or 70% are male in the present study.

A study of schizophrenia done in the same hospital (1) showed that of 200 schizophrenics chosen between 1934 and 1944 by the use of rigid criteria (4) for schizophrenia, 51.5% were male and 48.5% were female. Thus, there is a marked difference from the equality of males and females which is seen in schizophrenia, with males showing marked predomination in delusional disorder. Of considerable interest is the fact that Rimón et al. (9) found that in Helsinki 47.5% of the diagnoses of paranoia were made in men and 52.5% in women. For the diagnosis of schizophrenia there was a much larger preponderance of women. This was also true of the sex ratio in the general population (58% women, 42% men). Thus, the differences in the Achté study, the Kraepelin material, and the present study are all in the same direction. All indicate that men are either more likely to have paranoia or delusional disorder than women or that there is at least a relative preponderance of men when compared to schizophrenia. There is no clear reason to explain the difference in sex ratio between paranoia and schizophrenia.

Age of Onset and Age at Index Admission

This material is given in Table 2. As may be seen, the onset occurs equally between 20 and 29, 30 and 39, and 40 and 49. Relatively few patients be-

TABLE 2. Age of onset and age at index admission

Age	Age of onset N	%	Age at index N	%
10–19	1	3	—	—
20–29	8	28	3	10
30–39	10	35	11	38
40–49	9	31	10	35
50–59	1	3	5	17

come ill before 20 and relatively few become ill after 50. One of the exclusion criteria in this group is that the patient could not be over 60. If there was a large increase in delusional disorder after the age of 60 after the relatively small frequency between 50 and 60, such a dichotomous frequency curve would force one to question whether the over 60 delusional illnesses were to be considered the same illness as those occurring earlier in life.

Length of Illness at Index Admission

This material is seen in Table 3. Three-quarters of the patients in this study had been ill 1 or more years prior to their admission, which was in almost all the cases their first admission to any hospital. Of some interest

TABLE 3. *Length of illness at index*

	N	%
Less than 6 months	7	24
6 months–1 year	1	3
1–2 years	4	14
2–3 years	2	7
More than 4 years	15	52

is the finding that 35% of the males but only 11% of the females were admitted to the hospital after being ill for only a year or less.

Major Theme

This material is seen in Table 4. As may be noted, delusions concerning marriage were common as were delusions concerning plots and being un-

TABLE 4. *Major theme*

	N	%
Conjugal	11	38
Law	2	7
Litigious	3	10
Sexual	2	7
Unfairly treated, plotted against	10	35
Scientific	1	3

fairly treated. All of the patients in whom the major theme was the law, litigation, or science were males (6/20, 30%).

Social Functioning and Personality

This material is seen in Table 5. Generally, patients with delusional disorder had a satisfactory work history. Precipitating factors were not striking. The patients were not considered to be fussy or rigid (obsessional). They were, however, considered to have been chronically jealous or suspicious.

Symptoms (Delusional)

This material is seen in Table 6. Delusions of reference, jealousy, and persecution were clearly the most common. The more exotic types of symptoms were rarely seen.

TABLE 5. Social functioning and personality

	N	%
Work history (lifetime)		
Satisfactory	22	76
Unsatisfactory	7	24
Withdrawn	8	28
Precipitating factors		
None	21	72
Less than 8th grade education	16	55
Some college or graduated	9	31
Embittered	13	45
Haughty	6	21
Fussy, rigid	5	17
Jealous or suspicious	19	66

TABLE 6. Symptoms (delusional)

	N	%
Reference	22	76
Jealousy	14	48
Persecution	24	83
Hypochondriacal	3	10
Grandeur, inventions	2	7
Grandeur, high descent	0	0
Grandeur, prophet, saints	0	0

Symptoms (Nondelusional)

This material is seen in Table 7. Patients showed a few depressive symptoms but, of course, did not meet criteria for an affective illness. They showed a high frequency of sexual problems. They frequently showed at least one manic symptom which generally was overtalkativeness or circumstantiality (30% of all cases). Ten percent of the cases showed an increased sex drive. They did not meet the criteria for mania.

TABLE 7. Symptoms (nondelusional)

	N	%
Some depressive symptoms	13	45
Significant drinking history	1	3
Sex problems	16	55
Suicide threats	2	7
Suicide attempts	4	14
1 Manic symptom	12	41
2 Manic symptoms	1	3.4
3 Manic symptoms	1	3.4

Type of Discharge

Almost all of the patients were discharged from the Iowa Psychiatric Hospital to the community (Table 8). This is in contrast to the schizophrenics which were studied as part of the Iowa 500 (1). It is true that schizophrenics do not cover the same years of admission as the patients with delusional disorder but even at that the reversal is striking. Of the 12 patients who were admitted during the same years as the schizophrenics, 9 (75%) were dis-

TABLE 8. *Discharged to community or hospital*

	Delusional disorder		Schizophrenics (Iowa 500)	
	N	%	N	%
Community	23	79	52	26
Hospital	6	21	148	74

charged to the community. Schizophrenics went on to a subsequent hospitalization. Patients with a delusional disorder went back to the community.

Follow-up

In the Iowa Psychiatric Hospital, patients were systematically followed up by a social worker. The follow-up material is presented in Table 9. The quality of the follow-up is such that in some cases it is impossible to determine whether or not the patients were absolutely asymptomatic. It was possible, however, to tell whether they were socially recovered, and in fact about a third of them had this kind of outcome. The remainder of those followed up were symptomatic in a similar way to when they had entered the hospital. What is particularly important is that no new diagnosis was given to 93% of the entire sample. One was subsequently diagnosed as schizophrenic and one had a diagnosis of affective disorder. This latter person was diagnosed manic-depressive, depressed. This diagnosis was made at a state hospital; but in fact the patient had been continuously delusional for 6 years. Of 9 women in whom there was a follow-up, 4 of 9, 44% were socially recovered; of 17 men, 24% were socially recovered.

Of 25 patients in whom it was possible to obtain a reasonable clinical picture in follow-up, only 4% or 1 had schizophrenic symptoms at follow-up. Such schizophrenic symptoms were the kind that were used in the selection criteria for rejection of cases from the study.

There is a series of studies by Retterstøl (7) which involve a personal follow-up of paranoic patients. Of 18 patients with jealousy, paranoic psychoses (16 males, 2 females) who were followed from 2½ to 18 years, schizophrenia developed in 2 patients. Of interest is the fact that at the time

TABLE 9. Follow-up

Number followed up (FU)	26	(90%)
FU 6 months or less	4	(14%)
FU 6 months–2 years	12	(43%)
FU 2–20 years	10	(34%)
Mean FU for entire group		2.6 years
Last known location of patient (27/29 known)		
Hospital	7	(26%)
Home	20	(74%)
Recovery (26/29 known)		
Chronically ill	18	(69%)
Socially recovered	8	(31%)
Last known diagnosis		
No new one	27	(93%)
Schizophrenia	1	(3%)
Affective disorder	1	(3%)
Productive work since discharge (23/29 known)		
Yes	14	(61%)
No	9	(39%)
Marriage stable (17/29)		
Yes	9	(53%)
No	8	(47%)
Schizophrenic symptoms in FU (25/29)		
No	24	(96%)
Yes	1	(4%)

they were originally seen, the jealousy delusions in these 2 patients had appeared "grotesque." Otherwise, the remaining patients were working. Of the 16 patients who did not develop schizophrenia, 11 were considered "reactive psychosis" and were evaluated as cured without relapse. Five were considered as chronic reactive psychoses. Thus, in this group the prognosis seems better than in the material which is presented in the present chapter.

Retterstøl (8) also presented a follow-up of 15 patients who had hypochondriac delusions as their main delusional idea. Of these 10 were male and 5 female. Six patients were considered reactive psychosis, cured in follow-up. One patient was registered as reactive psychosis cured with one relapse, and two patients were considered psychosis, chronic. The remaining six patients were considered to have a schizophrenic outcome.

One patient who was rejected for the present study was delusional about having a bad odor. He was rejected because it was impossible to determine whether this was delusional or whether, in fact, he had a hallucination of the odor. The possible hallucination was enough to make him not eligible for the present study.

Treatment

Most patients in the study had no treatment, but seven had psychotherapy and five were given neuroleptic drugs (Table 10). Of the seven who were

TABLE 10. *Treatment*

	N	%
None	16	55
Psychotherapy	7	24
Neuroleptics	4	14
ECT	1	3
Neuroleptics and ECT	1	3

given some kind of psychotherapy, three were considered improved at the time of discharge. In follow-up, however, one of these was clearly chronically ill. Thus, two out of seven were considered improved at discharge and at least socially recovered at follow-up.

Of the five patients who were given neuroleptic drugs, three were considered improved at discharge. Of these three there is no follow-up in one. In another the patient was clearly chronically ill after a follow-up of 6 months; and after a follow-up of 2 to 3 years, the third patient was at least socially recovered.

Mooney (6) presented the results of treatment with chemotherapy on patients who had pathologic jealousy. The patients are relatively few in number ($N = 12$) but after initial treatment the author considered 67% much improved. He concluded that phenothiazine drugs had an initial favorable effect on delusional jealousy and its associated symptoms. On follow-up 42% were considered much improved.

Family History

As part of the social and medical evaluation of patients admitted to the Iowa Psychiatric Hospital, a systematic family history was obtained on almost all of the patients (Table 11).

What is noteworthy is the minimal amount of major remitting illness (2.4%). This figure is not corrected for age. If one simply looks at the number of parents who have a major remitting illness, one finds that the prevalence goes up to 3.4%. This is probably a more reasonable figure in light of the fact that the sibs have not all passed through the age of risk, whereas the parents almost certainly have traversed this. In family history study of manics, depressives, and schizophrenics, we have reported morbidity risks

TABLE 11. *Family history*

	N	Major remitting illness	Major chronic illness	Soft paranoid syndromes
Parents	58	2	1	1
Sibs	110	2	3	3
Parents and sibs	168	4 (2.4%)	4 (2.4%)	4 (2.4%)

for affective disorder in parents and sibs of the probands of between 12% and 15% (10). Morbidity risks for affective disorder in parents and sibs of schizophrenic probands varied between 4% and 7%. Although the data are few in number, it would be reasonable to conclude that there is little familial association between delusional disorder and affective disorder.

Family risks for schizophrenia are another matter. In the above-mentioned study, the morbidity risks for schizophrenia in the parents and sibs of schizophrenic probands varied between 1.8% and 2.6%. In the parents and sibs of affective probands, the risk was lower (0.3% to 0.8%). The prevalence from Table 11 shows parents and sibs ill with chronic illness at the rate of 2.4%; whereas in the evaluation of 200 schizophrenic probands, the morbid risk for schizophrenia in parents and sibs was 2.11%. The rates between delusional disorder patients and schizophrenics are similar even taking into account the different methodology for calculation (morbid risk versus prevalence). All of these figures are probably low because we are dealing with a family history methodology rather than a family study methodology. What is important is not the absolute numbers but the comparison of the two groups.

Certainly the delusional disorder patients will meet the criteria presented by Feighner et al. (4) for the diagnosis of schizophrenia. In a previous communication, we have pointed out that there is a likelihood that two kinds of schizophrenic-type illnesses exist (11). One of these is paranoid and the other nonparanoid schizophrenia. If there were a relationship between these two types, one would expect that there should be an increase in nonparanoid schizophrenia in the relatives of the paranoid schizophrenias over what one would expect in the general population. In fact, from the material present in the charts, this is not found. All four of the relatives diagnosed as having a major chronic illness had paranoid syndromes. The one mother had a similar delusion to that which the patient exhibited. She then had paranoia. There were three ill sisters among the sibs. One sister was diagnosed as having paranoid schizophrenia and another sister was called chronically paranoid and a third sister had "paranoia." Thus, it would appear that in the first-degree family members the illness was breeding true. There was no evidence for nonparanoid schizophrenia in the known first-degree ill relatives.

No sib or parent was known to have committed suicide, a finding in favor of a lack of relationship between delusional disorder and affective disorder or schizophrenia. Several soft diagnoses were mentioned in the first-degree family members. In the four cases noted in Table 11, one father "feels cheated," two sisters were "suspicious," and one brother was "suspicious." These are presented only for the sake of interest in that there is no way to compare them to any other data.

In the extended family notations were made on four of the delusional disorder probands. In one case a paternal aunt had "simple schizophrenia." In another case, an aunt was peculiar in late life and an uncle was considered mentally unbalanced. In a third case it was noted that there was paranoid illness on the paternal side of the family, and in the fourth case a half-sister was diagnosed as having an involutional paranoid syndrome.

One can conclude from the material that there is little reason to support a familial connection with affective disorder. There is some reason to believe that the illness was breeding true in the families of the delusional patients. This would suggest a qualitative difference from nonparanoid schizophrenia.

DISCUSSION

It really is true that viable research ideas spring from clinical practice and from seeing patients. The idea of studying delusional disorder and defining it in such a specific way as has been done here to a large extent springs from having seen an occasional patient who looks like the description. Such patients are very striking clinically. However, the most important thing about them is their relationship to the more frequently occurring illnesses such as affective disorder and schizophrenia. Are they in any way related to these highly prevalent illnesses? Are they part of the schizophrenia spectrum? These are matters of considerable importance. Prior to trying to answer some of these questions, however, we might attempt to reach reasonable conclusions from the material which has been presented.

From the data what can we say for sure? Given the rigid diagnosis, it seems certain that delusional disorder as defined is a relatively uncommon syndrome. Nevertheless, it does exist. As an illness it is unrelated to the intelligence level in probands.

What is likely to be true? It is likely that it is more frequent in men than in women. It exists for a considerable time prior to the admission to a hospital for treatment. It does not destroy the ability to function in the environment. Most commonly it manifests itself by delusions concerning marriage, plots, and being unfairly treated. Delusions of reference, jealousy, and persecution are common. It is not associated with any marked number of depressive or manic symptoms although the patients are frequently circumstantial and overtalkative.

Generally patients are discharged back to the community and this makes them unlike the vast majority of schizophrenics. In follow-up, they remain symptomatic but some become socially recovered. It is likely that some patients become totally recovered, although that material must be obtained from studies other than the present one. Treatment by psychotherapy or chemotherapy is of unknown value.

Family history is likely to show major chronic illness in excess of what might be expected ordinarily. These illnesses are similar in kind to the illness in the proband. No evidence exists for any relationship between affective disorder (major remitting illnesses) and delusional disorder.

What is apparent from the above is that the things which are sure are considerably fewer than the things which are likely or possible. The things which are likely or possible are in fact considerably more important than the things which are sure, and this poses a significant problem.

Probably the most important problem is related to the genetic or family background of these patients. Very little information exists on this matter. A recent paper by Debray (2) compared two groups of patients. One of these was *delire chronique paranoiac* (paranoia) and the other was *psychose hallucinatorie chronique* (chronic hallucinatory psychosis). All of the patients were interviewed and "in most cases one or several members of their families." Taking into account schizophrenia and personality disorder in the first-degree relatives of probands, significantly more were seen in the paranoia patients than in the chronic hallucinatory psychotic patients. The type of schizophrenia in the family members is not presented. The paranoia group is more likely to have psychiatrically ill family members than the general population. This seems not true of the chronic hallucinatory psychosis group. In any event, the Debray study to a large extent is a family history study rather than a family study and more information is needed.

We have recently presented some material which suggested the possibility that there were two types of paranoid schizophrenia. One of these was related to hebephrenia and the other existed independently. A recent paper by Depue and Woodburn (3) indicated that about half of paranoid schizophrenics remained paranoid across 10 years of illness whereas the other half changed to a nonparanoid status about 6 years after the first admission. To this one would like to have information as to how many nonparanoid (hebephrenic and chronic catatonic) changed to paranoid. In the present sample of delusional disorder patients, there was no reason to believe that the patients would develop typical schizophrenic symptoms.

Not only would it be valuable to have a systematic blind family study of delusional disorder patients, but it would also be valuable to have a follow-up study of the course of the illness in these patients. To this should be added a group of matched controls who have nonparanoid schizophrenia.

From the material which is certain about delusional disorder, namely, its relative uncommonness, it is clear that such a blind follow-up and family study can probably be done only by using a multicentered protocol. No one psychiatric center will obtain enough patients in the course of a couple of years to settle the issue. However, five or six large psychiatric facilities with active inpatient and outpatient services should be able to offer enough material for both the delusional disorder patients as well as the nonparanoid schizophrenic controls. It would seem that if this is a subject of importance, some planning should be put into formulating such a study.

SUMMARY

A definition of delusional disorder is given. This definition comes from clinical practice and is quite rigorous. Delusional disorder exists but is uncommon. It is likely to be called schizophrenia (paranoid schizophrenia) because it fills published criteria for such a diagnosis. It is more likely seen in men than women. It bears no relation to IQ. It does not destroy the ability to function socially but does create problems in living because of interpersonal conflicts. Familially it bears no relation to affective disorder. It seems to breed true within families but this is not proven. What is necessary to settle major issues is a multicentered systematic blind family study and follow-up with a group of nonparanoid schizophrenia as controls.

ACKNOWLEDGMENT

This study was supported in part by NIMH Grant #24189.

REFERENCES

1. Clancy, J., Tsuang, M., Norton, B., and Winokur, G. (1974): A comprehensive study of mania, depression and schizophrenia. *J. Iowa Med. Soc.*, 64:394–396.
2. Debray, Q. (1975): A genetic study of chronic delusions. *Neuropsychobiology,* 1:313–321.
3. Depue, R., and Woodburn, L. (1975): Disappearance of paranoid symptoms with chronicity. *J. Abnorm. Psychol.*, 84:84–86.
4. Feighner, J., Robins, E., Guze, S., Woodruff, R., Winokur, G., and Munoz, R. (1972): Diagnostic criteria for use in psychiatric research. *Arch. Gen. Psychiatry,* 26:57–63.
5. Kraepelin, E. (1921): *Manic-Depressive Insanity and Paranoia.* E. S. Livingstone, Edinburgh.
6. Mooney, H. (1975): Pathologic jealousy and psychochemotherapy. *Br. J. Psychiatry,* 111:1023–1042.
7. Retterstøl, N. (1967): Jealousy-paranoiac psychoses. *Acta Psychiatr. Scand.,* 43:75–107.
8. Retterstøl, N. (1968): Paranoid psychoses with hypochondriac delusions as the main delusion. *Acta Psychiatr. Scand.,* 44:334–353.
9. Rimón, R., Stenbäck, A., and Achté, K. (1964): A sociopsychiatric study of paranoid psychoses. *Acta Psychiatr. Scand. [Suppl. 180],* 40:335–347.
10. Winokur, G., Morrison, J., Clancy, J., and Crowe, R. (1972): The Iowa 500. II. A blind family history comparison of mania, depression and schizophrenia. *Arch. Gen. Psychiatry,* 27:462–464.
11. Winokur, G., Morrison, J., Clancy, J., and Crowe, R. (1974): The Iowa 500: Clinical and genetic distinction of hebephrenic and paranoid schizophrenia. *J. Nerv. Ment. Dis.,* 159:164–171.

Critical Issues in Psychiatric Diagnosis,
edited by Robert L. Spitzer and Donald F. Klein.
Raven Press, New York © 1978.

Projective Testing and Psychiatric Diagnosis: Validity and the Future

Margaret Thaler Singer

University of Rochester School of Medicine and Dentistry, Rochester, New York; and University of California, Berkeley, California 94705

In recent years, the techniques for assessment of patients by psychologists using psychological tests and the psychiatric diagnostic conclusions drawn by psychiatrists based on interviews have both come under a storm of criticism. The question we face here is whether this criticism addresses itself to valid objections in such a way that ultimately both assessment techniques and psychiatric diagnostic procedures can profit from an examination of the serious questions and problems that have been raised.

I do not intend to examine each of the critical review articles on either projective techniques or psychiatric diagnosis, because all of you know the general positions stated by reviewers such as Blatt (2), Buros (3), Frank (6), Goldfried et al. (7), Holt (8), Jensen (11), Mayman (17), Weiner (51,52), and Zubin (71,72).

The reactions of professional reviewers run the gamut of moral attitudes. However, many of the critics tend to become what theater people would term the "heavy." They range from the fire-and-brimstone spouting perjorative attacks on psychiatry calling it a game, a mythology, or a form of witchcraft (47,49); or equally vituperative attacks on projective techniques, such as "The rate of scientific progress in clinical psychology might well be measured by the speed and thoroughness with which it gets over the Rorschach" (11).

Some of the attacks on both psychiatric diagnosis and projective techniques have been so vitriolic that when I came upon the marvelously refreshing humor of writers such as Klopfer and Taulbee (15) and McArthur (18) I felt a need to share their sense of fun with you. Klopfer, Taulbee, and McArthur combined light-hearted phrasing with good scholarship when they wrote recent reviews which point up the central past problems in both psychiatric diagnosis and projective techniques.

Klopfer and Taulbee (15, p. 544) commented: "Frequently a sophisticated psychological instrument was correlated with the off-the-wall opinion of a first-year psychiatric resident."

McArthur (18, p. 443), commenting on the way the Rorschach, in particular, among the projective techniques has been used, wrote: "The variety of its applications and misapplications is wonderous; since the last *Mental Measurements Yearbook* it has been applied to facial disfigurement, reading disability, gang rape, shamanism, children on a holiday, murderers, married couples, left-handers and Athenians to name a few."

Not only have the psychiatric diagnosis against which tests were validated been off-the-wall, and the tests themselves inappropriately used, but sometimes psychologists have gone wild inventing new projective techniques. A recent survey of the 1971 to 1974 literature on projective techniques revealed the following new offerings: Draw-a-Dog Scale, Draw-a-Member of a Minority Test, and Draw-a-Person in the Rain Test. "Such exercises contribute little to producing the acceptable body of knowledge needed for establishing the reliability and validity of projective instruments" (15, p. 544). They also do little to advance the idea that psychology is, indeed, a science.

Klopfer, Taulbee, McArthur and others (2,6–8,14,15,17,18,51,52) have summed up what has happened. I am going to join them in noting not only have there been grossly inappropriate uses of projective techniques, but psychiatric diagnoses also have been poorly made or misused. But looking at the future, I feel there is cause for cautious optimism that recent trends in psychiatric diagnostic methodology indicate awareness that better definitions of psychiatric syndromes, attention to delineating subgroups within syndromes, and the developing of structured interview schedules for eliciting more reliable evaluations will continue. Also, recent work in assessment techniques has shown the need to correlate the psychiatric *constructs* with the test *constructs*. For example, the construct of clinically observed anxiety can be related to those features of Rorschach behavior which can be construed as anxiety which is not reflected in the traditional scoring procedures, but which has been conceptually validated.

Both projective techniques and psychiatric diagnosis based on interviews are not precisely refined tools. Yet despite the criticisms and challenges put to both fields, those working in both psychiatric and psychological research and patient care realize that assessment procedures are needed for: (a) administrative purposes, (b) treatment planning, and (c) research purposes. No matter who says what, patients will continue to be interviewed, tested, and evaluated for administrative purposes, treatment, and research because better ways to do it are not available. Nevertheless, the critics have made us think more clearly about what we are doing and how we are doing it. Historically, treatment and research techniques are not given up until something better has been found. Some of my older colleagues will remember the search for filterable viruses and the confusion which ensued when middle-aged patients were found to be suffering from a disease called dementia praecox. That is why the condition is now called schizophrenia.

The major task at this point is not to keep on compiling bibliographies of articles which reveal that projective techniques and psychiatric diagnostic procedures are fallible. Alas, we know. Nor is it necessary for us to feel chagrin or to look upon sterile logical positivistic analysis as being somehow related to superior scientific research. The task now is to delineate the conceptual problems underlying the entire field of personality assessment, clinical diagnosis, and treatment. With better concepts we can begin to answer the questions why and how should we assess which people for what ends. Clarity and consistency of diagnostic concepts and assessment concepts will produce more valid and reliable assessment and diagnostic results. The logical links need to be spelled out between why we test and diagnose and what the appropriate treatment procedures will be. Space prevents a discussion of correlates between diagnosis and various methods of treatment.

Certain features of psychiatric diagnosis and projective techniques need to be described before we can talk about future developments and directions in the two fields.

PSYCHIATRIC DIAGNOSIS

Psychiatric diagnosis is a process by which collection, selection, and matching are done. First, the clinician goes through a lengthy period of collecting information about the patient's past and present behavior. A study is made of both inner cognitive and emotional traits and states, as well as outwardly demonstrated signs and symptoms. Certain historical material and observations obtained from the family, from the patient, and from other observers as well as the psychiatrist's own impressions are gathered. Then the psychiatrist selects among these materials. He has to selectively attend to only portions of this material and attempt to organize it into a composite to match against diagnostic stereotypes. (Although the word stereotype has been and is almost exclusively used nowadays to connote a negative or false image, e.g., all professors are absent minded, we use it here to mean the ideal of its type.) As Spitzer and Endicott (45, p. 645) wrote:

> In the usual diagnostic manual, such as the American Psychiatric Association's Diagnostic and Statistical Manual (DSMII), diagnostic stereotypes are described under each category. The task of the diagnostician then becomes one of selecting the diagnostic category in which the stereotype most closely resembles the characteristics of the patient being diagnosed.

Spitzer went on to point out that many stereotypes listed in the diagnostic manuals have never been established as entities which can be distinguished one from another. Yet the practicing clinician has to sort through a vast array of stereotypes and attempt to match certain behavior patterns detected in patients who seem to match one or more stereotypes, some of which may not actually exist in real life, but have merely been passed on over generations of manuals.

One group, Feighner's (5), has limited itself to research only those conditions where strong evidence exists that specified conditions are diagnosable entities. This group's most merciful contribution to the field has been to legitimize that category we all know so well—"undiagnosed psychiatric disorder"—to classify those patients who do not fit the diagnostic manual stereotypes, yet who have undefinable psychopathological behavior.

Thus, the essential processes in diagnosis are (a) collecting historical and observational material, (b) selectively organizing portions of it in terms that come as close to listed stereotypes as possible, and (c) choosing the one or closest matching labels under which the patient will be diagnosed. At best, the final label (diagnosis) assigned to the patient is almost always experienced by the clinician as "not really telling the whole story." The psychiatrist has had to select those bits of behavior, signs, and symptoms which fit current diagnostic criteria, and ignore many features about the patient which he feels are important but which do not "fit" existing diagnostic categories.

Psychiatric observation has been a multilevel, multivariate study procedure, but the diagnosis is a unitary, unidimensional label often felt to be too simplistic and reductionistic. Psychiatric diagnosis is multilevel in the sense that past and present behavior and inner feelings are considered. It is multivariate in the sense that for any aspect of personality under consideration, the clinician inquires about and investigates a number of traits, states, and features. For example, at the overt behavior level, how the patient reports his own behavior, how his family reports it, and how the psychiatrist's observations of signs and symptoms are made are all taken into consideration. In the final stage, however, the multilevel, multivariate explorations of one personality are all condensed into a single diagnostic label.

Of the many comments made about the diagnostic procedure, Frank's (6, p. 167) overview distills the viewpoints of many:

> A review of some of the research in this area indicates that the current system of diagnosis of psychopathology does lack a sufficient degree of reliability and validity so as to suggest that its use in clinical work and research is not advised. Moreover, the review of this research leaves one with the uncomfortable feeling that the results of all the studies that have utilized psychiatric diagnosis as a dependent or independent variable are of questionable validity. The data reviewed . . . suggest that an entirely new system of classification is needed, one which can encompass the many variables that define psychological functioning and behavior in the human, including the viewing of these functions from a developmental frame of reference. Research bearing on this latter hypothesis is . . . promising and suggestive of further research endeavors.

Frank does not say what developmental aspects should be included in a new classification system nor how one would relate those developmental aspects to psychopathology. Nevertheless, this kind of reasoning represents a forward step in the ongoing efforts to enrich theoretical concepts and extend measurable dimensions of behavior.

CURRENT TRENDS

Trends in Psychiatric Diagnosis

From surveying the critiques of both projective testing and psychiatric diagnosis, and comparing them with those made in other areas of the behavioral sciences, it seems only fair to point out that the state of the literature in these two domains of psychology are neither more nor less confusing nor contradictory than the states which typify most areas of human behavioral research. Think of the state of the art in intelligence testing, psychotherapy research, assessment of teaching methods, and certain areas of political science.

However, research in psychiatric diagnosis and projective techniques has progressed. Current trends in psychiatric diagnostic research using semistructured interview schedules—Schedule for Affective Disorders and Schizophrenia, Spitzer et al. (45,46), and the World Health Organization Psychiatric Assessment Schedules (4,54,55)—represent steps toward the development of reliable and valid measures for assessing psychopathology. These two interview schedules permit assessment of patients' mental states to be standardized: (a) in the scope and style of collecting information, and (b) in the analysis and synthesis of discrete items from the interviews in order to relate them to diagnostic categories. Additionally, glossaries are provided which define precisely the diagnostic labels used in both schedules. Such efforts to secure reliable ratings of patients on critical dimensions of behavior will permit the testing of concepts about behavior from projective techniques to be integrated into the total assessment of a patient's status so that better selection of treatment or assistance can be provided to the patient.

As efforts grow to make psychiatric diagnosis more reliable, the task becomes how to spell out explicitly the behaviors the psychiatrist is to detect, observe, and rate. Paralleling these psychiatric efforts, there seems to be a trend in the use of projective techniques to relate them to the behavioral levels that are usable directly in many forms of interaction therapy. Before getting into those developments, it is useful to trace past efforts to validate projective techniques.

Trends in Projective Techniques

After it was discovered that skillful, experienced clinical psychologists used the procedure well, eager graduate students decided to dissect the Rorschach, much as the beginning pathology student might study laboratory reports. Just as the slides of tissue and blood chemistry reports did not convey the essence of the living person, neither did bits and pieces, such as single scores extracted from a Rorschach record, equal the end-product that skilled clinicians using the procedure had produced.

The history of research on the validity of the Rorschach has gone through four major phases (52). First came the development of empirical sign lists. This approach was a dead end for three reasons. First, the signs did not hold up well in cross-validation samples. Second, research was conducted on samples which did not reflect the actual clinical application needs of test users, that is, studies of signs which differentiate schizophrenics from normals are interesting, but not likely to yield indices that are useful in clinical practice where the clinician needs help in differentiating borderline syndrome persons from acute schizophrenics. Third, diagnostic groups contain heterogeneous collections of persons. For example, the class, schizophrenia, tells us little because a wide range of conditions are subsumed under the label. That is, schizophrenia occurs in acute and chronic forms, in patterns such as paranoid and nonparanoid, and has phases such as incipient, overt, and remitting. Other diagnostic categories such as neurosis and brain damage similarly are composed of persons who differ greatly from one another on important dimensions. Consequently, there is overlap between diagnostic categories as well as remarkable within-group variation that tend to cancel out all but the most extreme differences among groups.

Thus a sign approach to Rorschach validation was discarded in favor of a second approach: cluster and configurational scoring. However, the better configurational scoring methods which have proved valid, such as the Delta Index (50), the Communication Deviance manual (31), and the Rorschach Prognostic Rating Scale (13), require the scorer to learn specific and detailed scoring manuals and neither the busy clinician nor the novice researcher can always acquire the discipline to learn these methods. Additionally, certain configurational patterns (48), although reliable and valid, actually occur rarely. Finally, configurational patterns are felt to be mechanistic and of far less value than the fuller skillful clinical interpretations often made in actual practice.

The third major approach to validation, the global, was developed by those who felt the sign and pattern methods were confining and artificial. Hunt (10) had claimed that the examiner, not the tests, is the crucial clinical instrument. This hypothesis supported the use of global ratings. Primarily Zubin (71,72) argued that Rorschach users should abandon their "atomistic" attention to traditional scoring categories and use the test to validate global impressions. But the global approach also has its pitfalls, as do the sign and cluster methods. According to Weiner (52):

> The instrument and the examiner cannot be separated when the global impression approach is employed. When validating studies with this approach yield positive results, both the instrument and the examiner's judgments are proved useful. When negative results emerge, there is no way of determining whether the fault lies with weaknesses in the instrument or shortcomings of the examiner.

The fourth and best approach to validating the Rorschach is the testing of concepts. In such an approach, personality processes are offered as constructs, and the modes in which they appear in the Rorschach and in other behavior samples are studied. The research or prediction questions are: What personality variables or dimensions account for the behavior? Then, one asks, what features of a person's Rorschach behavior reflect or measure these personality variables?

When this kind of selecting and defining of personality-based concepts in the Rorschach and in the criterion behavior are not properly done, some poorly thought out research ensues. Two of the studies which cast doubt on the validity of the Rorschach resulted from studies in which it was used to predict success in graduate psychology training programs and success in pilot training. Success in neither of these endeavors is dependent solely on psychological factors, other variables of a nonpersonality type are paramount. As Holt (8) commented:

> On research project after project, it was shown conclusively that diagnostic skill did not enable a man to predict, for example, who would make a good clinical psychologist. . . . That . . . was a damaging failure; there was no *rational* reason why being a clinician oneself should enable one to predict whether a first-year graduate student would succeed, yet the failure of even recognized and respected masters of diagnostic testing to perform this form of prophecy made it look as if they were hardly better than poseurs.

Another glaring example of misguided efforts using the Rorschach was to ask testers to predict success in pilot training (9). Success or failure in pilot training did not hinge solely on psychological and personality variables. Rather, factors which caused failure were often extraneous to anything the Rorschach measured. For example, failure to complete pilot training often had more to do with budget problems, the number of pilots actually needed at particular times, and transactional breakdowns between instructor and student—the teacher just did not like the student and had the power to drop him. All these variables not only are extraneous to the Rorschach, but could never possibly be measured by it.

Blatt (2) posed three questions which appear central in evaluating research using projective techniques: Was the research methodology appropriate for validating inferences about psychological processes? Have the projective techniques been used in ways which reasonably approximate the distinction an experienced clinician would make in evaluating the phenomenon? Are the validating criteria carefully defined, reasonably reliable, and under sufficient control so that extraneous and unknown variables have minimal influence?

PROJECTIVE TECHNIQUES AND THE MAJOR DIAGNOSTIC CATEGORIES

We have pointed out that the criteria used in many studies involving projective techniques have often been nonpsychological in nature and dependent on factors not predictable from personality. But the usual psychiatric diagnostic categories against which test findings have been compared also suffer from murky definitions, overlapping usages, and unstable applications. The very fact that the Rorschach and findings from other projective techniques correlate with major diagnostic categories such as neurosis, schizophrenia, and brain damage suggest that with better diagnostic classification and clearer delineation of the significant psychological dimensions involved in clinical diagnosis, assessments will produce better and more useful and selective findings for the clinician.

Neurosis

It seems illogical that after attention focused on how useful the Rorschach and other projective techniques were in the hands of skilled clinicians, researchers did not attempt to use the very features which made the devices helpful as the starting points of research. That is, the skillful Rorschach interpreter is able to spell out some very personal and clinically useful inferences from the percepts and communication of the individual patient's Rorschach responses. The personal attributes, the concerns, the stylistic features of his communication are attributes on which treatment can be planned.

After learning that the skillful clinician could delineate specific aspects of individual neurotic functioning, then the researchers of the Rorschach proceeded to try to study gross clumps of "neurotics." That is, research lumped together very diverse subgroups of neurotics into one large class—neurosis.

The term "neurosis" sometimes refers to a state such as "neurotic depression" or "anxiety neurosis." Yet the term "neurosis" is also applied to ongoing trait level, enduring personality formations, as in the term "obsessive-compulsive personality." The term "neurosis" is used to refer to both states and traits. Further, the very symptoms used to define neurotic states are symptoms which also appear in psychotic patients. For example, the traditional neurotic symptoms of anxiety, conversions, phobias, depression, compulsive acts, and obsessive ruminations are all phenomena which appear in psychotic persons as well as in neurotics. Not only do features of neurotic and psychotic conditions overlap, those between neurosis and character disorders also overlap. Those traits of character termed immaturity, rigidity, low anxiety tolerance, and minor distortions of reality are characteristics of both character and neurotic disorders. "Perhaps symptom neuroses and character disorders should both be considered neurotic behavior; however, there is no general agreement that such is the case, and the point here is not to resolve such complex classification issues but rather to highlight the nosological morass against which intrepid Rorschach investigators set out to develop, validate, and apply indices of neurosis" (7, p. 253).

The inconsistency with which neurosis, maladjustment, and character problems are diagnosed from one clinician to the next and from one institution to another, and from one country to another has caused the several efforts to develop checklists and systems for scoring Rorschach indices of these conditions to fail when cross-validation attempts were tried. Five systems for scoring "neurotic or maladjustment" signs in the Rorschach, those of Miale and Harrower-Erickson, Munroe, Davidson, Muensch, and Fisher (7) have had various successes and failures, and have been criticized:

> Because "neurosis" is such a broad and imprecise concept, there are no adequate criteria against which Rorschach scores presuming to measure it can be compared; because these five indices were compiled largely from clinical consensus, rather than from conceptual analysis or empirical sifting of potential test indices, there was never any solid basis for expecting them to differentiate adjustment levels or predict behavior. The failure thus lies with the indices themselves, crippled by the methods used to construct them, rather than with the Rorschach in general. (7, p. 287)

Thus in future work attempting to study neurotic behavior and its Rorschach correlates, very specific subgroups of neurotics should be delineated against which to analyze the proper conceptual levels of those psychological and communicational aspects of Rorschach performance.

Brain Damage

In a lengthy review of the state of the art of applying the Rorschach to the diagnosis of brain damage signs, Goldfried et al. (7, p. 378) concluded that:

> No definitive statement can be made as yet about the efficacy of the Rorschach in the diagnosis of organicity, primarily because the research on organic signs has characteristically failed to provide either an adequate definition of the nature of the organic involvement in the experimental group or careful exclusion of organicity in the controls. Studies in this area have furthermore consistently failed to consider the relationship of organic signs to such critical subject variables as age, intelligence, and size, locus and duration of the lesion.

These same authors note that the best of the brain damage sign lists is that of Piotrowski (22,23). This list, however, fails to differentiate chronic schizophrenics from brain damaged patients, and also yields a high rate of false-negative indications (failing to detect brain damage signs in known cases). However, in settings in which chronic schizophrenia was not a highly likely diagnostic possibility, such as in a medical or neurological ward, a high score on the Piotrowski index is a strong suggestion of the possible presence of brain damage. But this approach to Rorschach validation needs the same work that is needed in the area of diagnosing neurosis. Here, in the realm of brain damage assessment through the study of Rorschach behavior, much detailed subgrouping on the basis of age, education, and types and durations of lesions is needed. When the medical subgroups are better defined, then the study of the perceptual and language behavior found on the Rorschach can be better tested.

Schizophrenia

The efforts to use the Rorschach to diagnose schizophrenic conditions have been among its most successful research ventures.

Probably the best work has grown out of the astute observations of Rapaport et al. (25). These workers writing about deviant verbalizations on the Rorschach pointed the way for those who followed them and who tried to take those verbalizations and attempt to make their scoring reliable. The work of Watkins and Stauffacher (50) followed by that of Powers and Hamlin (1955), Pope and Jensen (24), Singer, and Miller (19) indicate that this approach to using the Rorschach verbalizations is more valid and more promising than most uses of traditional scoring methods.

Why is this so? One of the central diagnostic features which clinicians use to diagnose the various forms of schizophrenia is to evaluate the language and reasoning procedures of a patient during a psychiatric interview. When a patient is deemed to show signs of "thinking disorders," which Wynne and Singer (65) noted should best be labeled communication and experience disorders, the psychiatrist has detected one of the agreed upon characteristics said to define a number of schizophrenic persons: namely, the presence of peculiar communication, the so-called thought disorder sign. This is a conceptual level characterization of a feature central to schizophrenia. *The ways patients phrase their ideas and the kinds of ideas and reasoning expressed during the Rorschach, as outlined in Rapaport's list of deviant verbalizations, are the behavioral counterparts during the Rorschach procedure of the same types of behavior which the psychiatrist would be paying attention to in a clinical interview.* Relevant aspects of the communicative behavior elicited by the Rorschach should be studied and compared with the conceptualized characteristics of communicative behavior during an interview. In this way the Rorschach procedure is a semistructured interview in which the patient is given an opportunity to display his or her use of language and reasoning to another person.

The Rorschach should be defined as a semistructured interview. The stylistic features of communication in this semistructured procedure should be analyzed along specific dimensions. These dimensions should be related to the more precise new methods in psychiatric diagnosis. This use of the Rorschach and the newer methods of psychiatric research augur well for future developments of ways to classify the communication problems of schizophrenics of various types. This definition of what the Rorschach procedure is and the good results found with this type of use of the technique have already had promising research results in related fields.

Rorschach Prognostic Rating Scale

Since one of the aims of using projective techniques in psychiatric diagnosis is to better plan therapy, how has the Rorschach fared on this specific task? Goldfried et al. (7) noted that among the various efforts to develop prognostic rating scales, that of Klopfer et al. (13) has been most successful in predicting success in therapy. Its scores have correlated with overt behavior changes in office and hospital patients due either to therapy or to spontaneous improvement, and the scores have related to a person's skill at adjusting to new and difficult situations. But it also has limitations: it correlates negatively with severity of personality disorder and correlates positively with educational level and good premorbid history. There has been concern that the Prognostic Rating Scale scores might predict response only to "traditional insight-oriented" therapies. More recent reports (20,21) found the scale to predict outcome correctly for (a) neurotic patients in behavior modification and (b) rational-emotive psychotherapy. This scale which became available in 1951 had early encouraging results. Recent findings on groups undergoing other than traditional insight-oriented psychotherapy suggest that the scale may continue to be useful in predicting and assessing outcome in forms of psychotherapy other than those that are insight oriented.

Trends in Personality Assessment

Based on the history of how man has studied man, I think the interview will remain a central procedure in such endeavors. Zubin et al. (72, p. 622) refer to the clinical interview as "our ultimate criterion of psychopathology." I think that the various projective techniques will come to be seen best as semistructured and structured interview procedures which induce special, standardly acquired behavior samples which can be used to test specific concepts. In the foreground will be those aspects of the Rorschach, TAT, and Sentence Completion procedures which can be conceptually defined along with other less frequently used methods that will be validated against conceptually defined personality attributes, behaviors, or theoretically predicted correlations. Many of the traditional scoring methods applied to the Rorschach and other projective techniques which have proved ineffective will be dropped whereas theoretically derived concepts of psychological behavior will be tested. Thoughtful critics (2,6–8,15,17,18,51,52) have been pointing out that when researchers test concepts about verbal interactions from the material gathered by projective techniques and checked against equally clearly outlined theoretically derived concepts, the findings add reliable and valid bits of data to the study of personality, cognition, and psychopathology.

PROJECTIVE TECHNIQUES AS TRANSACTIONAL COMMUNICATION

The study of the communication between the subject and the tester during the assessment transaction has revitalized certain research with the Rorschach and TAT (16,27,28,31–33,35,36,43,44,59):

The most promising use of projective tests for measuring behavior directly is probably a form of interaction testing or consensus administration of the Rorschach and other projective techniques. This has been used in groups, with couples, with families, and with teams of co-workers. It enables the examiner to get simultaneously intrapsychic information based upon the content and style of the responses, and at the same time have a direct view of the interaction between people who have real-life relationships. (15, p. 562)

The aim of much of our work (26–44,53,56–70) has been to illustrate how techniques such as the Rorschach, TAT, proverbs, and other standardly administered assessment devices can be used in other than traditional ways of scoring and interpretation not with primary emphasis on the prediction of an individual's intrapsychic experiences, but with an emphasis on predicting his interpersonal impact on others.[1] Test behavior interpreted in this manner can be used to plan individual, couple, and family therapy as well as used in research. However, a shift must be made from using the test behavior primarily to diagnose, to trying to predict the impact or effect of this person on others who must deal with him or her in intimate, ongoing relationships. In work over the years with Dr. Lyman Wynne, we have felt that this contrast between arriving at a person's clinical psychiatric diagnosis and attempting to sketch out predictively his or her personal impact on others is central in a productive use of tests in family research and family therapy (26–44,53, 56–70).

Perhaps with this shift in interpreting psychological test behavior, there may be further progress toward the continued validation of projective techniques because this use of the tests places interpretations into the realm of viewable, verifiable behavior. When the focus moves from looking inside the person to looking at how his behavior may affect the behavior of those around him, then perhaps we will be better able to assess the devices themselves. For we shall be attempting to correlate two measures of observable transactional behavior. That is, the interpretations will predict what kinds of behaviors are evoked or called forth by certain acts and attitudes.

For some years we have used various psychological tests and assessment data in ways which both appear close to traditional approaches but yet are different from such traditional uses. At first glance to a casual listener or reader, we may seemingly be making only a slight change in perspective and vantage point for interpretation, but in actuality we are making a major change in interpreting test behavior. In family research and family therapy, tests permitting one to conclude what a person's possible impact on other people may be is more useful than using tests primarily to diagnose or label.

Although using a very different orientation to test *interpretation,* we have

---

[1] We use the term "predict" in the sense Benjamin (1) used it, that of predicting from one set of data to another, and not in the folk-sense of forecasting behavior yet to come.

elected to stay with well-known devices such as the Rorschach, TAT, Wechsler, proverbs, and other familiar techniques in order to draw on the existing body of knowledge of what to look for in the way of good and poor performance features of subjects on those procedures. Experienced clinicians are familiar with these devices and will more willingly respond to new ways of looking at familiar tests than to learn about unknown devices. More important is that these testing techniques can be regarded as prototypes of a number of frequently performed tasks in which parents and children engage. These various techniques exemplify those frequent daily exchanges in the formative years of children's lives in which parents demonstrate how to view a situation, show their own styles of attending and communicating, and attempt to relate past experiences and knowledge to the current task. When parental test behavior is regarded as samples of parents' enduring, stylistic ways of transacting, we reason that studying their behavior from the point of view of its inferred impact on family members will help us to assess, at least in the current scene, how they attend and communicate, and permit retrospective speculation about the impact or effect of their styles of responding over the years on one another and especially on their children. This focuses on the behaviors fed into the family system, as to both stylistic and content features by all members (26–44,53,56–70).

OVERVIEW

This discussion has ranged from noting the dire predictions of critics of both psychiatric diagnostic procedures and projective techniques to noting the hopeful outlooks for the future expressed by many observers. It appears that not only our own views but the consensus of critics of both assessment and psychiatric diagnostic fields is that the efforts to make psychiatric interviews more reliable and valid procedures are an advance for assessment itself, assessment researchers, and therapists planning treatment with patients. Stepping back from efforts to validate the Rorschach and other projective devices against any will-of-the-wisp criterion offered has occurred. The new look in clinical psychological research with projective techniques is clearly coming to focus on testing theoretically derived concepts within far more sophisticated research designs than have been previously used.

Projective techniques are being seen as having many dimensions, having aspects of perceptual-cognitive communication tasks. They can be regarded as a semistructured interview; a stimulus to fantasy production; a starting point for transactional behavior.

At all times the user of projective devices needs to ask: Is the variable being studied both clinically and with the Rorschach or other projective technique a behavioral variable, a conscious content, a self-concept, a symbolic content, or a transactional remark with its impact on a listener? Depending on what is being studied, different aspects of a person's responses will be analyzed and scoring procedures used which reflect the concepts being studied.

Both psychiatric diagnostic methods and the uses of projective techniques have profited from the critiques made of them. Although progress may be slow, the future lies, if the past has been a forecaster, in the direction of better conceptualized research in clinical psychiatry and clinical psychology.

REFERENCES

1. Benjamin, J. D. (1959): Prediction and psychopathological theory. In: *Dynamic Psychopathology in Childhood,* edited by L. Jessner and E. Pavenstadt, pp. 6–77. Grune & Stratton, New York.
2. Blatt, S. J. (1975): The validity of projective techniques and their research and clinical contribution. *J. Pers. Assess.,* 39:327–343.
3. Buros, O. K. (1972): *Seventh Mental Measurements Yearbook.* Gryphon Press, Highland Park, N.J.
4. Carpenter, W., Strauss, J., and Bartko, J. (1973): Flexible system for the diagnosis of schizophrenia. Report from the WHO International Pilot Study of Schizophrenia. *Science,* 182:1275–1278.
5. Feighner, J. P., Robbins, E., Guze, S. B., Woodruff, R. A., Jr., Winokur, G., and Munoz, R. (1972): Diagnostic criteria for use in psychiatric research. *Arch. Gen. Psychiatry,* 26:57–63.
6. Frank, G. H. (1969): Psychiatric diagnosis: A review of research. *J. Gen. Psychol.,* 81:157–176.
7. Goldfried, M. R., Stricker, G., and Weiner, I. B. (1971): *Rorschach Handbook of Clinical and Research Applications.* Prentice-Hall, Englewood Cliffs, N.J.
8. Holt, R. R. (1967): Diagnostic testing: Present status and future prospects. *J. Nerv. Ment. Dis.,* 144:444–465.
9. Holtzman, W. H., and Sells, S. B. (1954): Prediction of flying success by clinical analysis of test protocols. *J. Abnorm. Soc. Psychol.,* 49:485–498.
10. Hunt, W. A. (1959): An actuarial approach to clinical judgment. In: *Objective Approaches to Personality Assessment,* edited by B. M. Bass and I. A. Berg. Van Nostrand Reinhold, New York.
11. Jensen, A. R. (1964): The Rorschach technique: A re-evaluation. *Acta Psychol. (Amst.),* 22:60–77.
12. Kelly, E. L., and Fiske, D. W. (1951): *The Prediction of Performance in Clinical Psychology.* University of Michigan Press, Ann Arbor.
13. Klopfer, B., Kirkner, F. J., Wisham, W., and Baker, G. (1951): Rorschach prognostic rating scale. *J. Proj. Technol.,* 15:425–428.
14. Klopfer, W. G. (1968): Current status of the Rorschach test. In: *Advances in Psychological Assessment,* edited by P. McReynolds, pp. 131–149. Science and Behavior Books, Palo Alto, California.
15. Klopfer, W. G., and Taulbee, E. S. (1976): Projective tests. *Annu. Rev. Psychol.,* 27:543–567.
16. Loveland, N. T., Singer, M. T., and Wynne, L. C. (1963): The family Rorschach: A new method for studying family interaction. *Fam. Process,* 2:187–215.
17. Mayman, M. (1973): If projective testing hasn't yet died, shouldn't we let it just fade away? Unpublished manuscript.
18. McArthur, C. C. (1972): The Rorschach. In: *Seventh Mental Measurements Yearbook,* edited by O. K. Buros. Gryphon Press, Highland Park, N.J.
19. Miller, J. S. (1976): The communication of meaning. Unpublished thesis, University of California, Berkeley, California.
20. Newmark, C. S., Finkelstein, M., and Frerking, R. A. (1974): Comparison of the predictive validity of two measures of psychotherapy prognosis. *J. Pers. Assess.,* 38:144–148.
21. Newmark, C. S., Hetzel, W., Walker, L., Holstein, S., and Finkelstein, M. (1973):

Predictive validity of the Rorschach Prognostic Rating Scale with behavior modification techniques. *J. Clin. Psychol.,* 29:246–248.

22. Piotrowski, Z. A. (1937): The Rorschach inkblot method in organic disturbances of the central nervous system. *J. Nerv. Ment. Dis.,* 86:525–537.

23. Piotrowski, Z. A. (1940): Positive and negative Rorschach organic reactions. *Rors. Res. Exchange,* 4:147–151.

24. Pope, B., and Jensen, A. R. (1957): The Rorschach as an index of pathological thinking. *J. Proj. Technol.,* 21:54–62.

25. Rapaport, D., Gill, M., and Schafer, R. (1946): *Diagnostic Psychological Testing, Vol. II.* Year Book Medical Publishers, Chicago.

26. Singer, M. T. (1963): A Rorschach view of the family. In: *The Genain Quadruplets,* edited by D. Rosenthal, pp. 315–325. Basic Books, New York.

27. Singer, M. T. (1967): Family transactions and schizophrenia: I. Recent research findings. In: *The Origins of Schizophrenia,* edited by J. Romano, pp. 147–164. Excerpta Medica International Congress Series No. 151, Amsterdam.

28. Singer, M. T. (1968): The consensus Rorschach and family transactions. *J. Proj. Technol.,* 32:348–351.

29. Singer, M. T. (1969): Proberb Scoring Manual. Unpublished, 21 pp.

30. Singer, M. T. (1969): Position statement. NIMH Workshop on Methodological Issues in Research with Groups at High Risk for Development of Schizophrenia: Measuring Verbal Behavior: Reasoning, Roles and Scoring Rationale. NIMH, Washington, D.C.

31. Singer, M. T. (1973): Scoring manual for communication deviances seen in individually administered Rorschach. Revision. Unpublished, 100 pp.

32. Singer, M. T. (1974): Impact versus diagnosis: A new approach to assessment techniques in family research and therapy. Presented, Cumana, Venezuela.

33. Singer, M. T. (1976): Schizophrenia, families and communication disorders: I. Overview of research findings. Stanley R. Dean Award Lecture.

34. Singer, M. T. (1977): Attentional problems in schizophrenia. In: *The Origins of Schizophrenia, Second Rochester International Conference on Schizophrenia,* edited by L. C. Wynne and R. Cromwell. John Wiley & Sons, New York.

35. Singer, M. T. (1977): Family transactional styles and schizophrenia. In: *The Origins of Schizophrenia, Second Rochester International Conference on Schizophrenia,* edited by L. C. Wynne and R. Cromwell. John Wiley & Sons, New York.

36. Singer, M. T. (1977): The Rorschach as a transaction. In: *Rorschach Psychology,* edited by M. A. Rickers-Ovsiankina, pp. 455–485. John Wiley & Sons, New York.

37. Singer, M. T. (1977): The psychological test features of borderline patients. In: *The Borderline Patient,* edited by P. Hartocollis. International Universities Press, New York.

38. Singer, M. T., and Wynne, L. C. (1963): Differentiating characteristics of the parents of childhood schizophrenics, childhood neurotics, and young adult schizophrenics. *Am. J. Psychiatry,* 120:234–243.

39. Singer, M. T., and Wynne, L. C. (1964): Stylistic variables in family research. Presented at Marquette University and Milwaukee Psychiatric Hospital.

40. Singer, M. T., and Wynne, L. C. (1965): Thought disorder and family relations of schizophrenics: III. Methodology using projective techniques. *Arch. Gen. Psychiatry,* 12:187–200.

41. Singer, M. T., and Wynne, L. C. (1965): Thought disorder and family relations of schizophrenics: IV. Results and implication. *Arch. Gen. Psychiatry,* 12:201–212.

42. Singer, M. T., and Wynne, L. C. (1966): Communication styles in parents of normals, neurotics and schizophrenics: Some findings using a new Rorschach scoring manual. *Am. Psychiatr. Assoc. Res. Rep.,* 20:25–38.

43. Singer, M. T., and Wynne, L. C. (1966): Principles for scoring communication defects and deviances in parents of schizophrenics: Rorschach and TAT scoring manuals. *Psychiatry,* 29:260–288.

44. Singer, M. T., Wynne, L. C., Levi, D., and Sojit, C. (1968): Proverbs interpretation reconsidered: Transactional approach to schizophrenics and their families. Presented at Symposium on Language and Thought in Schizophrenia, Newport Beach, California.

45. Spitzer, R. L., and Endicott, J. (1975): Attempts to improve psychiatric diagnosis. *Ann. Rev. Psychol.,* 26:643–648.
46. Spitzer, R. L., Endicott, J., Fleiss, J. L., and Cohen, J. (1970): The psychiatric status schedule: A technique for evaluating psychopathology and impairment in role functioning. *Arch. Gen. Psychiatry,* 23:41–55.
47. Szasz, T. S. (1962): *The Myth of Mental Illness.* Secker and Warburg, London.
48. Thiesen, J. W. (1952): A pattern analysis of structural characteristics of the Rorschach test in schizophrenia. *J. Consult. Clin. Psychol.,* 16:365–370.
49. Torrey, E. F. (1972): *The Mind Game.* Bantam Books, New York.
50. Watkins, J. G., and Stauffacher, J. C. (1952): An index of pathological thinking in the Rorschach. *J. Proj. Technol.,* 16:276–286.
51. Weiner, I. B. (1972): Does psychodiagnosis have a future? *J. Pers. Assess.,* 36:534–546.
52. Weiner, I. B. (1977): Approaches to Rorschach validation. In: *Rorschach Psychology,* edited by M. A. Rickers-Ovsiankina, pp. 575–608. John Wiley & Sons, New York.
53. Wild, C., Singer, M. T., Rosman, B., Ricci, J., and Lidz, T. (1965): Measuring disordered styles of thinking: Using the Object Sorting Test on parents of schizophrenic patients. *Arch. Gen. Psychiatry,* 13:471–476.
54. Wing, J. K., Cooper, J. E., and Sartorius, N. (1974): *The Measurement and Classification of Psychiatric Symptoms.* Cambridge University Press, London.
55. World Health Organization (1968): *Psychiatric Assessment Schedules.* World Health Organization, Geneva.
56. Wynne, L. C. (1966): Overview of the conference proceedings. *Am. Psychiatr. Assoc. Res. Rep.,* 20:224–234.
57. Wynne, L. C. (1967): Family transactions and schizophrenia: II. Conceptual considerations for a research strategy. In: *The Origins of Schizophrenia,* edited by J. Romano, pp. 165–178. Excerpta Medica International Congress Series No. 151, Amsterdam.
58. Wynne, L. C. (1968): Methodologic and conceptual issues in the study of schizophrenics and their families. *J. Psychiatr. Res. [Suppl.],* 6:185–199.
59. Wynne, L. C. (1968): Consensus Rorschach and related procedures for studying interpersonal patterns. *J. Proj. Technol. Pers. Assess.,* 32:352–356.
60. Wynne, L. C. (1969): Hearing a different drummer: Sources of schizophrenia in the family. Frieda Fromm-Reichman Memorial Lecture, Washington School of Psychiatry.
61. Wynne, L. C. (1970): Communication disorders and the quest for relatedness in families of schizophrenics. *Am. J. Psychoanal.,* 30:100–114.
62. Wynne, L. C. (1971): Family research on the pathogenesis of schizophrenia: Intermediate variables in the study of families at high risk. In: *Problems of Psychosis, Vol. II,* edited by P. Doucet and C. Laurin, pp. 401–423. Excerpta Medica, Amsterdam.
63. Wynne, L. C., Caudill, M., Kasahara, Y., Kuomaru, S., Singer, M. T., and Higa, M. (1971): Translation problems in the cross-cultural study of psychopathology: A comparison of Japanese and American disorders of thinking and communication. In: *Mental Health Research in Asia and the Pacific.* University of Hawaii, Honolulu.
64. Wynne, L. C., and Singer, M. T. (1963): Thought disorder and family relations of schizophrenics: I. A research strategy. *Arch. Gen. Psychiatry,* 9:191–198.
65. Wynne, L. C., and Singer, M. T. (1963): Thought disorder and family relations of schizophrenics: II. A classification of forms of thinking. *Arch. Gen. Psychiatry,* 9:199–206.
66. Wynne, L. C., and Singer, M. T. (1963): The transcultural study of schizophrenics and their families. *Folia Psychiatr. Neurol. Jpn. [Suppl.],* 7:28–29.
67. Wynne, L. C., and Singer, M. T. (1964): Thinking disorders and family transactions. Presented at Joint Meeting of the American Psychiatric Association and the American Psychoanalytic Association, Los Angeles, California.
68. Wynne, L. C., and Singer, M. T. (1966): Schizophrenic impairments of shared

focal attention: A strategic concept for research and therapy. Tenth Annual Bertram Roberts Memorial Lecture, Yale University, New Haven, Conn.
69. Wynne, L. C., Singer, M. T., Bartko, J., and Toohey, M. L. (1977): Schizophrenics and their families: Research on parental communication. In: *Developments in Psychiatric Research,* edited by J. M. Tanner. Hodder and Stoughton, Sevenoaks, Kent, England.
70. Wynne, L. C., Singer, M. T., and Toohey, M. L. (1975): Communication of the adoptive parents of schizophrenics. In: *Schizophrenia 75: Psychotherapy, Family Studies, Research,* edited by J. Jorstad and E. Ugelstad, pp. 413–451. Universitetsforlaget, Oslo, Norway.
71. Zubin, J. (1967): Classification of the behavior disorders. *Annu. Rev. Psychol.,* 18:373–406.
72. Zubin, J., Salzinger, K., Fleiss, J. L., Gurland, B., Spitzer, R. L., Endicott, J., and Sutton, S. (1975): Biometric approach to psychopathology: Abnormal and clinical psychology—statistical, epidemiological and diagnostic approaches. *Annu. Rev. Psychol.,* 26:621–671.

Critical Issues in Psychiatric Diagnosis,
edited by Robert L. Spitzer and Donald F. Klein.
Raven Press, New York © 1978.

Validity of Projective Tests for Psychodiagnosis in Children

Rachel Gittelman-Klein

Queens College, City University of New York, Flushing, New York 11367; and Child Development Clinic, Long Island Jewish-Hillside Medical Center, Glen Oaks, New York 11004

Are we beating a dead horse or belaboring the obvious by examining critically the contribution psychological tests make in the diagnosis of childhood disorders? Although it is tempting to answer in the affirmative, to do so seems unwise. The horse is still alive, although perhaps not well. At the risk of seeming self-serving, I should like to summarize briefly some of the reasons that justify a review of the topic at this time.

First, in all the many reviews on projective psychological tests, findings obtained from children and adults are treated interchangeably. As a matter of fact, it has been stated explicitly that the Rorschach, for one, requires interpretative adjustments to take into account only a child's incomplete emotional development and that, otherwise, "The psychological significance of each of the Rorschach features remains the same for clients of all ages, and in general, the same interpretative postulates can be derived from the series of scores, configuration, ratios, and such" (23).

However, it is reasonable to assume that disturbed children differ from adults and adolescents in important respects that preclude the assumption that various age groups represent a homogeneous psychopathological population. It therefore seems unjustified to generalize to children from studies performed with adults. There has been no recent attempt to distill data pertinent exclusively to children from the vast literature on projective testing.[1] Since it is generally easier to study adult psychiatric patients than children (adult patients are more numerous and are more often institutionalized, which makes them more easily accessible), many more studies have been done with adults than with children; and failure to distinguish the sources of clinical data inevitably exaggerates the amount of accumulated knowledge regarding the usefulness of projective tests in children.

---

[1] A review of the Rorschach in emotionally disturbed children has appeared (7); but in view of its totally uncritical nature, it is of little value to the reader interested in the current state of the art.

Second, the recent textbook on psychiatry edited by Freedman, Kaplan, and Sadock, probably the single most influential resource for psychiatric residents, contains two articles on psychological testing (3,15), neither of which offers critical overviews of projective testing. In one (15), the value of personality tests is emphasized, with claims that many characteristics of patients that are of key concern to the diagnostician, such as level of reality testing, and prognosis can be learned through psychological tests. No attempt is made to support these views with empirical findings. The other article (3) mentions projective tests only briefly and concludes, "The large majority of available projective techniques cannot be evaluated independently of the skill of the clinician using them" (p. 2084). This statement implies that skillful clinicians can obtain meaningful clinical information from projective tests. The type of information derivable is not specified, no clues are given to help one identify skillful clinicians, and no data are advanced to support the author's statement. The two articles might lead readers relatively unsophisticated in the use of psychological tests (among whom I would include psychiatrists in general and, especially, psychiatrists in training) to conclude that projective tests have considerable merit. From Carr's article (15) one would judge the payoff to be very great; from Anastasi's (3), nebulous but nonetheless present. Given the potential formative impact this textbook has on professionals specializing in psychodiagnosis, a more critical review would seem warranted.

Finally, the American Psychiatric Association will soon publish a new diagnostic manual that will depart considerably from its predecessor. It is hoped that the very extensive revisions in the nomenclature for childhood disorders will facilitate assigning children to specific diagnostic groupings. No one claims that the process of finding the best diagnostic fit for a patient is an easy one, and we need all the help we can get. If psychodiagnostic testing can also offer some assistance in the nosological decision-making process with regard to children, it should not be ignored.

The above considerations are among the reasons that seem to justify reviving a topic many of us may feel has been commented on *ad nauseam*.

It is generally assumed by many theoreticians of differing views that there are meaningful relationships between certain personality characteristics, or levels of personality organization, and mental disorders. To the extent that this conceptual model is accurate, the identification of personality features should provide meaningful information for purposes of diagnosis; and in this endeavor, psychological tests should be useful.

I shall deal first with findings regarding personality characteristics, and then with attempts at classification. Several projective techniques will be considered: the Rorschach, the Human Figure Drawing or Draw-a-Person test (DAP) (62), the Thematic Apperception Test (TAT), the Bender-Gestalt (B-G) (52), and the Children's Apperception Test (CAT) (5,6). All are widely used in clinical settings. Since interest scatter has been employed for psychodiagnosis, I shall also review relevant studies of the Wechsler Intelligence Scale for Children (WISC), and data on some less commonly used projective techniques.

Except for the Bender-Gestalt test, no special scoring has been proposed for projective tests used with children. The Bender-Gestalt test as used in adults applies psychodynamic interpretations to the overall execution of drawings, in which, to use the simplest and most obvious example, circular figures are symbolic of the female body and sharp angular ones, of masculine characteristics. Along these lines, overlap between a round and pointy figure has been interpreted as the "hurtful penetration of the feminine by the masculine" (56, p. 21). Studies on children's Bender-Gestalt tests have shunned this approach in favor of more quantitative ones that rely on formal characteristics of the drawing (49).

It is customary for reviews to summarize empirical findings for each test separately. This approach certainly has advantages—it enables the reader to assess easily the overall status of any measure. But I consider it more relevant to examine how well various personality characteristics are tapped by the tests. The clinician is more likely to ask himself, "Is the child aggressive, depressed, anxious, psychotic? How can I find out?" rather than "I have a Rorschach test. What can I possibly use it for in this child?" Consequently, in this review, research findings are organized around clinical themes rather than tests.

A large body of research consisting of abstracts of papers presented at professional meetings and doctoral dissertations available only in abstract form have been omitted deliberately, because of the lack of opportunity to evaluate the designs of investigations presented in such form.

Moreover, no study that failed to include comparison groups has been included. This exclusionary criterion has greatly reduced the number of studies. In comparing disturbed youngsters with normal children, some investigators have made use of normative data obtained either from standardization samples or from other studies rather than concurrent control groups. Such a practice is obviously unacceptable, since other study samples and normative samples may differ with respect to characteristics that affect the test scores studied (i.e., age, sex, IQ, socioeconomic status). Consequently, studies that have not made use of concurrent controls are not included (10,59,64, 72,98,100,102). An illuminating case in point is a Rorschach study that compared hard-of-hearing children with matched controls and with test norms (25). A significant difference was found between the subjects and the published norms, but not between the former and their matched controls.

Among the studies with concurrent control groups, the appropriateness of the controls was not a selection factor. Neither was the issue of whether or not the study was "blind" a criterion for inclusion. If all reports that did not specifically indicate that the test scorers were blind with respect to the subjects' group membership had been omitted, remarkably few studies would have been included.

PERSONALITY CHARACTERISTICS

Aggression

Several investigators have studied whether children's aggressive tendencies could be determined by projective tests. Kagan (45) found that among 118 public school, middle class boys, classified according to five groups on the basis of teacher ratings of degree of aggressiveness, the more aggressive youngsters produced significantly more themes of fighting on the TAT than did the less aggressive ones. However, the difference in mean frequency of fighting themes between the two extreme groups, the aggressive and very nonaggressive, was only one. (Children rated most aggressive had 2.62 themes of aggression compared with 1.42 themes for the least aggressive group.) Therefore, the clinical usefulness of the score in individual cases is questionable. Four other TAT themes of aggression did not differentiate among the levels of aggression reported by the teacher.

In another study (57), the level of fantasy aggression on the TAT failed to correlate with level of peer-rated, overly aggressive behavior ($r = 0.07$) in 44 normal children. However, the author found that mothers' attitudes toward the overt expression of aggression mediated the relationship between fantasy and overt aggression. There was a significant positive ($r = 0.43$) relationship between the two measures of aggression in children whose mothers encouraged aggression, but a significant negative ($r = -0.43$) association in the group without such maternal attitudes. The difference between the two coefficients was highly significant.

These results suggest that the relationship between TAT fantasy aggression and overt aggression in normal children is influenced by maternal concerns. It is not known whether the same relationships would exist for pathological groups; if they did, this would complicate the interpretation of TAT fantasy themes. This particular study is of considerable significance, and it is unfortunate that no further investigations along its lines have been conducted.

Using human figure drawings, 31 aggressive children were compared with shy children matched for age, sex, and IQ (51). The test administration and scoring were done with some time between them to minimize the likelihood of contamination by knowledge of group membership. No specific predictions were advanced, and no mention was made of whether the drawings of both groups of children were equivalent in quality of performance.

Of 33 characteristics studied, 6 differentiated between the shy and the aggressive children. The shy group drew a significant excess of figures with cut-off hands and missing mouths: the aggressive children showed a significantly greater tendency to draw figures with asymmetry of limbs, prominence of teeth, long arms, and big hands.

Although significant, the differences are unimpressive. For example, the greatest single difference between the groups in frequency for a drawing feature is for 8 of 31 subjects. Therefore, the overlap between the groups is very large, and the findings cannot be applied meaningfully for clinical purposes.

Handler and McIntosh (37) classified 49 third grade boys in public school classes as either aggressive, withdrawn, or neither (controls) on the basis of teacher and peer ratings. There was no IQ or age difference among the three groups. The children were given a 2-min clinical interview, on the basis of which, also, the child was assigned to one of the three clinical groups. Each child completed a Bender-Gestalt and a Draw-a-Person test. Further, each child was asked to select the most congruent description of himself from personality sketches portraying a normal, an aggressive, or a passive boy. All test ratings were made independently, but it is not reported whether group membership was known to the raters. The test protocols were dichotomized according to low versus high aggression and withdrawal levels. The technique and rationale for determination of cut-off scores are not given.

The authors predicted that responses evaluated as aggressive would be significantly more frequent among the children rated as aggressive by teachers and peers than among withdrawn and control children and that test ratings indicating withdrawal would be more frequent among withdrawn children. Moreover, the projective data were expected to have greater classificatory accuracy than the 2-min clinical interview and the children's self-ratings. In fact, Bender-Gestalt test ratings of aggression were significantly more frequent among the aggressive children than the controls, but those of the withdrawn children did not differ significantly from the controls. The results of the contrast between the aggressive and the withdrawn children are not reported. DAP ratings of aggression and withdrawal did not discriminate among the groups. The B-G test also failed to identify the withdrawn children.

In toto, of 12 comparisons, only 1 was significant in the predicted direction. The authors claim that the projective tests were better than the self-ratings or the very brief clinical assessment in categorizing the subjects. They report that the B-G test classified 80% of the aggressive children. Unfortunately, they do not indicate how many of the nonaggressive children were identified as aggressive, thus rendering interpretation of the 80% hit rate in one group difficult. No appropriate statistical analyses of the differences in predictive accuracy were undertaken. Curiously, combining the two projective tests decreased the predictive value of each.

The level of aggression in 63 severely disturbed, institutionalized boys of average or near average IQ was assessed by social workers (95). The ratings dichotomized the sample into low and high aggression levels. No differences in IQ or frequency of Rorschach response were found between the two groups. Five of the test determinants differed significantly between the aggressive and nonaggressive groups. If the presence of two signs was used as a criterion of level of test-elicited aggression, 82% of the aggressive boys, but only 64% of the nonaggressive boys, were accurately identified. As is often the case in measures of pathology, the presence of signs was more predictive than their absence.

The same sample as Townsend's was used by Davids (18) to study the relationships among (a) ratings of overt aggression, (b) aggressive test content on the TAT, and (c) total psychological assessment. The TAT fared poorly. Of four scoring systems applied, two differentiated significantly between the groups, but marginally. The psychologist's global clinical predictions were significantly correlated with the children's aggressive behavior. The contrast between a quantified test score and an overall psychological judgment is an important one. It has been claimed by some that the use of scores, or the statistical approach, as it is called, does not reflect the ecology of psychodiagnosis as practiced by clinical psychologists and that, therefore, little can be expected of it. In this case it would indeed appear that the clinical assessment approach might be better than some of the objective test scores for predicting aggressive behavior. However, it would be erroneous to conclude that the predictions made on the basis of the total testing procedure emanated from insights obtained during the evaluation, or from the tests. It is conceivable that the testers were predicting children's future behavior solely on the basis of their knowledge of past behavior. If so, a considerable degree of accuracy could be expected, regardless of the evaluation. Without controls for sources of information used by the clinicians, no conclusions can be reached regarding the merits of the formal psychological evaluation procedure.

A more recent study (12) investigated the ability of the DAP and the Hand Test[2] to predict aggressive behavior in 40 youngsters in a school for emotionally disturbed children. The children were rated by teachers for aggressive behavior 6 months after having been tested. Interrater reliability of aggressive content was within acceptable limits ($r = 0.75$). The children were retested at the time of the teacher evaluations, and the findings were negative in all respects. The levels of aggression on the two projective tests showed no significant association. Neither measure correlated with future or with concurrent level of aggressive behavior.

Self-Esteem and Self-Image

Body image (whatever the term means) and self-esteem have also been examined, typically with the DAP test. Three drawings (a person, opposite sex, and self) done by children with residual orthopedic difficulties from polio could not be differentiated from the drawings of normal children, matched for IQ, by clinicians who did not know which drawings had been done by which group ("blind") (91). Of a total of 165 signs (55 on each of the

---

[2] The child is presented pictures of a hand and is asked to relate what the hand is doing.

three drawings), 13 differed significantly between the two groups, 3 in the opposite direction from that predicted. The discrimination rate of the DAP in this study did not exceed chance.

Using global clinical judgments, investigators obtained similar results in a "blind" study of the DAP (16): Expert clinicians were unable to distinguish between the human drawings of children with upper limbs missing and normal children matched for sex, age, and mental age. Only drawings produced by the children when instructed to draw a picture of themselves were classified at a rate 17% above chance. The findings suggest that to infer a child's "body image" from his drawing of a person is fallacious. The fact that a child fails to reveal his own obvious physical defects in the drawing of "a person" does not indicate that he is unaware of these defects.

Other investigators (78) postulated that since self-esteem had been shown to be influenced by the presence or absence of parental figures, the figure drawings of orphans in institutions should differ from those of children (matched for age and IQ) from intact homes. It was predicted that the drawings of the orphans would be smaller. The findings did not corroborate the hypothesis. The study was not a blind one and suffers also from failure to obtain objective, independent measures of self-esteem.

The figure drawings of chronically obese children, treated in an outpatient clinic, were compared with those of normal public school children matched for sex, IQ, and socioeconomic status (75). Three age groups were studied: 7-, 10-, and 13-year-olds. Significant differences in body image were found in the 10- and 13-year-olds, but not in the younger group. The conclusion is drawn that obese children have more immature body images. However, the control group was inappropriate: the obese patients should have been compared with other children brought to the hospital for a reason other than obesity. Since the obese children had been brought by parents dissatisfied with them, the difference between the groups might have been related to the obese children's other difficulties (such as parental disappointment) rather than to overweight *per se*.

Thirty boys referred for evaluation because of cross-gender behavior were compared on the DAP with "masculine" boys matched for age and socioeconomic status (32). The "feminine" boys (57%) drew a female figure first significantly more often than the "masculine" boys (24%), giving support to the notion that the gender represented in the first drawing reflects sexual identification. This study was partially replicated in 19 boys referred for gender role abnormality (92). Compared with 35 noneffeminate school and learning-problem boys matched for age, the effeminate boys of young age (4 to 7 years) drew a female figure first significantly more often than the controls. The difference did not occur in boys from 8 to 10 years of age, however. In other groups this characteristic has been found to be unreliable. Therefore, the finding may not be valid in clinical groups other than the one studied. Differences in other aspects of the drawings were found between the groups, such as amount of clothing drawn on the female figure and the proportions of the figures. But as the authors point out, the within-group score variability for these measures is very large, and the DAP characteristics cannot be interpreted clinically with confidence.

The concept of body perception inferred from the Rorschach test was examined in 80 normal schoolchildren classified as socially well adjusted or poorly adjusted on the basis of convergent ratings in teacher, peer, and school personnel reports, and direct school observations (60). Contrasting the highest and lowest quartiles in overall adjustment, the authors found no differences among 6-year-olds, but significantly better body boundary perception among the better adjusted older subjects. The results for what is referred to as "body penetration awareness" were inconsistent. At some ages the better adjusted children produced more such themes; at other ages, the reverse was found. Consequently, the relevance of this dimension is of dubious significance in evaluating social adjustment. The number of responses was controlled to some extent, since a child had to give three responses to each card, but IQ was not taken into consideration.

Using the Blacky test and self-ratings, Davids and Lawton (19) found that 30 middle class normal children had better self-concepts than 25 middle and lower class children, unmatched for IQ, in residential treatment.

Other Personality Characteristics

The personality characteristics of aggression and self-image have received the most attention; only a few explorations of other personality characteristics have been conducted.

Themes of loss have been investigated among orphaned children by means of Rorschach, and/or TAT, or CAT responses (40). A large group of children who had lost one or both parents were compared with controls. As predicted, themes of loss (which had satisfactory interrater reliability) were significantly more frequent in children who had experienced a loss.

Another study, conducted in Britain, used the CAT and Rorschach to investigate the personality of grossly deprived children and to identify children who could not adjust successfully to fostering in normal homes (99). The deprived group consisted of children removed from an adequate foster home because of severe friction between the foster parent and the child; the controls were children awaiting foster placement. The "foster failures" produced more themes of loneliness and desertion on the CAT and fewer stories depicting normal families and realistic parental attitudes. Several differences were found on the Rorschach, but they varied according to age. For instance, the 5- to 6-year-old deprived youngsters had more color responses, whereas the 7- and 8-year-olds had fewer such responses compared with their controls. Moreover, even when significant differences occurred, the mean frequency for specific signs was very low (e.g., although the 7-year-old "foster failures" had more "blackness" on the Rorschach than the controls, the respective frequencies were 0.83 and 0.22). Obviously, the absence of such a sign is not informative; and there was a great deal of overlap between the groups, even when significant differences occurred.

The study has many flaws. The controls differed from the experimental subjects in a variety of important ways: the two groups were separated from their families for different reasons; they had significantly different IQs; the amount of separation experienced by each group was very different. No attempt was made to reconcile contradictory findings at different ages. [For further critical comments, see Gross (33).] But in spite of the limitations of the study, the author concludes that the Rorschach and CAT "should be given weight in reaching a judgment as to whether a child should be fostered or would be more appropriately cared for in a children's home" (p. 19). It is clear that no such claim can be made on the basis of the results.

TAT records of 12 children in foster homes were compared (blindly) to those of controls matched for age, sex, race, and academic achievement (77). Surprisingly, the fostered children gave significantly longer stories. They expressed more need for affiliation, and had more words revealing sad affect. The two groups did not differ on themes of death, separation, anger, or aggression.

The needs of normal third graders as expressed in nondirective play interviews were compared with the children's needs expressed on the TAT and CAT (9). A "significant" association was reported between needs expressed in the play sessions and on the tests for 5 of the 26 needs. The authors conclude that "the animal pictures and TAT are valid instruments for revealing manifest needs of children." Given the fact that the sample size was very small (eight subjects), this statement is somewhat overconfident. But much more serious is the flawed data analysis. The authors intercorrelated the three ratings of each of the 26 needs for each child, using nonindependent measures in single subjects as scores for deriving correlation coefficients. There is no way of interpreting such results, and no way of obtaining levels of probability.

Although need achievement has been studied extensively among normal children, it has received scant attention in groups of patients. In a blind study, Lifshitz (61) used TAT cards to tap need achievement in 64 nonpsychotic, nonretarded, non-brain-damaged children in psychotherapy. The patients had lower need achievement, regardless of sex, when compared with normal girls, but not when compared with normal boys. The results are therefore weak with regard to the relevance of this personality characteristic in disturbed children.

Some personality characteristics as inferred from TAT stories in underachieving and achieving fifth graders matched for IQ were investigated (73). The underachievers were rated as more passive-aggressive than the controls by their teachers. On the TAT, the underachievers expressed significantly more hostility but did not differ in need for independent action. The results are presented in the form of mean differences between the group, and it is not possible to assess the degree of overlap between the underachievers and achievers for the teachers' ratings of passive-aggressive behavior nor for amount of hostility on the TAT.

Lehmann (54) studied CAT responses given by kindergarten subjects of low socioeconomic status from broken or intact homes. In addition, the CATs of children of low, middle, and high socioeconomic status were contrasted. A number of personality and other factors such as sibling rivalry, aggression, fear, toilet habits, and others were measured. Children from broken homes did not differ from those from intact homes. The only significant difference found was a greater number of fear responses in the children of high socioeconomic status. However, the overlap among the groups was very large.

Various physical deficits of children have been viewed as reflections of psychopathology. This notion has been applied to children with nonorganic hearing disorders (24,82) and those with nonorganic articulation problems (27). Of two "nonblind" studies investigating personality characteristics in small samples of hard-of-hearing children and controls matched for sex and age, one (24) found no group differences either in Rorschach-response determinants or in pattern of scores. The other (82) reports significant differences between hard-of-hearing and normal children on three Rorschach scores. Here again, though significantly different, the groups overlap greatly.

First grade children with diffuse, nonorganic, articulatory problems were compared with controls matched for age, IQ, and sex (27). Measures obtained "nonblind" consisted of teacher ratings, the CAT, and an interview with the mother. Both the teachers and the mothers reported more behavioral disturbance in the experimental subjects, who also produced more themes of aggression and anxiety on the CAT. The authors erroneously conclude that the data support a psychogenic hypothesis. Although group membership and test responses were correlated, it is difficult to establish a cause-and-effect sequence. Alternatively, both phenomena—speech defect and deviant test responses—might be the outcome of another independent factor, such as brain injury (the subjects with language disorders had significantly more birth difficulties). The data are further interpreted in *non sequitur* fashion as pointing to the limitation of symptomatic treatments in speech pathology.

In a blind study, Aaron (1) obtained TAT stories from two types of allergic children, one group with asthma and one without, and a control group. There were no age or IQ differences among the groups. Only two measures differentiated the groups. More asthmatics (4 out of 16 children) than normals (none out of 20) mentioned the gun on a card. On a depression score, the asthmatic children had significantly more elevated scores than the allergic nonasthmatic children and than the normals. The latter two groups did not differ. Assuming that differences between children with physical ailments and other children are reliable, difficult interpretational problems arise from correlational studies such as the ones summarized. Are asthmatic children more likely to become secondarily depressed, or are depressed children more likely to develop respiratory allergies? Each causal relationship has clinical importance, but each carries very different theoretical and treatment implications.

DIAGNOSTIC CLASSIFICATION

The bulk of the research in psychodiagnosis has attempted to differentiate between normal children and children either in treatment or referred for treatment. This is the least specific classification possible. It makes no distinction among diagnostic groupings, and the approach may well be meaningless if different pathological groups have contrasting response patterns. Combining characteristics which are opposite in nature could lead to negative results in mean differences between disturbed and normal groups, and only the score variances might reveal group contrasts.

Comparisons Between Patients and Normal Children

In spite of the heterogeneity of the groups of patients, all the studies performed have found significant differences between patients and controls.

Surprisingly, the Bender-Gestalt test has been the measure most frequently used for assessing differences between "emotionally disturbed" youngsters and normal children.

Byrd (14) found that 150 nonretarded preadolescents without organic brain lesions, who were diagnosed as needing psychotherapy, differed significantly from 200 well-adjusted children on 4 of 15 scores of the B-G, the rater being aware of to which group the children belonged. The best discrimination could predict group membership for 85% of the normal subjects and 58% of the children needing therapy. Other measures led to either too many false-positive or too few true-positive assignments. Thus, there was either a large overlap between the groups or a low hit rate for each score.

A large group of inpatients were found to be significantly different from normal children on the Bender-Gestalt, Draw-A-Person, and Rorschach tests (94). However, the two groups' IQs differed significantly, obscuring the diagnostic significance of these differences.

Similar interpretational difficulties because of group IQ differences occurred in another "nonblind" study in which schizophrenic children differed significantly from normal subjects on the Bender-Gestalt test (30). Since the schizophrenic children and mentally retarded subjects matched for IQ did not differ, the author concludes that the B-G test scores are primarily a function of IQ.

A study by Clawson (17) revealed significant differences on the Bender-Gestalt and Rorschach tests between children in outpatient treatment (those diagnosed as psychotic, retarded, or suffering from organic disorders were excluded) and IQ-matched controls. The scores that Byrd (14) had found differentiated significantly between the groups were replicated in this study. Further, ratings of constriction and aggression on the Rorschach were significantly associated with Bender scores assumed to tap similar functions. The IQ determination was not uniform for the groups: the Stanford-Binet or WISC was used for IQ testing of clinic patients; the Draw-a-Person test, for controls. Although these two sets of measures correlate significantly, they differ considerably, and cannot be construed to be equivalent. Moreover, the test rater knew to which group a child belonged and his other test scores as well.

Koppitz (49), in a "nonblind" study, scored B-G tests of 136 controls and 136 children referred because of emotional problems for developmental level and indicators of emotional difficulties. The index patients made significantly more immature drawings and displayed more "emotional indicators." When classified by age, only one sign discriminated between the groups at all ages. With a minimum cut-off score of three signs, 13% of the controls and 44% of the patients could be identified as disturbed. Although the rate of false positives is relatively low, the hit rate among the emotionally disturbed children is not sufficiently high to warrant clinical use of the test scores.

Several studies have made use of the DAP to assess psychopathology. In a group of 622 kindergarten children, those rated by the teachers as having poor adjustment had significantly more deviant drawings (i.e., more grotesque figures, and more "body missing") (96). Of this large group, 42 of the well and poorly adjusted children could be matched for performance on a vocabulary test which was used as an IQ estimate. The significant association between behavioral adjustment and DAP test characteristics remained even with IQ controls. Forty-five percent of the 21 children rated as having poor school behavior had one or more signs on the test; none of the 21 normal children did. One year later, 150 of the children were rated again by their teachers. The consistency in teacher-rated behavioral deviance was moderate. Unfortunately, the data are not presented in a fashion enabling an estimate of the predictive ability of the DAP—a moderate but significant association appears to be present between early presence of signs and later school difficulties.

Both emotionally disturbed and brain-damaged youngsters matched for age and IQ were found to have significantly more signs on the DAP than normals (34). The affected groups did not differ. The classificatory accuracy of the test is not reported; however, from the means and standard deviations presented, it seems that there was a large overlap between the normal and disturbed children.

Dillard and Landsman (20) evaluated 117 fourth and fifth graders who had been given DAPs in kindergarten. The children also had received group

IQ tests in second grade. Of the original group, 36 (30%) had been referred for treatment. These children had performed significantly worse on the DAP in kindergarten. Since the IQs of the referred children were significantly lower than those of the children not referred for treatment, a subsample of 20 pairs of children matched for IQ was selected from the total group. The results were identical to those obtained from the overall sample; namely, the referred children were significantly worse on the DAP than their IQ-matched controls. Unfortunately, the authors do not present score distributions which could indicate the accuracy of the DAP in predicting the nonspecific event of referral. It is further regrettable that no description of the referred children is offered. A 30% prevalence of behavior problems is very high, although not inconceivable in some populations. The absence of some descriptive clinical data renders interpretation of the results difficult.

Using the DAP, two "nonblind" studies (29,51) found that formal, objective aspects of the drawings discriminated significantly between clinic patients and controls. In one case (51), use of two signs or more identified 60% of the patients and only 5% of the controls as disturbed. In the other study (29), the same criterion identified 58% of the patients and 18% of the controls as disturbed. There is remarkable consistency between the studies in the identification of true positives. The difference in number of false positives may result from the fact that Koppitz (51) selected children identified by teachers as having good social, emotional, and academic adjustment, whereas Fuller et al. (29) randomly chose controls from lists of children evaluated by teachers as having no emotional problems. These studies were not reported to be "blind," but test protocols were rated by independent raters with good reliability. On the negative side, however, there is no reported attempt to equate the groups for IQ. It is possible that this factor contributed to the differences reported.

In a "nonblind" Rorschach study (81), the mean frequencies of nine test determinants were significantly different in 100 children with behavior problems and 100 controls equivalent in IQ and in number of responses. The samples overlap greatly. Although highly significantly different ($p < 0.001$), the following means indicate that distributions of group scores do not allow for individual assignment, i.e., for the index subjects and controls, respectively: pure color, 0.1 versus 0.0; F + %, 64% versus 78%; F%, 62% versus 51%.

Scoring the Rorschach for barrier scores, Fisher (26) found in a "nonblind" study that 46 children referred because of extreme impulsivity and restlessness had significantly fewer barrier scores than normal subjects of equivalent IQ drawn from the same school.

In two investigations (39,97) that contrasted normal and emotionally disturbed children on the CAT but failed to equate the groups for IQ, the responses of the disturbed children were found to be more deviant than those of the normal subjects.

The study by Walton (97) compared 47 institutionalized boys with 328 normal children. The accuracy rate is not reported. With such a large number of subjects, significant differences may account for relatively little variance and can have little, if any, clinical relevance.

The study by Haworth (39) is most interesting since the results on the CAT correlated with a rank order of disturbance in three groups of children. Thirty early elementary grade normal children were classified as deviants and nondeviants on the basis of their responses to a specially designed film. The two subgroups of normal children were compared with 15 children with emotional problems matched for school grade and sex. Significant differences were found in the number of CAT critical scores among the three groups, the nondeviant normal children having the fewest, the disturbed children the most. If a cut-off score of 5 critical scores (of a possible 10) was applied, 93% of the clinic subjects, 53% of the deviant normal children, and 0% of the nondeviant normal subjects were identified. This study offers the best evidence available of the CAT's ability to uncover deviance. Unfortunately, no "blinding" and no IQ matching are indicated in the report.

Register and L'Abate (80) compared 175 school children with 61 youngsters referred for help, matched for age, sex, IQ, and socioeconomic status. This is the only study in which all these important variables were balanced in the study samples. All the children had taken the Missouri Children's Picture Series (MCPS) twice, 10 days apart. The scales' reliability on the test-retest was poor to acceptable (0.38 to 0.78). Three years later, teachers and psychologists rated the children as normal or abnormal. No criteria are given for the ratings. Of seven MCPS scales, three (the hyperactivity, aggression, and inhibition scales) discriminated in the expected directions among the subgroups. Although the authors claim that the psychologists' ratings of abnormality were more strongly associated with deviant MCPS responses than the teachers' ratings, they did not perform the appropriate statistical analyses to test this contention.

The Register and L'Abate study (80) supports the hypothesis that, at least on this test, performance on a personality test is predictive of ratings of difficulties. However, as in many other cases, the overlap among the groups is very large; and strong exception must therefore be taken to the authors' statement that the MCPS "will make possible early detection of disturbance even in very young children" (p. 387).

Comparisons Among Diagnostic Groups

It is self-evident that discriminating among various syndromes has greater clinical value than distinguishing nonpatients from patients. However, the latter comparison has methodological advantages in that one is not faced with problems of criterion validity. A child either is or is not in treatment. The accuracy of the event predicted is not in serious question.

Obviously, the same is not true when one is assessing personality constructs or membership in a diagnostic class. The degree to which tests will be able to predict a phenomenon is necessarily influenced by the accuracy or validity of subjects' assignment to the various diagnostic groupings. Should the clinical diagnostician or the test be indicted if no relationship between the two assessments is found? The question is unanswerable unless independent validation data are offered for the variable predicted. There is not a single study in which this effort has been made. As a matter of fact, nowhere are figures indicating the reliability of the diagnoses presented, nor are the reported diagnostic classifications ever based on objective, identifiable, reproducible clinical criteria.

Do we stop here and disregard the available literature? Perhaps we should. Yet a number of studies have used groups so grossly different in psychopathology that it is justifiable to examine the findings. Of course, whether it is correct to assume that phenomenological differences among diagnostic groups are sufficiently obvious to warrant the premise that the groups are truly different is a matter of subjective judgment. No evaluation of the diagnostic meaningfulness of the literature is offered: all studies are reported. Let the reader beware.

The Rorschach test has been used by several investigators to identify types of childhood behavior patterns. Goldfarb (31) in a "nonblind" study contrasted 15 hospitalized schizophrenic children in institutional placement, and 15 children in foster homes. The schizophrenic and institutionalized children did not differ from each other, both having a more deviant Rorschach scores than the children in foster homes. The Rorschach results are interpreted by the author as reflecting differences in anxiety level between the groups. The significant IQ superiority of the foster children makes clear interpretations problematic.

"Blind" judges were unable to classify, beyond chance expectation, the Rorschachs of 42 children with reading disabilities and 42 children with various kinds of behavior problems (90). This study is a good example of the kind of study that has provoked criticisms of the empirical literature, because the experimenter asks a question no reasonable clinician should be expected to answer.

A "nonblind" French study (11) contrasted the Rorschachs of 20 children with obsessive fears, ideas, and rituals to those of 20 other psychiatric patients and 20 normal subjects. It was hypothesized that the test protocols of the children with obsessions would contain more sadistic and aggressive content, since these are the kinds of unacceptable repressed impulses typical of such children. Several such Rorschach indices appeared significantly more often in the children with obsessions than in the other two groups.

Significantly more "power concern" in TAT stories among 10-year-old paranoid schizophrenics as compared with four clinical groups—nonparanoid schizophrenics, passive-aggressives, anxiety neuroses, and psychoneuroses—

and normals of the same age has been reported (101). The five nonparanoid groups did not differ among themselves. The authors suggest that power concerns are the cause, rather than the result, of paranoid disorder in children. I must deviate from the promise not to comment on the diagnostic validity of groups studied in the case of this study. Schizophrenia, as found in adults, is very rare in children. This study is one in which objective criteria for diagnosis are essential. Their absence renders the results meaningless.

Some Rorschach determinants have been found to be significantly associated with outcome in psychotherapy in adults, but very little work on this subject has been done with children. An early study by Lessing (58) revealed a significant relationship between the mean number of human movement responses on the Rorschach and the outcome in individual psychotherapy as rated by the therapist. Of 19 children rated improved, 90% had given M responses, whereas only 60% of 14 children rated as unimproved had done so. None of the remaining 16 Rorschach signs were related to improvement. In addition, the author found that the independent evaluations of initial severity of disturbance by three psychologists correlated with outcome ratings. As might have been anticipated, the children considered mildly or moderately disturbed were more likely to be regarded as improved than the severely disturbed ones.

Lessing undertook a truly unique and laudable effort: she cross-validated the predictive value of the Rorschach finding and replicated the psychologists' ratings on an independent sample of 53 children. The two findings originally obtained disappeared in the replication study. Furthermore, the author failed to find a difference between senior and junior staff in ability to predict outcome.

Leitch and Schafer (55) used the TAT to contrast the perceptual and affective disturbances in 15 psychotic compared with 15 maladjusted youngsters. However, the IQs of the two groups were so different (respective mean IQs, 99 and 121) that the results have little significance.

Of 23 scores on the DAP, 2 were found to differ significantly in 27 neurotic children and 27 with behavior disorders (67). The ratings were not "blind," no predictions of specific differences were made, and obtaining 2 significant findings in 23 is not much better than chance, if better at all.

McConnell (65) studied the relationship of Bender-Gestalt test scores to organic disorders and to emotional problems in children. The children were classified according to three levels of severity of organic disorder and four of emotional disturbance, from situational reaction to psychotic. Mental age was controlled for each comparison. Three Bender-Gestalt scores were derived without knowledge of the children's diagnoses: developmental scores, brain injury indicators, and emotional indicators. Both the developmental scores and the brain injury indicators differentiated significantly between the organically impaired children and those without such disability, but not among the diagnostic groups. The emotional indicators were not related to severity of emotional problems or to brain damage.

The Bender-Gestalt was administered to 64 inpatient children, 43 of whom were discharged with a diagnosis of psychosis (8). The author does not report IQs or other descriptive data, but merely indicates that mean IQ, sex, and age of the two diagnostic groups were not significantly different. Five Bender-Gestalt factors were examined, of which four discriminated between the groups. In one instance the nonpsychotic subjects' performance was significantly worse than that of the psychotic subjects. Many measures tapping cognitive development and central nervous system (CNS) differentiated the groups, always to the disadvantage of the psychotic children. Therefore, it would appear that Bender-Gestalt differences reflect contrasting levels of organic disorder or CNS damage rather than specific psychopathological traits.

Although the DAP drawings of emotionally disturbed and brain-damaged youngsters were found to differ significantly from normal children's, the patient groups were indistinguishable (34). If consistent, these results might suggest that significant differences obtained between normals and emotionally disturbed children on graphomotor tasks such as the B-G and DAP might be due to the presence of unidentified CNS dysfunctions in some of the children included in the broad category of emotional disturbance.

Five investigations (28,38,66,86,89) have tried to relate WISC subtest score scatter to psychodiagnosis, but all have failed.

Discussion

There are some conspicuous omissions in the above summary. For instance, the Minnesota Multiphasic Personality Inventory (MMPI) is not mentioned. It has not been used in children except in a single study, by Marks et al. (63), in which a few 9-year-olds were included in a very large sample of adolescents; but the data on the young subjects are not presented separately. However, this study indicates that in some cases it is possible to use the MMPI in preadolescents. Of course, the issue of scale validity in this age group would have to be examined.

In addition, the Rosenzweig Picture-Frustration Study (83) is not discussed. Much was expected from this test, because it was thought to be a rational application of projective principles. For example, shortly after the test appeared, it was described as "a brilliant example of the fact that respect for projective subtleties and respect for sound experimental procedures need not be mutually exclusive. Moreover, the method is unusual . . . in that it constitutes a direct application of carefully developed theory" (93). Little work has been done with this measure, however. More importantly, its reliability is considered too poor to warrant serious consideration as a diagnostic tool: in 88 children tested 3 months apart, correlation coefficients for ratings ranged from 0.26 to 0.69 (84); and in another report (85), test-retest correlations of a group of 45 children yielded coefficients from 0.22 to 0.55.

Test reliability is problematic for all tests and requires consideration.

RELIABILITY

This discussion of reliability is not meant to be a comprehensive review of the topic. The subject is treated briefly only to highlight the findings obtained in children for the tests reported. Empirical results indicate marginal test-retest reliability of the "projective" characteristics of the DAP test. In a study of over 1,300 children, Hammer and Kaplan (36) accepted a 0.05 significance level as criterion for adequate reliability of tests administered 1 week apart. Contingency tables are not presented. In such a large group, a significant correlation may account for very little variance (e.g., a correlation coefficient of 0.06 is significant beyond the 0.05 level of chance in a sample size of 1,000). Even when such a weak criterion as 11 DAP test scores was used, only 6 were found "reliable."

The Bender-Gestalt scores have fared better, with test-retest correlations averaging about 0.6 (52).

TAT test-retest reliability of scores over time has not been found to be adequately reliable to warrant the assumption that the test measures stable, enduring personality dimensions. In correlations of eight TAT content areas in 86 children tested three times on seven TAT cards, only two areas were found to be significantly associated over time, but weakly so, accounting for only 10% of the variance (46). A further attempt led to better, but still not impressive, results (47). The test-retest reliability of the CAT in young children seems quite variable across measures, from very low ($r = 0.1$) to relatively high (0.8) (79).

The Rorschach test-retest reliability in normal children is positively related to age. The test-retest reliability over a few years' span is low for children under 8 years old, but quite good above that age (2). Some data, although contradictory, suggest that there may be a heritability factor for Rorschach determinants (4,35,74). If these preliminary and less than well-executed studies are replicated in careful investigations, strong support will be given to the notion that the Rorschach taps some meaningful human characteristics, at least in young adults. The validity problem that will remain is: Meaningful for what?

Another consideration is that test-retest reliability cannot be assumed to exist for all groups if it has been established on the basis of a specific group. If a test has been found to be reliable for normal subjects, its reliability for any other group under study still needs to be determined.

Interrater reliability poses fewer problems. With adequate training, any number of individuals can usually obtain a reasonable degree of agreement.

Yet such reliability cannot be taken for granted. Interscorer reliability is almost never reported. The work of Koppitz (50) and Haworth (39,40) is exceptional in this regard.

INTERVENING FACTORS

There is ample and consistent evidence that test results are associated significantly with a variety of factors. The most prominent characteristics of patients that must be controlled to ensure that test responses can be properly interpreted are age and IQ, which have been found to affect Rorschach content, the DAP test, the B-G test, and the TAT (13,21,22,44,76), and socioeconomic status (25) (it is not clear whether the latter relationship is independent of IQ).

Given that claims have been advanced, and some support obtained, for certain experiential factors being related to test responses, care should be taken to assure that study samples are equivalent in terms of parental loss, self-esteem, and level of aggression if characteristics other than these are being investigated.

Ideally, one should control for any variable previously found to affect test results. This process would probably make it unduly cumbersome to obtain enough subjects for study. However, there is no justification for lack of control for IQ, age, sex, and socioeconomic status.

In specific instances certain other controls are necessary, such as the number of responses on the Rorschach and the quality of drawing on the DAP. Although both these characteristics are correlated with IQ, control for IQ alone will not remove their influence, since they may still contribute to features of test responses independently of IQ level.

The issue of whether or not studies are "blind" is obviously crucial. It is shocking that "nonblind" studies find their way into peer review journals. This practice does considerable disservice to the credibility of psychologists as concerned clinicians.

AN OVERVIEW

In the entire literature only a handful of studies have the characteristics of being "blind" and controlled for IQ—a sad state of affairs. Giving the tests the benefit of the doubt, within the limits of the research, I should be willing to conclude that children with a host of behavior disorders differ from normal children on projective test measures. The situation in this area is somewhat similar to that with regard to clinical neurological signs: the latter are often present with increased frequency in some child psychopathological groups, but no single abnormality is specific to a diagnostic grouping. It would be incorrect to assume, therefore, that brain dysfunction is unrelated to these states. Rather, I think we should conclude that it is related, but in ways that are phenotypically heterogeneous.

The same arguments can be made for projective testing. The empirical data are poor in ways more numerous than those touched on in this review. Yet there may very well be something there. On the other hand, the tests do not appear to have diagnostic specificity.

It is clear that anyone who still claims that WISC subtest scatter is relevant to personality diagnosis or psychopathology has to catch up on some reading.

As for personality correlates, the DAP test, the TAT, and the Hand Test emerge as invalid measures. Very little work has been done with the Rorschach in this area.

It is important to remember that even when statistically significant differences are reported, the overlap among groups has been so large that the clinical significance of the findings is nil. The poor showing of the tests is in a context in which the group membership is already established. There is no way to estimate whether the same level of discrimination can be anticipated when the tests are used in clinical situations whose base rates for the characteristics investigated are very different from those in the samples studied.

Further interpretational problems exist. If overtly aggressive children regularly produce a specific test response, can we then assume that the response is indicative of potential aggression in nonaggressive children? No, we cannot. Thus, even when test differences are found, their meaning cannot be generalized to different groups. Only prospective studies can answer the question whether similar test responses can predict clinical events in nonclinical groups. Of the four prospective studies which give statistical data regarding test predictability, two are negative with regard to predicting outcome in psychotherapy (58) and aggression (12). A third study (80) is positive in predicting "abnormality," but is clinically meaningless. The fourth study (20) was able to predict the event of referral beyond chance expectation, but its actual hit and miss rates are not provided.

A recent review of projective testing by Klopfer and Taulbee (48) claims good efficacy for Rorschach indices in predicting events. Certainly, in children this is far from being the case. The current status of projective tests in children can be summarized succinctly: sometimes they tell us poorly something we already know.

COMMENT

It is possible to be nihilistic about the merits of diagnosis, and consequently to point a finger at diagnosis as an invalid, meaningless concept. If so, why should tests be associated with diagnostic characteristics? Some time ago this argument might have been convincing, but it no longer is. In children as well as in adults, diagnostic classification is associated with a host of reliably predictable events. Therefore, the argument that since nothing is related to diagnosis, projective tests cannot be, is untenable.

No investigation in children has dealt with the issue of the incremental validity of the tests: the type of validity that refers to information accrued above and beyond what is already known. Once a diagnosis is established, can the use of projective tests add to our understanding in ways that will be important in the management of the patient? Unfortunately, there is nothing on which to base a rational view of the incremental validity of projective tests in children. Those who affirm that it exists are expressing a faith, nothing more.

Holt (41) has claimed, quite rightly, that investigators have asked clinicians to make absurd predictions that do not reflect the psychologists' expertise, such as predicting college grades. This limitation, at least, has not been typical of the literature here reviewed.

The point that skill and talent are crucial to the predictive process is undocumented and self-damning. The greater the need to rely on undefinable, artistic talents, the more difficult it is to justify the need for clinical psychological services. Who is to be the final arbiter of competence? Can objective means of establishing talent be found? I strongly suspect that the standards used are akin to those that guide our choice of literary or art critics: if they agree with us, they must be good.

The purposes to which psychological testing can be put have been outlined by Holt (42). They are quite ambitious, and include etiology (functional versus organic), prognosis, and optimal form of treatment. This is so because of the assumption that, as Holt has put it, "There are stable and pervasive characteristics in personality (generally called structural) which enable us to predict that people will respond differently to the same stimuli, press or treatment" (p. 456). This view is based on theoretical tenets that there is continuity between the agglomeration of traits we call personality, and symptoms, which we call diagnosis. The fate of both is related to treatment. The logic is flawless, but the premises are unproven, and may very well be false. If so, even if a clinical psychological evaluation revealed accurately the psychodynamic process, the genetic processes of the individual's core personality, it might be totally irrelevant to the diagnosis of many (not necessarily all) disorders. There is no evidence that psychogenetically determined personality characteristics are related to specific mental disorders. The likelihood of discontinuity between traits and syndromes needs to be considered. If discontinuities exist between intrapsychic processes, such as drive-defense configurations, and mental disorders, tapping the former domain, although interesting, will tell us nothing about the latter.

As Holt (43) has stated, prediction is a means in science, not an end in itself, understanding being the ultimate stage of knowledge. The projective tests, although perhaps not very good at predicting, are offered as tools that deepen our understanding. It is obviously true that one can often make a prediction without understanding the mechanism that accounted for the phenomenon predicted. However, there is no instance in which understanding does not facilitate prediction. One must therefore be suspicious of techniques that promise understanding but fail to deliver.

In 1970 Holt (43) argued that appropriate research had never been done on clinical psychological testing because of the formidable complexities and difficulties inherent in such undertakings. Many of us have been involved in evaluation and treatment research. As one so engaged, I would be the last to say that it is easy; but it is not so complex as to preclude trying. Many excellent treatment studies have appeared. Therefore, the argument that the investigation of the clinical validity of projective tests is too complex to permit empirical clarification is unacceptable. I have recently learned of an ongoing effort to assess the predictive validity of the MMPI that documents the feasibility of predictive investigations. Dr. Gottesman and his co-workers (*personal communication*) have related MMPI scores of the 14-year-old, members of the original standardization sample of the test, to hospitalization in adulthood. The subjects later hospitalized had had significantly more elevated scores at 14 on all the test scales except one. Similar studies could be done with existing clinical records, so that the ability of projective tests to predict a variety of life events in children could be explored.

Methodological issues have been discussed with great lucidity and charm by Meehl (68–71) and others (53,87,88). Perusal of these writings seems essential to anyone seriously concerned about the use of projective tests.

Over a decade ago, Zubin et al. (103) pointedly questioned how long a promising approach could remain so. The same can be asked today with regard to the use of projective tests in children.

Resources in the mental health field are limited. On the basis of empirical data, it is clear that the use of projective testing in children does not deserve a high priority.

Has the horse been finished off? Not quite. He refuses to die, but hardly even places in the money. A cautious gambler would not bet on him. The status of the research is reminiscent of the joke about the gambler who, returning from the track, was asked how he had done. He replied, "I broke even, and boy did I need it!"

ACKNOWLEDGMENTS

The preparation of this paper was supported in part by Public Health Service Grant No. MH-18579–05. The author wishes to acknowledge Dr. Howard Rombom's help in the literature search. Special gratitude is expressed to Dr. Howard Abikoff for his assistance.

REFERENCES

1. Aaron, N. S. (1967): Some personality differences between asthmatic, allergic, and normal children. *J. Clin. Psychol.,* 23:336–340.

2. Ames, L. B., Métraux, R. W., Rodell, J. L., and Walker, R. N. (1974): *Child Rorschach Responses: Developmental Trends for Two to Ten Years.* Bruner/Mazel, New York.
3. Anastasi, A. (1975): Psychological testing of children. In: *Comprehensive Textbook of Psychiatry, Vol. 2,* edited by A. M. Freedman, H. I. Kaplan, and B. J. Sadock, pp. 2070–2087. Williams & Wilkins, Baltimore.
4. Basit, A. (1972): A Rorschach study of personality development in identical and fraternal twins. *J. Pers. Assess.,* 36:23–27.
5. Bellak, L. (1971): *The T.A.T. and C.A.T. in Clinical Use.* Grune & Stratton, New York.
6. Bellak, L. (1975): *The T.A.T., C.A.T. & S.A.T. in Clinical Use.* Grune & Stratton, New York.
7. Bergman, A., and Schubert, J. (1974): The Rorschachs of normal and emotionally disturbed children: A review of the literature. *Br. J. Proj. Psychol. Pers. Stud.,* 19:7–13.
8. Berkowitz, P. H. (1961): Some psychological aspects of mental illness in children. *Gen. Psychol. Monogr.,* 63:103–148.
9. Bills, R. E., Leisman, C. J., and Thomas, R. W. (1950): A study of the validity of the TAT, and a set of animal pictures. *J. Clin. Psychol.,* 6:293–295.
10. Bosquet, K. T. (1956): Discriminative powers of Rorschach determinants in children referred to a child guidance clinic. *J. Consult. Clin. Psychol.,* 20:17–21.
11. Bouras, A. (1973): Contribution à l' étude du Rorschach chez les enfants obsessionnels. *Psychol. Fr.,* 18:233–249.
12. Breidenbaugh, B., Brozovich, R., and Matheson, L. (1974): The Hand Test and other aggression indicators in emotionally disturbed children. *J. Pers. Assess.,* 38:332–334.
13. Broadhurst, A., and Phillips, C. J. (1969): Reliability and validity of the Bender-Gestalt test in a sample of British school children. *Br. J. Soc. Clin. Psychol.,* 8:253–262.
14. Byrd, E. (1956): The clinical validity of the Bender-Gestalt with children: A developmental comparison of children in need of psychotherapy and children judged well-adjusted. *J. Proj. Techniques,* 20:127–136.
15. Carr, A. (1975): Psychological testing of intelligence and personality. In: *Comprehensive Textbook of Psychiatry, Vol. 1,* edited by A. M. Freedman, H. I. Kaplan, and B. J. Sadock, pp. 736–757. Williams & Wilkins, Baltimore.
16. Centers, L., and Centers, R. (1963): A comparison of the body images of amputee and non-amputee children as revealed in figure drawings. *J. Proj. Techniques Pers. Assess.,* 27:158–165.
17. Clawson, A. (1959): The Bender Visual Motor Gestalt test as an index of emotional disturbance in children. *J. Proj. Techniques,* 23:198–206.
18. Davids, A. (1973): Aggression in thought and action of emotionally disturbed boys. *J. Consult. Clin. Psychol.,* 40:322–327.
19. Davids, A., and Lawton, M. J. (1961): Self-concept, mother concept, and food aversions in emotionally disturbed and normal children. *J. Abnorm. Soc. Psychol.,* 62:309–314.
20. Dillard, H. K., and Landsman, M. (1968): The Evanston Early Identification Scales. Prediction of school problems from the human figure drawings of kindergarten children. *J. Clin. Psychol.,* 24:227–228.
21. Dudek, S. Z. (1972): A longitudinal study of Piaget's developmental stages and the concept of regression: II. *J. Pers. Assess.,* 36:468–478.
22. Edelstein, R. (1973): Verbal aptitudes of disturbed children from thematic protocols. *Percept. Mot. Skills,* 36:1194.
23. Exner, J. E., Jr. (1974): *The Rorschach: A Comprehensive System.* John Wiley & Sons, New York.
24. Fiedler, M. F., and Stone, J. L. (1956): The Rorschachs of selected groups of children in comparison with published norms: I. *J. Proj. Techniques,* 20: 273–275.
25. Fiedler, M. F., and Stone, J. L. (1956): The Rorschachs of selected groups of children in comparison with published norms: II: The effect of socioeconomic status on Rorschach performance. *J. Proj. Techniques,* 20:276–279.

26. Fisher, R. L. (1966): Failure of the conceptual styles test to discriminate normal and highly impulsive children. *J. Abnorm. Soc. Psychol.,* 7:429–431.
27. FitzSimons, R. (1958): Developmental, psychosocial, and educational factors in children with nonorganic articulation problems. *Child Dev.,* 29:481.
28. Frost, B. P. (1960): An application of the method of extreme deviations to the Wechsler Intelligence Scale for Children. *J. Clin. Psychol.,* 16:420.
29. Fuller, G. B., Preuss, M., and Hawkins, W. F. (1970): The validity of the human figure drawings with disturbed and normal children. *J. Sch. Psychol.,* 8:54–56.
30. Goldberg, F. H. (1957): The performance of schizophrenic, retarded, and normal children on the Bender-Gestalt Test. *Am. J. Ment. Defic.,* 61:548–555.
31. Goldfarb, W. (1949): Rorschach test differences between family-reared, institution-reared, and schizophrenic children. *Am. J. Orthopsychiatry,* 19:624–633.
32. Green, R., Fuller, M., and Rutley, B. (1972): It-Scale for children and Draw-A-Person Test: 30 feminine vs 25 masculine boys. *J. Pers. Assess.,* 36:349–352.
33. Gross, S. Z. (1963): Critique: Children who break down. *J. Child Psychol. Psychiatry,* 4:61–66.
34. Hall, L. P., and Ladriere, M. L. (1970): A comparative study of diagnostic potential and efficiency of six scoring systems applied to children's figure drawings. *Psychol. Sch.,* 7:244–246.
35. Hamilton, J., Blewett, D., and Sydiahia, D. (1971): Inkblot responses of identical and fraternal twins. *J. Genet. Psychol.,* 119:37–41.
36. Hammer, M., and Kaplan, A. M. (1966): The reliability of children's human figure drawings. *J. Clin. Psychol.,* 22:316–319.
37. Handler, L., and McIntosh, J. (1971): Predicting aggression and withdrawal in children with the Draw A Person and Bender Gestalt. *J. Pers. Assess.,* 35:331–335.
38. Hartlage, L. C. (1970): Differential diagnosis of dyslexia, MBD, and emotional disturbance in children. *Psychol. Sch.,* 7:403–406.
39. Haworth, M. R. (1963): A schedule for the analysis of CAT responses. *J. Proj. Techniques,* 27:181–184.
40. Haworth, M. R. (1964): Parental loss in children as reflected in projective responses. *J. Proj. Techniques Pers. Assess.,* 28:31–45.
41. Holt, R. R. (1958): Clinical and statistical prediction: A reformulation and some new data. *J. Abnorm. Soc. Psychol.,* 56:1–12.
42. Holt, R. R. (1967): Diagnostic testing: Present status and future prospects. *J. Nerv. Ment. Dis.,* 144:444–465.
43. Holt, R. R. (1970): Yet another look at clinical and statistical prediction: Or, is clinical psychology worthwhile. *Am. Psychol.,* 25:337–349.
44. Jacobs, J. C. (1971): Rorschach studies reveal possible misinterpretations of personality traits of the gifted. *Gift. Child Q.,* 15:195–200.
45. Kagan, J. (1956): The measurement of overt aggression from fantasy. *J. Abnorm. Soc. Psychol.,* 52:390–393.
46. Kagan, J. (1959): The stability of TAT fantasy and stimulus ambiguity. *J. Consult. Clin. Psychol.,* 23:266–271.
47. Kagan, J. (1960): Thematic apperceptive techniques with children. In: *Projective Techniques with Children,* edited by I. Rabin and M. R. Haworth, pp. 105–129. Grune & Stratton, New York.
48. Klopfer, W. G., and Taulbee, E. S. (1976): Projective tests. *Annu. Rev. Psychol.,* 543–567.
49. Koppitz, E. M. (1963): *The Bender Gestalt Test for Young Children.* Grune & Stratton, New York.
50. Koppitz, E. M. (1966): Emotional indicators of human figure drawings of children: A validation study. *J. Clin. Psychol.,* 22:313–315.
51. Koppitz, E. M. (1966): Emotional indicators on human figure drawings of shy and aggressive children. *J. Clin. Psychol.,* 22:466–469.
52. Koppitz, E. M. (1975): *The Bender-Gestalt Test for Young Children, Vol. 2.* Grune & Stratton, New York.
53. Lanyon, R. I., and Goodstein, L. D. (1971): *Personality Assessment.* John Wiley & Sons, New York.

54. Lehmann, I. J. (1959): Responses of kindergarten children to the children's Apperception Test. *J. Clin. Psychol.*, 15:60–63.
55. Leitch, M., and Schafer, S. (1947): A study of the Thematic Apperception Tests of psychotic children. *Am. J. Orthopsychiatry*, 17:337–342.
56. Lerner, E. A. (1972): *The Projective Use of The Bender Gestalt.* Charles C. Thomas, Springfield, Ill.
57. Lesser, G. (1957): The relationship between overt and fantasy aggression as a function of maternal response to aggression. *J. Abnorm. Soc. Psychol.*, 55:218–221.
58. Lessing, E. E. (1960): Prognostic value of the Rorschach in a child guidance clinic. *J. Proj. Techniques*, 24:310–321.
59. Levitt, E. E. (1957): Alleged Rorschach anxiety indices in children. *J. Proj. Techniques*, 21:261–264.
60. Liebetrau, C. E., and Pienaar, W. D. (1974): The relation between adjustment and body image at various age levels. *J. Pers. Assess.*, 38:230–233.
61. Lifshitz, M. (1974): Achievement motivation and coping behavior of normal and problematic preadolescent kibbutz children. *J. Pers. Assess.*, 38:138–143.
62. Machover, K. (1949): *Personality Projection in the Drawing of the Human Figure.* Charles C. Thomas, Springfield, Ill.
63. Marks, P. A., Seeman, W., and Haller, D. L. (1974): *The Actuarial Use of the MMPI with Adolescents and Adults.* Williams & Wilkins, Baltimore.
64. Maxwell, A. E. (1961): Discrepancies between the pattern of abilities for normal and neurotic children. *J. Ment. Sci.*, 107:300–307.
65. McConnell, O. L. (1967): Koppitz's Bender-Gestalt scores in relation to organic and emotional problems in children. *J. Clin. Psychol.*, 23:370–374.
66. McHugh, A. F. (1963): WISC Performance in neurotic and conduct disturbances. *J. Clin. Psychol.*, 19:423–424.
67. McHugh, A. F. (1966): Children's figure drawings in neurotic and conduct disturbances. *J. Clin. Psychol.*, 22:219–221.
68. Meehl, P. E. (1956): Wanted—A good cookbook. *Am. Psychol.*, 11:263–272.
69. Meehl, P. E. (1959): Some ruminations on the validation of clinical procedures. *Can. J. Psychol.*, 13:102–128.
70. Meehl, P. E. (1960): The cognitive activity of the clinician. *Am. Psychol.*, 15:19–27.
71. Meehl, P. E., and Rosen, A. (1955): Antecedent probability and the efficiency of psychometric signs, patterns on cutting scores. *Psychol. Bull.*, 52:194–215.
72. Morgan, A. B. (1968): Some age norms obtained for the Holtzman Inkblot Technique administered in a clinical setting. *J. Proj. Techniques Pers. Assess.*, 32:165–172.
73. Morrison, E. (1969): Underachievement among preadolescent boys considered in relationship to passive aggression. *J. Educ. Psychol.*, 60:168–173.
74. Murawski, B. J. (1971): Genetic factors in tests of perception and the Rorschach. *J. Gen. Psychol.*, 119:43–52.
75. Nathan, S. (1973): Body image in chronically obese children as reported in figure drawings. *J. Pers. Assess.*, 37:456–463.
76. Nickols, J. (1963): Rorschach z scores on disturbed subjects. *J. Consult. Clin. Psychol.*, 27:544–545.
77. North, G. E., and Keiffer, R. S. (1966): Thematic productions of children in foster homes. *Psychol. Rep.*, 19:43–46.
78. Prytula, R. E., and Leigh, G. G. (1972): Absolute and relative figure drawing size in institutionalized orphans. *J. Clin. Psychol.*, 28:377–379.
79. Reddy, P. V. (1960): A study of the reliability and validity of the Children's Apperception Test. *Br. J. Educ. Psychol.*, 30:182–184.
80. Register, M., and L'Abate, L. (1972): The clinical usefulness of an objective nonverbal personality test for children. *Psychol. Sch.*, 9:378–387.
81. Robbertse, P. M. (1969): Personality structure of socially adjusted and socially maladjusted children, according to the Rorschach Test. *Psychol. Monogr.*, 55:1–20.
82. Rodman, F., and Waters, J. E. (1961): Rorschach responses of children exhibiting psychogenic auditory symptoms. *J. Clin. Psychol.*, 17:305–306.
83. Rosenzweig, S. (1945): The picture-association method and its application in a study of reactions to frustration. *J. Pers.*, 14:3–23.

84. Rosenzweig, S. (1960): The Rosenzweig Picture Frustration Study, Children's form. In: *Projective Techniques with Children*, edited by I. Rabin and M. R. Haworth, pp. 149–176. Grune & Stratton, New York.

85. Rosenzweig, S., Ludwig, D. J., and Adelman, S. (1974): Fidélité test-retest du test de frustration de Rosenzweig et de techniques semi-projectives analogues. (Test retest reliability of the Rosenzweig Picture Frustration Study and analogous semi-projective techniques). *Rev. Psychol. Appl.,* 24:181–196.

86. Rowley, V. N. (1961): Analysis of the WISC Performance of brain damaged and emotionally disturbed children. *J. Consult. Clin. Psychol.,* 25:553.

87. Sawyer, J. (1966): Measurement and prediction, clinical and statistical. *Psychol. Bull.,* 3:178–200.

88. Schneidman, E. S. (1959): Suggestions for the delineation of validational studies. *J. Proj. Technol.,* 23:259–262.

89. Schoonover, S., and Hertel, R. (1970): Diagnostic implications of WISC scores. *Psychol. Rep.,* 26:967–973.

90. Siegel, M. (1954): The personality structure of children with reading disabilities as compared with children presenting other clinical problems. *Nerv. Child,* 10: 409–414.

91. Silverstein, A., and Robinson, H. (1956): The representation of the orthopedic disabilities in children's figure drawings. *J. Consult. Clin. Psychol.,* 20:333–341.

92. Skilbeck, W. M., Bates, J. E., and Bentler, P. M. (1975): Human figure drawings of gender-problem and school-problem boys. *J. Abnorm. Child Psychol.,* 3:191–199.

93. Stone, L. J. (1950): Recent developments in diagnostic testing of children. In: *Recent Advances in Diagnostic Psychological Testing*, edited by M. R. Hanover, pp. 73–98. Charles C. Thomas, Springfield, Ill.

94. Taturka, J. H., and Katz, J. (1955): Study of correlations between encephalographic and psychological patterns in emotionally disturbed children. *Psychosom. Med.,* 17:62–72.

95. Townsend, J. K. (1967): The relation between Rorschach signs of aggression and behavioral aggression in emotionally disturbed boys. *J. Proj. Technol. Pers. Assess.,* 31:13–21.

96. Vane, J. R., and Eisen, V. W. (1962): The Goodenough Draw A Man test and signs of maladjustment in kindergarten children. *J. Clin. Psychol.,* 18:276–279.

97. Walton, D. (1959): A children's Apperception Test—An investigation of its validity as a test of neuroticism. *J. Ment. Sci.,* 105:359–370.

98. Watkins, J. M., and Watkins, D. A. (1975): Comparison of normal and emotionally disturbed children by the Plank scoring system for the Bender Gestalt. *J. Clin. Psychol.,* 31:71–74.

99. Williams, J. M. (1961): Children who break down in foster homes: A psychological study of patterns of personality growth in grossly deprived children. *J. Child Psychol. Psychiatry,* 2:5–20.

100. Willis, J. W., and Gordon, D. (1974): The Missouri Children's Picture Series: A validation study with emotionally disturbed children. *J. Clin. Psychol.,* 30:213–214.

101. Wolowitz, H. M., and Skorkey, C. (1969): Power motivation in male paranoid children. *Psychiatry,* 32:459–466.

102. Zehrer, F. A. (1951): Investigation of Rorschach factors in children who have convulsive disorders and in those who present problems of adjustment. *Am. J. Orthopsychiatry,* 21: 292–302.

103. Zubin, J., Eron, L. D., and Schumer, F. (1965): *An Experimental Approach to Projective Techniques.* John Wiley & Sons, New York.

Critical Issues in Psychiatric Diagnosis,
edited by Robert L. Spitzer and Donald F. Klein.
Raven Press, New York © 1978.

Psychological Tests and Psychodiagnosis

Loren J. Chapman and Jean P. Chapman

Psychology Department, University of Wisconsin, Madison, Wisconsin 53706

Psychological tests have been widely used for psychodiagnosis in two senses. One has been that of describing the personality functioning, usually the psychodynamics, of the individual. The second is diagnosis in the sense of assigning a patient to a category of illness, in particular a category of the *Diagnostic and Statistical Manual* of the American Psychiatric Association. We shall focus here on this second use of tests to diagnose patients.

Research on the ability of clinicians to use psychological tests for either diagnostic purpose has been extremely discouraging. This story is, of course, an old one. Study after study has found that when the performance of clinicians using tests is checked against other criteria, the clinicians are found to perform only a little bit better than chance either in assigning patients to diagnostic categories or in describing their personality functioning. The one bright exception in the description of personality functioning has been Margaret Singer's success in blind matching of the Rorschach protocols of patients and their parents. But the findings on prediction of diagnostic category have been more nearly univocal. A classic study on this topic was that of Little and Schneidman (7). They asked prominent psychodiagnosticians each to interpret blind protocols of his favorite psychological test and predict the patient's diagnostic category. These diagnosticians agreed on diagnostic category only slightly above chance either with one another or with psychodiagnosticians who relied on case history.

Clinicians who use psychological tests invariably believe that they do much better with tests than is indicated by objective data. One reason for their belief is that human beings are subject to systematic illusions in judging whether one class of events is correlated in its occurrence with a second class of events. For example, clinicians who use the Draw-A-Person Test have often reported that patients who draw human figures with large or elaborate eyes more often have paranoid symptoms and that patients who elaborate the genital area more often have sexual conflicts. Such statements of correlation are central to the use of any psychodiagnostic test to make inferences about individuals. The clinician bases such statements in part on published literature but to a much larger extent on his own experience of the correlation between test responses and characteristics of patients. Observers often report erroneous relationships between test responses and characteristics of patients.

We have offered the term "illusory correlation" for systematic illusions in the perception of such relationships. Because this is our own area of research, we shall summarize some of these findings.

ILLUSORY CORRELATION

One of our earlier investigations of illusory correlation (1) focused on the Draw-A-Person Test. We chose the Draw-A-Person Test for several reasons. It is a widely used test. Writers who discuss this test have almost invariably done so in terms of correlates of individual signs in test performance, rather than complex configurations of signs. Also, despite the popularity of the test and of the signs, research reports on the validity of these signs have been more consistently negative than for most other tests.

Our first step was to ask practicing clinicians to tell us how they use the Draw-A-Person Test in their clinical practice. We presented brief statements of six clinical problems and asked 110 experienced psychodiagnosticians to tell us what drawing characteristics they had seen in patients with each of these problems. The six statements of problems were:

1. He is worried about how manly he is.
2. He is suspicious of other people.
3. He is worried about how intelligent he is.
4. He is concerned with being fed and taken care of by other people.
5. He has had problems of sexual impotence.
6. He is very worried that people are saying bad things about him.

We asked the diagnosticians to assume that each patient was a man drawing a picture of a man.

In the 44 questionnaires returned to us, the diagnosticians generally concurred on their descriptions of drawing characteristics they had seen made by patients with each kind of problem. For example, 91% said that in their experience suspicious patients draw large or atypical eyes, and 82% said that a person worried about his intelligence tends to draw a large or emphasized head. In general, the 44 diagnosticians agreed on two or three characteristics of drawings that are made by each type of patient.

We wondered if these same correlations between drawings and clinical problems could be produced as illusions in materials in which the correlations were objectively absent. To answer this question, we obtained 45 drawings of male figures. We measured head size, eye size, etc. in each drawing and rated more subjective characteristics of the drawings, such as atypical eyes and elaboration of the genital area.

We attached to each picture two of the six statements of problems that we had sent to clinicians. For example, to one picture we attached the statement: "The man who drew this (a) is suspicious of other people, and (b) has had problems of sexual impotence." We used each symptom statement on 15 of the 45 drawings and assigned the symptom statements systematically so that no correlation existed between the symptom statements and the diagnostic signs reported earlier by our experienced clinicians. For example, the statement "He is worried about how intelligent he is" was attached as often to pictures with relatively small heads as to pictures with relatively large heads.

We then presented these drawings and symptom statements to 108 college students who said they had not heard of the Draw-A-Person Test and knew nothing about its interpretation. We tested the students in groups. We summarized for each group of students the rationale of the Draw-A-Person Test. We told the students they would see a series of drawings along with brief statements about the men who drew them, that many of the men had the same problems, and that the students should examine the pictures and statements of problems carefully to find characteristics shared by drawings done by men with each type of problem. We then passed the pictures around in a prearranged random order, allowing 30 sec viewing time for each picture.

The results were as follows. We found that although we had carefully intermixed the pictures and the statements so that no objective correlations between them existed, illusory correlations were seen by nearly all subjects. Further, the illusory correlations that the students found were much the same as those that the diagnosticians reported from their clinical practice. For example, 76% of the students and 80% of the diagnosticians reported that patients who were worried about their manliness drew pictures with broad shoulders. Fully 91% of the clinicians and 58% of the students reported that patients who were suspicious of others drew atypical eyes. Every one of the 15 most frequently reported drawing characteristics was reported most often for the same statement of problem by the students as by the diagnosticians. The research literature fails to support the clinical validity of these signs (10,11). And in the students' case we know the signs were illusions, because they were not in the data. We must suspect, therefore, that the comparable reports by the diagnosticians were influenced by illusory correlations.

We also gathered evidence that the illusory correlation is accounted for by the verbal associative connection between symptom and drawing characteristics. We made a word-association questionnaire to determine how much the symptoms (suspiciousness, intelligence, impotence, etc.) suggest various parts of the body (eyes, head, sexual organs, muscles, etc.). Questions took the following form: "The tendency for SUSPICIOUSNESS to call to mind HEAD is (1) very strong, (2) strong, (3) moderate, (4) slight, (5) very slight, (6) no tendency at all." We gave this questionnaire to 45 students who had not participated in other parts of the experiment. The verbal associations these students reported neatly paralleled the illusory correlations that our earlier groups of students had seen between symptoms and drawing characteristics. The verbal associations were an even closer match with the correlations reported by practicing clinicians. The findings lead us to believe that many common but erroneous beliefs of diagnosticians concerning the correlates of psychological test performance arise as associatively based illusory correlations.

WHY PSYCHOLOGICAL TESTS FAIL

Let me return now to the broader question of the failure of test users to predict diagnostic category of the patient taking the test. This failure is not due solely to the inability of the human brain to process the available information efficiently, but is also due to an inherently modest relationship between test responses and our diagnostic categories. Actuarial prediction of diagnosis from test responses, as by a computer, does only a little better than human test interpreters. Goldberg (3) examined the relationship of responses on the Minnesota Multiphasic Personality Inventory (MMPI) to the clinical diagnostic distinction of psychosis versus neurosis. Goldberg compared the predictive validity of 65 different actuarial systems for combining the 11 MMPI Scale scores. He found that the best among these systems predicted with 70% accuracy. Although 70% accuracy is better than the best clinician in his study could do using the same 11 scale scores, it is a modest improvement on chance, which was about 50%. Prediction of membership in diagnostic categories more refined than psychosis or neurosis is usually even worse. However, the MMPI is not really a very good test for predicting diagnostic category, and a better test should yield better prediction. A better test for differential diagnosis could probably be achieved by writing items with particular diagnostic distinctions in mind.

Yet one cannot expect any test to predict membership in our present diagnostic categories with high accuracy. The failure is not entirely the fault of the tests and is at least partly because the categories are of such uncertain meaningfulness. Our current psychodiagnostic categories, and any new ones that we are likely to adopt in the near future, are only a matter of temporary convenience and will probably be altered when we learn more about the state of nature. This brings us to what is perhaps the most promising use of psychodiagnostic tests, that of discovering more meaningful diagnostic categories for emotionally disturbed patients.

TESTS AS A MEANS OF IMPROVING THE
DIAGNOSTIC SYSTEM

Let us consider the case of schizophrenia. Many psychopathologists believe that schizophrenia is very likely more than one disorder, regardless of whether one takes the broad American definition of schizophrenia or a more narrow European definition. But if schizophrenia truly consists of more than one disorder, how is one to discover those disorders? One promising approach is to measure the symptoms, and to look for groupings of patients who do and do not have certain symptoms. Then we can look for different antecedents, different courses, and different outcomes for patients with the different symptoms. One can look for different genetic loading and different biochemical abnormalities in patients with the different symptoms. Convergences in such studies would support the view that different disorders had been found. But how can we measure the symptoms? Psychological tests are primarily an attempt to measure symptoms. A test has the advantage of focusing on specific symptoms of interest which are difficult to isolate using only clinical observation or interview.

A modest relationship between test performance and psychodiagnostic categories may not necessarily mean that the test is of little diagnostic validity. Such findings may actually point the way toward discovery of more meaningful categories. Possibly the test is sometimes better than the diagnostic category that it is intended to predict. The patterns of test response may correspond to diagnostic distinctions which have greater validity than the official diagnostic distinctions. We wish to develop the argument that this may be the case for the relationship between the diagnosis of schizophrenia and some of those kinds of Rorschach performances that are conventionally viewed as indicative of schizophrenia. There is a good relationship between the diagnosis of schizophrenia and Rorschach responses such as fabulized responses, contamination, confabulation, perseveration, vagueness, and overly elaborate symbolic response. Nevertheless, some patients who appear clearly to be schizophrenic do not show these Rorschach signs. Moreover, some people who show these Rorschach signs are not clinical schizophrenics but instead have a milder disorder or even appear clinically normal. Both of these failures of perfect correspondence between Rorschach performance and diagnosis may point toward improvement of the diagnostic system. Let us consider first the finding that some schizophrenics give nonschizophrenic Rorschach performances.

THE RORSCHACH TEST AND THE DIAGNOSIS OF SCHIZOPHRENIA

Kantor et al. (5) found that process schizophrenics give Rorschach responses that clinicians recognize as schizophrenic but that reactive schizophrenics do not. Since that time more than a dozen investigators have similarly found that process schizophrenics give deviant Rorschach responses but that reactive schizophrenics do so much less. Numerous other investigators have similarly reported differences on other psychological tests between process and reactive schizophrenics. Such findings are consistent with the possibility that process and reactive schizophrenia are different disorders. The findings of Kety et al. (6) in the Danish Adoption Studies further support this contention, in that their chronic schizophrenics, who might be labeled process schizophrenics, showed a clearer genetic risk for the disorder than their acute schizophrenics, who might be called reactive. Process and reactive schizophrenia may be different disorders.

The observation of schizophrenic-like Rorschach performance in persons who show no clinical schizophrenia may also point toward possible changes in our nosological system. Patients who appear schizophrenic on the Rorschach but are not clinically schizophrenic are often included in the borderline category. Rapaport et al. (8) divided their preschizophrenics into two types, the coarctated or inhibited and the overideational. Rapaport et al. found that the overideational preschizophrenics showed schizophrenic-like Rorschachs, in fact, even more so than full-blown clinical schizophrenics. Gunderson and Singer (4) have reviewed a number of other investigations with findings of borderline schizophrenics showing schizophrenic-like Rorschachs. It may be that at least some borderline schizophrenics share a common disorder with one subset of those patients whom we recognize as clinical schizophrenics. However, borderline schizophrenia may itself consist of more than one subdisorder.

OUR TESTS FOR SCHIZOTYPY

My co-workers and I at the University of Wisconsin have been developing a series of true-false tests to measure symptoms of schizotypy as described by Paul Meehl. Schizotypy is Meehl's term for borderline patients. This chapter will focus on two of these tests. One is a true-false scale of anhedonia, the reduced ability to experience pleasures. Examples of such items are "The beauty of sunsets is greatly overrated" (true) and "I have always loved having my back rubbed" (false). The second scale is one of body image aberration. Examples of items are "Sometimes my feet seem far away" (true) and "The boundaries of my body always seem clear" (false). We have developed these scales through a series of testings and revisions, using students as subjects, administering separate scales of acquiescence and social desirability to screen out items which have these two kinds of method variance. We have already published a full description of the development of the Anhedonia Scale (2) and will soon do so for the Body Image Aberration Scale. Clinical schizophrenics as a group score higher than normal subjects on both of these scales, but their heightened performance is contributed by only a portion of the total schizophrenic sample. About a third of hospitalized schizophrenics are deviant on the Anhedonia Scale and about two-thirds not. We have been able to rule out depression as a source of this distinction by using the Beck Inventory of Depression. We had made a considerable effort, in constructing the test, to measure long-standing anhedonia rather than the relatively transient anhedonia of depression. A group of depressed patients, especially characterological depressives, might score more anhedonic on our scale than normal subjects, but among schizophrenics the difference in anhedonia is not due to depression. The schizophrenic subjects appear to fall into two clusters, one cluster corresponding to the performance of normal subjects and the second cluster scoring more anhedonic. This finding encourages us to believe that the Anhedonia Scale may separate out a distinct subvariety of schizophrenia.

The Body Image Aberration Scale identifies about one-sixth of hospitalized schizophrenics as deviant. However, the proportion is much higher among the more recently admitted patients. The Body Image Aberration Scale and Anhedonia Scale have an essentially zero correlation with each other even though they both have high reliabilities, .75 to 0.90, as estimated by the coefficient-alpha measure of internal consistency.

THE RORSCHACH AND SCHIZOTYPY

But to get back to the Rorschach, a student of mine, William Edell, has picked out college students who score at least two standard deviations above the mean on either Anhedonia or Body Image Aberration. He administered the Rorschach test to 24 anhedonic subjects, 24 subjects high on body image aberration and 24 control subjects. He found that male schizotypes, whether anhedonic or high on body image aberration, almost uniformly give schizo-phrenic-like Rorschach performance as measured by conventional indices. He used Watkins and Stauffacher's (12) Delta Percentage Index Score, which combines several conventional Rorschach indicators of schizophrenia as described by Rapaport et al. (8), such as confabulation, contamination, fabulized responses, and perseveration, and takes number of responses into account. For males, he found very little overlap between body image aberra-tion subjects and controls or between anhedonics and controls on the Delta Percentage Index Score. For female subjects, he found that the body image aberration subjects similarly showed almost no overlap with controls, but the anhedonics did not differ much from controls.

TYPES OF SCHIZOPHRENIA

I suggested earlier that the presence or absence of schizophrenic-like Rorschach performance may identify two kinds of schizophrenics. Now I wish to make the further suggestion that subjects with schizophrenic-like Rorschach performance may be of more than one type. As we mentioned before, anhedonia and body image aberration are uncorrelated within college students as well as within schizophrenics, despite a reliability of each scale that is high. The fact that different subjects are deviant on anhedonia and body image aberration may indicate that they correspond to different dis-orders. Of course, this kind of finding is only the starting point of an attempt to discover meaningful disorders. We must look at other characteristics of persons who appear to fall into these different clusters to see if they differ in other ways. We have begun such studies using interviews and other psychological measures. We have found thus far that college students who are deviant on either body image aberration or anhedonia are socially ineffective and somewhat isolated, as one would expect for individuals at high risk for schizophrenia. Our interview for psychotic symptoms is the relevant portion of Spitzer and Endicott's (9) Schedule for Affective Disorders and Schizophrenia—Lifetime Version. Many of the students who are high on body image aberration report on interview isolated psychotic symptoms, many of which are those used for a diagnosis of schizophrenia in the Research Diagnostic Criteria of Spitzer and Endicott. These symptoms include delusions of thought insertion and withdrawal, hallucinations, several kinds of other delusions, and robot-like behavior. Yet these are functioning college students. Dr. Arnold Friedhoff has agreed to examine the blood and urine of these subjects for some biochemical abnormalities that he believes may characterize schizophrenia.

CONCLUSION

Psychological tests are a promising approach to the discovery of meaningful subdisorders among emotionally disturbed patients, but findings using them are thus far only suggestive. Investigators using psychological tests have not yet pursued questions of nosology in a sufficiently systematic way to obtain strong support for the suggestion that different test score patterns correspond to different disorders. Such investigations should, of course, be collaborative, involving specialists in test construction, clinical observation, psychophysiological measures, therapy, and biochemical measures. I believe that within the context of such collaboration, specialists in psychological testing can hope to make a meaningful contribution toward the improvement of our diagnostic system.

ACKNOWLEDGMENT

The research reported in this chapter was supported by a research grant (MH-18354) from the National Institute of Mental Health, United States Public Health Service.

REFERENCES

1. Chapman, L. J., and Chapman, J. P. (1967): Genesis of popular but erroneous psychodiagnostic observations. *J. Abnorm. Psychol.,* 72:193–204.
2. Chapman, L. J., and Chapman, J. P. (1976): Scales for physical and social anhedonia. *J. Abnorm. Psychol.,* 85:374–382.
3. Goldberg, L. R. (1965): Diagnosticians versus diagnostic signs: The diagnosis of psychosis versus neurosis from the MMPI. *Psychol. Monogr.,* 79.
4. Gunderson, J. G., and Singer, M. T. (1975): Defining borderline patients: An overview. *Am. J. Psychiatry,* 132:1–10.

5. Kantor, R. E., Wallner, J. M., and Winder, C. L. (1953): Process and reactive schizophrenia. *J. Consult. Psychol.,* 17:157–163.
6. Kety, S. S., Rosenthal, D., Wender, P. H., and Schulsinger, F. (1968): The types and prevalences of mental illness in the biological and adoptive families of adopted schizophrenics. In: *The Transmission of Schizophrenia,* edited by D. Rosenthal and S. S. Kety, pp. 345–362. Pergamon Press, New York.
7. Little, K. B., and Schneidman, E. S. (1959): Congruencies among interpretations of psychological test and anamnestic data. *Psychol. Monogr.,* 73.
8. Rapaport, D., Gill, M., and Schafer, R. (1946): *Diagnostic Psychological Testing, Vol. II.* Year Book Medical Publishers, Chicago.
9. Spitzer, R. L., and Endicott, J. (1976): *Schedule for Affective Disorders and Schizophrenia—Lifetime Version.* New York State Psychiatric Institute, New York.
10. Swensen, C. H. (1957): Empirical evaluations of human figure drawings. *Psychol. Bull.,* 54:431–466.
11. Swensen, C. H. (1968): Empirical evaluations of human figure drawings: 1957–1966. *Psychol. Bull.,* 70:20–44.
12. Watkins, J. G., and Stauffacher, J. C. (1952): An index of pathological thinking in the Rorschach. *J. Proj. Techniques,* 16:276–286.

Critical Issues in Psychiatric Diagnosis,
edited by Robert L. Spitzer and Donald F. Klein.
Raven Press, New York © 1978.

Discussion: Role of Psychological Testing in Psychiatric Diagnosis

Joseph Zubin

V.A. Hospital, Pittsburgh, Pennsylvania; Department of Psychiatry, University of Pittsburgh; and New York State Psychiatric Institute, New York, New York 10036

About a quarter of a century ago our association first tackled the problem of the relation of psychological test to diagnosis. That symposium held in 1950 can serve as a base line from which to note the progress made in this field. But before delving into history, let us survey this present volume.

All the contributors seem to agree that at the present time the usefulness of psychological tests, especially of projective techniques in diagnosis, is rather limited. They also seem to agree that the use of individual signs of psychopathology in the form of specific Rorschach, TAT, and Draw-A-Man responses is not a valid procedure for making inferences regarding the presence of psychopathology. If there is any value in the use of projective techniques, it inheres in regarding the protocols not as tests but as interviews which, when analyzed for their content, yield the kind of information, perhaps less directly, that the usual clinical interview offers. This is the reason why scaling Rorschach responses for their content rather than for the alleged stimuli in the cards which evoked them may be a valuable approach. Such content scaling yields dimensions which are also tapped by the clinical interviewer, and hence one would expect considerable correlation between them. I had put forth this idea for the usefulness of the Rorschach in the early fifties. The last quarter of a century seems to have vindicated my contention.

By the way, Dr. Singer indicates that I suggested that "atomistic" approaches to the validation of the Rorschach be abandoned and that instead global impressions be used. I am equally opposed to both of these methods. Instead I proposed that careful scaling for content analysis, not global impressions, be used.

It is clear that the difficulties in relating the results of psychological testing to diagnosis are not inherent in the tests alone since the diagnostic schema is also faulty. It is fortunate, however, that as a result of the efforts of our Biometrics Research Unit, through the cooperation of my colleagues Burdock, Endicott, Fleiss, Gurland, Hardesty, Sharpe, and Spitzer, combined with the efforts of the Medical Research Council Social Psychiatry Research Unit at the Institute of Psychiatry, the Maudsley Hospital in London headed by John K. Wing, a group of systematic structured interviews of high reliability and some validity were developed.

It should be noted that systematic structured interviews represent a confluence of two disciplines—the psychological and the psychiatric, the former stressing the psychometric tradition of objectivity, reliability, and validity, the latter stressing the clinical tradition of understanding, insightfulness, and dynamic interaction. As is well known, the two disciplines had lived side by side in the halls of psychopathology—in hospitals and clinics—with but limited interaction. Until recently, the psychologist had limited himself to testing, eschewing the free-wheeling clinical interview, while the psychiatrist had limited himself to the interview in the search for a diagnosis. Only where psychologists and psychiatrists attained an equal footing could mutual interaction take place, and one of the places affording such free coalitions is the Biometrics Research Unit at the Psychiatric Institute. Here a series of structured interviews developed which combined the virtues of the two disciplines, mixing clinical relevance with psychometric precision. These interviews occupy the middle ground between psychological tests and clinical interviews, and in fact one of them—the Structured Clinical Interview of Burdock and Hardesty—actually regards itself as a test rather than an interview and provides standard norms for scoring the resulting dimensions and their profiles not unlike the way the Wechsler Bellevue Intelligence Test is scored. We undertook the development of the structured interviews when it was realized that the clinical interview, although unreliable and invalid, nevertheless was the only criterion available for determining the validity of tests in the clinical field. If it were to serve as a criterion, it had to be objectified and made reliable and valid.

The usefulness of these interviews has been fully demonstrated in the U.S.–U.K. Project on the Diagnosis of the Mental Disorders conducted by the Section on Diagnosis and Psychopathology of the Biometrics Research Unit headed by Barry Gurland (now Chief of the Department of Geriatrics at P.I.), with the help of Larry Sharpe in the United States and John E. Cooper, Robert E. Kendell, and John Copeland in the United Kingdom. A further evidence of their usefulness was afforded by the WHO International Pilot Study of Schizophrenia under the general guidance of Tsung Yi Lin, John K. Wing, and Norman Sartorius, and represented in the United States by Lyman Wynne, John Strauss, and William Carpenter.

But reliable interview results are not enough for arriving at a diagnosis, since the dimensional scores provided by these interviews have to be integrated into a typological schema before a diagnosis can be arrived at.

Now, with the help of the St. Louis group (Eli Robins, Sam Guze, and George Winokur), Drs. Spitzer and Endicott have succeeded in developing a set of operational definitions for the diagnostic categories in the form of Research Diagnostic Criteria which promise to provide a high level of reliability for the diagnostic labels themselves.

It is now possible to relate the dimensional profiles provided by the systematic structured interviews to the requirements demanded by the Research Diagnostic Criteria. It is even conceivable that a computer program could be developed for interdigitating the information from both sources, but it would probably be premature since the final diagnosis still requires some clinical flair.

We now have a much better base against which to judge the value of psychological tests in relation to diagnosis.

But why is diagnosis in the mental disorders fraught with so much difficulty? A comparison with diagnoses in the medical and social fields does not indicate that we are much worse off, but the troubles of others are only half a consolation. Our diagnoses depend primarily on overt behavior, and not on any external criteria independent of the gross deviant behavior in the form of neurophysiological or neurochemical or biological tests. We must realize that the behavior of the patient consists of three components: (a) his sytematic way of behaving which characterized him before the episode developed, i.e., his personality, (b) his systematic way of behaving after the episode began—his psychopathology, and (c) incidental unsystematic happenstance aspects of his behavior. We can dismiss the third source, since it should not be systematic enough to interfere with our judgment of the first two sources, but it often causes difficulties in the unwary clinician.

Since the patient had a personality long before he became a patient, it is important to try to assess its premorbid character in any diagnostic procedure. In fact, this premorbid personality complicates our diagnoses. If we ever succeed in getting external criteria independent of gross behavior, we could detect the presence of the focal disorder which the patient has without much difficulty, even as it can be done in such conditions as TB or PKU. However, as long as we depend on behavior, we will have an admixture of the effects of the focal disorder impinging on the premorbid personality to produce an episode of illness. I say illness advisedly because it differs from person to person even though they may have the same focal disorder. The diagnosis of mental disorders is so difficult because we are faced with a complex illness from which we have to dissect the underlying cause—the focal disorder.

Perhaps the failure of the MMPI to relate to diagnosis is at least partially a reflection of the fact that the MMPI is basically a test of personality and not of psychopathology.

What is the relation between the premorbid personality and psychopathology?

I have elsewhere discussed this question at length (4,5). Here let me briefly indicate that premorbid personality may be regarded as identical with the psychopathology of the patient, or as totally independent of it, with the middle ground held by an interaction between the two. The evidence in the literature is rather evenly divided between the tenability of any of these formulations, and to keep an open mind perhaps the second hypothesis—the null hypothesis—might be adopted tentatively.

Once we recognize the distinction between illness and focal disorder, we realize that we must also distinguish between the traits of the individuals and his states. A trait is a characteristic which persists throughout life with such modifications as the environment produces in it. A state is transitory, and the characteristic behavior during a state such as an episode disappears when the episode ends. This introduces another complication in diagnosis. Can we separate the traits which characterize the person both before and after the episode from the states—those behavioral characteristics which represent the psychopathology of the episode?

Thus far, this volume has dealt with traits that are highly subject to the modification of experience, and I wonder whether the scales of anhedonia and body image aberration developed by the Chapmans are trait or state related. Certainly many Rorschach responses are definitely state related, as I will argue later on the basis of recent evidence. Furthermore, even the trait-related behaviors are not uninfluenced by experience. That is why in our own studies of vulnerability we have stressed the use of techniques which involve responses that are relatively free of past experiences. We believe that neurophysiological responses and psychophysiological responses which occur within 1,000 msec following stimulation are relatively freer of the effects of prior environmental experiences and hence would show less variability and be more directly related to psychopathology.

Despite the influence of experience on such traits as anhedonia and perhaps even body image aberration, it would be well to consider whether individuals prone to schizophrenia have a lower threshold for these traits. If so, they could be used in detecting vulnerable individuals with a view to prevention as the Chapmans apparently are aiming at.

In general, in both the psychological tests as well as in the diagnostic arena, there has occurred a revolution which has broken through the mould of previous research and has provided reliable techniques. How valid they are requires another breakthrough. Content validity is relatively easy to get at, and has already been achieved in the interviewing area. Concurrent validity is really a form of reliability, and this type of validity has also been achieved. Predictive validity in psychopathology will have to wait for the development of good criteria for outcome which are now begging to be developed. How to integrate outcome as viewed by the patient, by his family, by the therapist, by changes observed in testing and interviewing, at the end of the episode, by the milieu he returns to, and by the system of health care is indeed a challenging question.

Even with today's fallible criteria of outcome, we nevertheless can point to what amounts to a law of prediction in psychopathology. Good premorbids tend to have a good outcome whereas poor premorbids have a poor outcome. This has held true since prognostic studies began. A survey of all prognostic studies in the world literature as of 1960 (8) indicated that of the approximately 300 studies (296 to be exact) dealing with premorbid personality, good premorbids had a good outcome in all but 2 studies, and these were in the area of psychosexual development, and 10 studies were neutral with regard to outcome. If those with sudden onset and those with shorter duration of illness are added, the number of favorable-to-good outcomes rises to 708 out of 740, with only 21 studies with unfavorable outcome and 11 studies with neutral outcome. One explanation that can be provided for this law is that schizophrenia is not a continuing but an episodic disorder occurring in vulnerable individuals when they are subjected to internal or external stress-producing life events. Only their vulnerability persists, like an allergy. But all patients recover from their episodes. When they do, they revert back more or less to their premorbid status. If they had a good premorbid status, and return to it, they are regarded as having a good outcome. If they had a poor premorbid status, they also return to it, but are regarded as having a poor outcome because they still can not cope adequately (5).

Others are so vulnerable that they recover only briefly before entering another episode, the brief interlude of recovery going unnoticed. There is probably another group of patients who have actually recovered but because of iatrogenic and hospitalization effects still appear to be in their episode. Finally, there may be a minority who remain continuously chronic, but according to recent studies (7), they are a rapidly vanishing group. This may be why, as Dr. Singer reports, the Rorschach Prognostic Rating Scale correlates negatively with severity of personality disorder and positively with educational level and good premorbid history. Here too, the good premorbids tend to have the good prognosis.

The great need now is to develop *construct* validity for our tests. The attempts at providing measures of anhedonia and of body image aberration are steps in this direction. We need more tests of this variety perhaps in the area of speech analysis, neurophysiological behavior, and other behaviors to see if some of the concepts abounding in psychopathology regarding diagnostic groupings can be validated. Could one provide, for example, an objective validation of Schneider's first rank symptoms? Look what REM did for the subjective clinical concepts regarding sleep. Can we provide objective indicators accompanying thought broadcasting, or feeling of being controlled? It is a challenge well worth considering.

The innovative approach of Dr. Singer to the consensus Rorschach is a good example of a productive approach to the construct validation of deficiency in communication in schizophrenics and their families. I wonder whether the recent critique of the success with which Dr. Singer can identify by their Rorschach protocol the parents of schizophrenic children could not be resolved by analyzing a consensus Rorschach in which both parent and child participated for a series consisting of parents with normal children and parents with schizophrenic children.

Perhaps the most insightful evaluation of the role of the Rorschach in detecting schizophrenia comes from the Bürgholzli where Rorschach himself worked. In a follow-up of 208 schizophrenic probands and their relatives, Manfred Bleuler tried to use the Rorschach to determine whether some of the clinically normal relatives of schizophrenics were latent schizophrenics and would yield protocols which best resembled the protocols of schizophrenics themselves and whether the resemblance to schizophrenic protocols was not found in a control group consisting of relatives of brain-disordered patients (organic brain syndrome cases who had no blood relatives with schizophrenia). This study is reported in a German volume entitled *The Schizophrenic Mental Disturbances in the Light of Long Term Patient and Family Histories* (1), which is now being translated at Yale University. The present report is based on a translation by David Zubin of a section written by A. Uchtenhagen entitled "Schizophrenia-like Rorschach results with the blood relatives of schizophrenics."

Uchtenhagen, who conducted this study for Manfred Bleuler, found the following:

1. In agreement with earlier studies, about a quarter of the blood relatives of schizophrenics react like schizophrenics on the Rorschach even though they are normal clinically.
2. Clinically normal relatives of brain-disordered patients who showed psychotic behavior without being schizophrenic also showed about 25% of their protocols to be schizophrenic-like, no different than the protocols of blood relatives of schizophrenics.
3. It is concluded that the presence of a schizophrenia-like Rorschach protocol does not mean the presence of schizophrenia in the subject. *The Rorschach test is not a definitive diagnostic device for the detection of a schizophrenic psychosis.*
4. Since about a quarter of the blood relatives showed abnormal protocols and at best only 6 to 12% of blood relatives develop schizophrenia phenotypically, a prognosis based on the abnormal Rorschach would be wrong in from 19 to 13% of the cases (or 14 to 8% when abnormal but nonschizophrenic personalities are removed from the sample).
5. The descendants of schizophrenia-like reacting subjects did not develop schizophrenia more often than the general population—hence, such parents can not be regarded as providing a schizophrenogenic milieu, nor should they be counseled not to propagate.

In view of these negative findings regarding the usefulness of the Rorschach in detecting latent schizophrenia, Uchtenhagen asks, Does the presence of a schizophrenic-like test result mean anything at all?

His answer is rather illuminating. He dismisses the possibility that the schizophrenia-like pattern is an unspecific reaction to the test situation by both schizophrenics and nonschizophrenics because of the high frequency with which such patterns are found in genuine schizophrenics and because there are many points of contact between the indicators in the schizophrenic-like response pattern and individual clinical symptoms such as stupor, unpredictable variation in control of reality, flightiness, and perception of cruel, sinister, cold world. He also dismisses the possibility that the deviant pattern results from the fear of being found mentally ill like the sick relative because although the fear is detectable and often directly expressed, its presence did not differentiate between those who showed schizophrenic-like patterns and those who did not. He similarly dismisses entanglement in a guilt-ridden fashion with the fate of the sick relative.

Uchtenhagen offers the following interesting hypothesis:

"The presence of a schizophrenia-like test result can mean that *the subject in question carries the possibility of schizophrenic experience and behavior in him, but that these do not show up in his accustomed niche in life.* This possibility manifests itself in him under a specific key stress, namely, the confrontation with the Rorschach test. Just as patients with a so-called schizophrenic reaction to an unbearable conflict specific for them decompensate psychotically (the conflict is more clearly recognizable and the frequency of psychoses in the family clearly smaller than in schizophrenia proper), so the *"schizophrenic reaction to the Rorschach test" is the psychosis-like breakdown in face of the specific unbearable conflicts activated in the projection test* (here the conflicts are clearer and the familiar concentration of psychoses is even smaller than with the schizophrenic reactions). The unconscious conflicts activated in the projection test mobilize fears and awaken defense mechanisms, which otherwise remain hidden under a more or less well-adapted behavior, and do not result in delusions and flightiness, as in the clinically ill.

The unconscious conflicts, the activation of which can lead to the picture of a schizophrenic psychosis or a schizophrenia-like attitude on a test, are by no means specific for the illness schizophrenia. They do not correlate with clinical pictures of illness, and often demonstrate to the contrary the closest similarity with the condition of normals. It is, therefore, to be recommended that *the interpretative attitude of the subjects be correlated less with their social behavior than with their inner state of conflict.* The apparently equal interpretative attitude of psychotics and the clinically normal clearly attests to this. Rorschach research will profit more from this than from an endeavor toward the diagnosis of illness pictures, which are clinically defined in terms of symptoms. Rorschach diagnosis will be able to ascertain its place in clinical practice and in the theory of schizophrenia all the more as it contributes to the understanding of inner states of conflict, rather than engaging in the prognosis of behavior."

In other words, at least some of the unaffected relatives of schizophrenics are vulnerable to schizophrenia to a sufficient degree so as to react to the Rorschach situation stressfully in a schizophrenic-like manner. Perhaps their vulnerability is of such a low degree that ordinary life exigencies and challenges are insufficient to elicit a full-blown episode, but their vulnerability is revealed by the miniepisode evoked by the Rorschach challenge. Furthermore, the schizophrenic-like pattern of responses seems to reflect a *state*-rather a *trait*-related behavior. Perhaps retesting under states in which the Rorschach is not such a stressful challenge such as would be provided by the more relaxed situation of vocational guidance or school counseling may yield a more normal Rorschach. That the role of the contingency in which the Rorschach (or any other test) is given is important has been demonstrated in many instances, but Bleuler's demonstration of the dependence of the results on the situation is most striking.

Dr. Gittelman's finding that the Rorschach discriminates between normal children and those with "emotional problems" may be similarly explained as reflecting a state rather than a trait which is elicited by the Rorschach situation. Her doubts about the utility of this finding may reflect this possibility. Her generalization about the failure of tests in prognosis may reflect the possibility that state-induced test results may be good for noting clinical change, i.e., serve as markers for the presence or absence of episodes but not good for traits related to prognosis.

Regarding her discussion of the continuity relationship between personality and psychopathology, it may hold true only for disorders in children whose personality has not yet developed fully so that it is difficult to separate the interaction effect between the two. It probably does not hold true for adults, as I indicated earlier.

SUMMARY

A quarter of a century ago, in June, 1950, the 40th annual meeting of this association was devoted to the topic: Relation of Psychological Tests to Psychiatry. The foreword to the 1950 symposium published in 1952 (3) reads as follows:

> The use of psychological tests in psychiatry is so widespread today that evaluation of their actual and potential contribution to diagnosis, prognosis and treatment is long overdue. With this in mind, the American Psychopathological Association invited a select number of experts in this field to discuss critically the role of tests in psychiatry. This volume summarizes the results of these discussions.
>
> A review of these contributions indicates that there is a great diversity of opinion regarding not only the clinical usefulness of the tests, but their nature, purpose and scientific value. Nearly all the contributors would like to see these tests improved. Some are hopeful that the quantification of these technics would lead to better understanding of the mind of the normal as well as that of the abnormal. Others do not hold out so much hope for them,

and regard them at best as ancillary tools. That the intelligence tests have provided a scientific basis for the measurement of mental function in school children and in the feebleminded is generally accepted. That they have served well as screening techniques and guides in selection of men for military, vocational and scholastic purposes is also generally accepted. That they can prove to be as useful in the field of mental disease and epilepsy has not yet been fully demonstrated.

Personality tests of both the inventory as well as of the projective type arouse the greatest diversity of opinion. According to some investigators they are on a much lower level of scientific development than the intelligence tests. While their clinical usefulness is undeniable, their scientific accuracy and precision leaves much to be desired. Others regard them as far superior to any of the other psychological technics and, although they are aware of their present shortcomings, hold out a bright future for their development.

Heretofore, the chief use of these tests has been for diagnostic purposes. Their use in the evaluation of therapy has only now begun and their use for prognostic purposes is in its early stages.

The encouraging progress made in the treatment of mental disorders by the somatotherapies as well as the psychotherapies, and the rather rapid alteration in patient behavior observed under and after these therapies has provided proving grounds for a crucial investigation of the reliability, validity and prognostic values of these tests. Some of these tests have proved their worth; others have been found wanting. Since the changes which these therapies bring about are chiefly in the sphere of affect, it is highly desirable for test makers to turn their attention to the development of this neglected area in psychological test construction. While waiting for such tests to be developed, it might be well to sharpen the interview technic, provide it with more scientific checks and counterchecks and standardize its procedures and the evaluation of its contents. Armed with the probe of the interview, the new tests that are being further developed will have a ready touchstone for their evaluation.

No apology need be made for the limited number of tests discussed in these papers. To have included all would have strained to the limit the publisher as well as the reader. It is hoped, however, that a sufficient sampling has been presented to give a fair cross-section of present day practice. (3)

What progress has been made since then?

1. One advance projected in 1950 has already taken place. We have sharpened the interview and converted it from a blunderbus to a sharp shooting rifle. The hope that this interview can become a touchstone for validating psychological tests can now be fulfilled.
2. Progress in personality tests of the inventory type and the projective type has been only modest in comparison. The provision of special diagnostic profiles for the MMPI is a notable advance, but they have not yet been generally accepted in diagnostic practice. In projective techniques, the tendency to regard them not as tests but as interviews is proving to be useful since the content analysis of the protocols correlates with diagnostic interview results.

3. The promise of prognostic tests has not yet paid off, but here again the improvement in diagnosis may lay the foundation for better prognosis.

4. The use of tests in evaluating outcome of treatment has turned out so poorly that rating scales had to be substituted.

5. The hope that tests of affect would be developed has not come to pass, and here again, rating scales have taken over.

6. The distinction between trait-related and state-related behavior has come to the fore, and this powerful distinction helps to explain why it is important to know the conditions under which test results were obtained. The impact of the test situation on the results obtained with the Rorschach by Manfred Bleuler on blood relatives of schizophrenics is a case in point.

7. The role that the premorbid personality plays in directing the expression of the focal disorder into a unique illness and the role that it plays in outcome are important developments. This helps explain why the cross-sectional test alone, without knowledge of the premorbid personality, may be of little help in either diagnosis or prognosis.

8. The discovery of test markers or other types of markers that will indicate the beginnings and ends of episodes, as well as markers that persist regardless of the presence or absence of episodes (markers characteristic of vulnerable individuals), is the next development to be expected. These markers can serve to validate diagnosis.

9. With regard to diagnosis, it seems that we have licked the problem of reliability with regard to the interview and the diagnostic categories. With regard to the validity of the interviews we have not been so fortunate. It is true that the response to lithium can serve as a confirmation of a diagnosis of manic-depressive psychoses and that similarly the effectiveness of some other drug treatments bolsters our belief in our diagnostic accuracy, but diagnosis by outcome has proved dangerous in the past.

10. Construct validity studies is the path we must take to consolidate our gains, and the Chapmans have shown us a good example in their attempt to establish the constructs of anhedonia and body image aberration for schizophrenia. At the present time there seems to be more activity and progress in the development of psychophysiological and neurochemical approaches to construct validity of our diagnoses than in the personality inventory and projective techniques approach. What we need to find are objective indicators of the presence of a given disorder by establishing the presence of markers which reflect the constructs on which the diagnoses rest.

11. Much of the literature on the role of psychological tests in diag-

nosis can be faulted on the ground that most of the tests indicated poorer performance in mental patients and few if any of the studies controlled for differences in motivation and interest between patients and normals. In order to eliminate the effect of these spurious influences, techniques in which patients excel or in which motivation is cancelled out need to be found (6).

12. The use of forced choice methods and of signal detection theory techniques in the investigation of psychopathology has indicated that many of the differences between patients, especially schizophrenics, and normal controls reflect not differences in sensitivity to incoming stimuli, but differences in the criterion which the patient adopts in his decisions regarding reporting or not reporting what he perceives. Thus, differences in critical flicker function between schizophrenics and normals have been found to be due not to differences in sensitivity to flicker, but to the reluctance of schizophrenics to report the transition from flicker to fusion until they are very sure of their judgment (2). For this reason many of our previous findings are suspect and need to be replicated with forced choice or signal detection methods before they can be of use in the construct validity of diagnosis.

REFERENCES

1. Bleuler, M. (1972): *Die schizophrenen Geistesstörungen im lichte langjähriger Krankenund Familiengeschichten* (*The Schizophrenic Mental Disturbances in the Light of Long Term Patient and Family Histories*). Intercontinental Medical Book Corporation, New York.
2. Clark, C., Brown, J., and Rutschmann, J. (1967): Flicker sensitivity and response bias in psychiatric patients and normal subjects. *J. Abnorm. Psychol.*, 72:35–42.
3. Hoch, P. J., and Zubin, J. (Eds.) (1952): *Relation of Psychological Tests to Psychiatry*. Grune & Stratton, New York.
4. Zubin, J. (1965): Psychopathology and the social sciences. In: *Perspectives in Social Psychology*, edited by O. Klineberg and R. Christie, pp. 189–207. Holt, Rinehart and Winston, New York.
5. Zubin, J. (1976): The role of vulnerability in the etiology of schizophrenic episodes. In: *Treatment of Schizophrenics: Progress and Prospects*, edited by L. J. West and D. E. Flinn, pp. 5–33. Grune & Stratton, New York.
6. Zubin, J., Salzinger, K., Fleiss, J. L., Gurland, B. J., Spitzer, R. L., Endicott, J., and Sutton, S. (1975): Biometric approach to psychopathology: Abnormal and clinical psychology—statistical, epidemiological and diagnostic approaches. *Annu. Rev. Psychol.*, 26:621–671.
7. Zubin, J., and Spring, B. (1977): Vulnerability—a new view of schizophrenia. *J. Abnorm. Psychol.* (*in press*).
8. Zubin, J., Sutton, S., Salzinger, K., Salzinger, S., Burdock, E. I., and Peretz, D. (1961): A biometric approach to prognosis in schizophrenia. In: *Comparative Epidemiology in the Mental Disorders*, edited by P. H. Hoch and J. Zubin, pp. 143–203. Grune & Stratton, New York.

Discussion

Dr. Zubin: On the matter of tests for organic disorders, there is the Reitan-Halstead battery, the primary tool that clinical neuropsychologists use for detecting the presence of brain damage. Such techniques had been thought to be useful in discriminating the various types of functional disorders in mental patients. Unfortunately, this did not turn out to be the case, as Gerald Goldstein's recent review indicates [Goldstein, G., and Halperin, K. M. (1977): Neuropsychological differences among subtypes of schizophrenia. *J. Abnorm. Psychol.,* 86:34–40].

Dr. Ming T. Tsuang: In reference to the EMI scans and psychometry, currently at The University of Iowa one of our residents, Dr. Luke Tsai, and I have been conducting a study entitled "Mini-Mental State and Computerized Tomography."

The Mini-Mental State (MMS) is a short series of questions assessing cognitive functions of a patient within 5 to 10 min. The MMS was published by Folstein et al. in the *Journal of Psychiatric Research,* 1975. We studied 63 patients who were referred for computerized tomography (CT) scans of the brain. The examiner had no knowledge of the patients' CT findings when administering the MMS and scored their answers immediately. Maximum score for the MMS is 30 points. These 63 patients were then divided into group A: 32 patients with negative CT findings, and group B: 31 patients with positive CT findings.

We found that group A had a mean total score of 26, which was significantly higher than the 20 of group B. When group B was subdivided into those with cerebral atrophy and those with focal lesions only, the patients with focal lesions had a mean total score of 25, which was significantly higher than the 18 of the patients with cerebral atrophy.

Therefore, from our preliminary findings we conclude that the MMS, although it requires future refinement and study, can be used to predict cognitive impairment due to cerebral atrophy.

Dr. Abrams: I wanted to mention neuropsychological testing as a potential aid in establishing the validity of psychiatric diagnoses. Dr. Michael Taylor and I have used the Aphasia Screening Test, a part of the Halstead-Reitan battery, for this purpose. The test significantly separates schizophrenic from manic patients diagnosed according to our rigorous criteria when both tests and research diagnoses are "blind."

In another series of patients we have employed Aaron Smith's test battery, which includes the WAIS, Raven's Matrices, Peabody Picture Vocabulary, Benton visual retention test, and a number of other evaluations. Schizophrenic patients performed significantly worse on this battery than manics, regardless of age, educational level, or drug administration. But, as others have found, schizophrenics were not significantly different from patients with organic brain disease.

Dr. H. E. King: Dr. Zubin, only a few years ago we were fond of saying such things as "intelligence is what intelligence tests measure" in the absence of a better definition. It seems to me that in your presentation your definition of what constitutes a "psychological test" might be: "something that is sold by the Psychological Corporation." Now, I realize that one has to limit discussion somewhere, but not everything not formally labeled a "psychological test" should therefore automatically go by the board. For example, I foresee a great wave of articles—soon to appear in the literature—on the subject of "tracking" performance. This will follow from advances recently made in solid state electronics which make it far easier to record a sample of this interesting form of behavior than it once was, and to observe the effects of experimental attempts to distract the subject while he is performing. Whether this is properly called a measure of attention, or of distraction, would you regard measures such as these as "psychological tests"? Why in your presentation was an approach based on measures of this kind systematically left out of the discussion?

Dr. Zubin: I am glad you pointed out that I neglected to stress sufficiently the role of psychophysiological and neurophysiological tests, but when I spoke about neurophysiopsychological tests being the wave of the future, that is what I meant.

I think you point to a breakthrough in the area of technology which makes it easier for us to measure things we cannot measure now, namely, monitoring continuous behavior on the part of the patient, something you have pioneered in.

Dr. Winokur: As I drifted in and out of the forest of verbiage this afternoon, I came across the idea that the closer the psychological tests approximated the kinds of things that one goes after in clinical interviews such as ways of communicating styles of behavior and styles of interacting, the better the tests, the more reliable the tests were in agreeing with the actual diagnosis.

I think I did conclude this mostly from Dr. Singer's comments. If this is true, then it is a terrible indictment, the reason being that it really does not provide us with any place to go. It fails to provide us with any new insights about the illness.

It simply gives us another way to find out the things that we already know; and, in fact, if that is all we get out of the psychological tests, why do them?

The question is: is there some reason to believe that the psychological tests will allow us to develop any new insights into the pathophysiology or the pathopsychology of the illness?

Dr. Zubin: There is more to it, perhaps, than appears on the surface. What is the difference between a clinical judgment and a psychological test result that bear on the same phenomenon? It is the difference between putting your hand on the patient's forehead to see whether he has a fever, and putting a thermometer in his mouth to see what the thermometer measures.

I think the more objective measures the psychological test offers, even when the clinician is aware of the phenomenon, the more valid the test is.

But there is one more thing which perhaps was not clear in the presentation, namely, that we are now working on techniques and methods which transcend clinical observation. For example, the fact that the critical duration for sensory integration in schizophrenics is different from that of depressives and normals is something we cannot test clinically yet. The reaction time studies also provide indicators which we cannot validate clinically. In short, where there is a similarity between clinical observation and the psychological tests, we are providing a better measure in the psychological test —a more objective and reliable one. Secondly, we are beginning to get markers in the psychophysical and psychophysiological and neurophysiological areas today which are independent of clinical observations and which nevertheless characterize the behavior of different diagnostic categories of patients.

Dr. Shagass: I heard someone make the "organic against functional" contrast. This comes up from time to time at clinical case conferences where a very good psychology group reports Halstead-Reitan test results, and they tell that the patient has a dysfunction of the left hemisphere, and perhaps which part of it, and so on.

The point I want to make is that all of these tests are functional tests. They indicate nothing about etiology except in terms of what can be derived from systematic studies of the probability that a particular kind of dysfunction, particularly in a certain population, may be connected with a certain kind of etiology. You can see the same kind of dysfunction on the basis of many different causes, whether it is a hole in the brain, a hemorrhage, or just an inability to answer questions, and it depends how the subject is tested and so on. I think perhaps this point needs to be emphasized.

Dr. Goodwin: I want to follow Dr. Winokur's nonteasing remarks. This bears on the practical problem that arises when the clinician's judgment disagrees with psychological test results. The Rorschach, for example, tells us the patient has "incipient" schizophrenia, maybe even advanced schizophrenia, but he does not appear to be schizophrenic.

Now, who is right? Since the psychiatrist usually has more clout than the psychologist, the former probably will decide. But have there been any follow-up studies indicating that psychological tests—*any* psychological tests —are more sensitive to early or obscure psychopathology than the clinician's judgment based on a clinical interview?

There are no such studies. And until such studies *are* done and demonstrate that psychological tests are superior predictors, psychological tests are virtually useless.

Critical Issues in Psychiatric Diagnosis,
edited by Robert L. Spitzer and Donald F. Klein.
Raven Press, New York © 1978.

Genetic Studies of Antisocial Personality and Related Disorders

Raymond R. Crowe

Department of Psychiatry, University of Iowa College of Medicine, Iowa City, Iowa 52242

Diagnostic validity has been referred to as predictability (16): Does the diagnosis tell us something about the patient that we did not know before making the diagnosis? The two methods which have been the most useful in validating psychiatric diagnoses have been follow-up and family studies. Thus, if a diagnosis predicts certain prognostic and family history features which were not used in making the diagnosis, then these facts substantiate the validity of the diagnosis. Of these two methods, the family study has been especially important because it can not only uncover genetic factors but also indicate a genetic relationship with other illnesses. If these familial findings can be substantiated by adoption studies, and thus proven to be indeed genetic, then this provides strong evidence for the validity of the original diagnosis.

The problem of diagnostic validity is especially acute with respect to the diagnosis of antisocial personality. This diagnosis is based on criteria, any of which may occur in psychiatrically normal persons. The question, then, is whether the aggregate of a number of these criterion symptoms defines a psychiatric syndrome which can be shown to be biologically valid. The literature contains a number of studies bearing on the question of the genetics of antisocial personality. The purpose of this chapter is to review the pertinent genetic studies on antisocial personality in order to determine whether they support the validity of that diagnosis and to examine the apparent association between antisocial personality and several other psychiatric disorders.

TWIN STUDIES

Unfortunately, no twin studies on antisocial personality *per se* are available, but the literature does contain 10 twin studies on adult criminality which have recently been reviewed by Dalgard and Kringlen (14). In view of the finding that 79% of a group of 223 convicted male offenders met research criteria for a diagnosis of antisocial personality (18), these twin studies on criminality are relevant to the question of genetics of antisocial personality. The pair-wise concordance rates reveal that in every study the concordance among monozygotic twins exceeds that found among dizygotic twins. The rates vary greatly from study to study ranging from 26 to 100% concordance among monozygotes and from 0 to 54% among dizygotes. Pooling the data yields an overall concordance rate of 51% among 252 monozygotic twins compared with 20% among 326 dizygotic twins. Finally, among the six studies which have compared same-sex with opposite-sex dizygotic twins, the concordance rate was found to be higher among the former in every case. This is to be expected with the disorder in which males are affected more frequently than females because index cases will be predominantly male, and therefore male co-twins will be at greater risk than females.

The degree of confidence which can be placed in these data is limited by a number of methodological problems including lack of personal interviews, lack of psychiatric diagnoses, nonsystematic selection of twins in the earlier studies, and among the older studies problems with zygocity determinations. Moreover, the cardinal assumption of the twin studies, that monozygotic and dizygotic twin pairs are treated equally by the environment, may not hold with respect to criminality. Nevertheless, these studies do point to a genetic influence in antisocial personality as a lead worth pursuing.

FAMILY STUDIES

A series of investigations by the Washington University group has provided excellent data on the families of antisocials (9,17,19), these data having the advantage of being based on (a) large numbers of subjects, (b) direct interviews, and (c) research criteria diagnoses. The data to be reviewed are based on personally interviewed first-degree relatives of convicted criminals, the majority of the latter diagnosed as antisocial personalities. There were 260 relatives of male probands and 106 relatives of female probands. Antisocial personality was greatly increased among these relatives compared with the general population expectation of 3 to 4% for males and 0.5% for females (10). When male probands were studied, 19% of their male and 3% of their female relatives were diagnosed as antisocial; and for the female probands the figures were 31% and 11%, respectively. Even more interesting was the spectrum of related disorders found among these relatives. Briquet's syndrome (hysteria) was found only among the female relatives, the prevalence figures being 31% and 5% among relatives of female and male probands, respectively. Alcoholism and drug dependency were likewise found more frequently in these families than would be expected in the general population. A third finding worth noting is the pattern found among these prevalence rates. The risk for each disorder was found to be greater among males than among females (with the exception of hysteria) and greater when the index subject was female than male.

Two other studies (6,23) found the same spectrum of disorders in the parents of children diagnosed as having the hyperkinetic child syndrome. Interviewing the parents of 59 hyperkinetic children, Morrison and Stewart (23) diagnosed antisocial personality in 5% of the fathers, hysteria in 10% of the mothers, and alcoholism in 20% and 5%, respectively. Likewise, Cantwell (6) found antisocial personality in 16% of the fathers, hysteria in 12% of the mothers, and alcoholism in 30% and 8%, respectively, of the parents of his 50 children. These rates are higher than the ones found among the parents of their control groups of nondisturbed children.

Thus, the family studies have solidly established the familial nature of antisocial personality, but, in addition, have demonstrated a spectrum of related disorders which includes hysteria, alcoholism, drug dependency, and the hyperkinetic child syndrome.

ADOPTION STUDIES

Although the family study is much broader than the twin study with respect to the kinds of information it can provide, it, in turn, suffers from one serious drawback in its inability to separate genetic and environmental influences in familial transmission. Thus, one cannot determine from the twin or from the family studies whether the familial nature of antisocial personality and its spectrum has a biological basis. The adoption study offers the unique advantage of focusing on individuals who have been separated from their biological background in every way except their heredity. Thus, similarities between adoptees and their biological relatives are assumed to be on the genetic basis and similarities between adoptees and their adoptive relatives are assumed to be on an environmental basis. Several types of adoption studies have appeared in the literature (27). The *adoptees study* is a follow-up of subjects born to affected biologic parents and reared by unaffected adoptive parents. The *adoptees family study* follows up both the biologic and adoptive relatives of affected adoptees. The *adoptive parents study* examines similarities between affected adoptees and their adoptive parents and is thus a variation of the family study.

The first relevant adoption study was an adoptees family study based on hospital records of the biologic and adoptive relatives of an index group of 57 psychopathic adoptees and an equal number of control adoptees (28). To facilitate comparison with other studies, the data have been reanalyzed to include first-degree relatives only. Also, the three groups of control relatives (the adoptive relatives of the index subjects and the adoptive and biological relatives of the control subjects) were found to have similar rates of illness and have been pooled. The first finding to emerge from the study was that the genetic hypothesis was supported. Of the 136 index biological relatives, 4.4% were diagnosable as psychopaths from their hospital records compared with only 0.5% of the 373 control relatives. Secondly, the validity of the "psychopathy spectrum" was likewise supported. The spectrum included definite and probable psychopathy, criminality, alcoholism, drug abuse, hysterical character disorder, and other character deviations. This spectrum was found in 17.6% of the index relatives compared with 5.6% of the control relatives. If the psychopaths are excluded in order to look at the other spectrum disorders, the figures are 13.2% and 5.1%, respectively, again supporting the validity of the spectrum. Although these numbers are considerably smaller than those found in the family studies, it should be remembered that these data are based on hospital records and therefore represent only a minimum estimate of the true amount of pathology present.

Hutchings and Mednick (21) have reported an adoptees family study of criminal records among the relatives of 143 criminal adoptees and an equal group of adopted controls. A multiple regression analysis of criminal outcome on a number of genetic and environmental variables revealed that a criminal outcome in the adoptee correlated independently with (a) criminality in a biological parent, (b) criminality in an adoptive parent, and (c) a psychiatric diagnosis in the biological mother. Thus, these data support both genetic and environmental factors as contributing factors in adult criminality, and by extension, antisocial personality. The correlation between criminal outcome and a psychiatric diagnosis in the biological mother provides more evidence in support of the spectrum. Of the 22 ill mothers, the illnesses were diagnosed as neuroses in 8, as "abnormal reactions" in 5, as psychopathy in 3, as attempted or completed suicides in 3, and as alcoholism, schizophrenia, and psychogenic psychosis in 1 each. Due to differences in nomenclature, it is difficult to compare this study with the Washington University work, but in view of the number of neuroses, it is certainly conceivable that a number of these mothers would fit the criteria for hysteria.

The study I conducted was an adoptees study of 52 subjects born to a group of women offenders who had been institutionalized in Iowa and 90% of whom were felons (12,13). Although the subjects were not separated from their mothers at birth, all but two were separated in the first year with a mean of 4 months. They were matched with an equal control group of adoptees on age and sex and turned out to match rather closely on age at maternal separation and age at placement as well. The preliminary follow-up was a study of arrest records on these adoptees, who at that time ranged in age from 15 to 45 with a mean of 25 years. I found that 15% of the index adoptees had arrest records totaling 18 arrests, compared with only 4% of the control group who totaled 2 arrests. Of the index group, 13% had been convicted of a crime, compared with only 2% of the control group; furthermore, 10% of the former had been incarcerated for an offense serving a total of 3½ years, whereas none of the controls had been incarcerated.

The final follow-up included both records and personal interviews and was based on 46 index subjects and 46 controls who were 18 or over by the end of the follow-up period. Information sufficient for a diagnosis was available on 40 index subjects and 35 controls, consisting of a personal interview in most cases. These records were evaluated blindly by a reviewer,[1] who made diagnoses according to the research criteria of Feighner et al. (15), and by three independent raters[2] using DSM-II, their consensus being taken as the final diagnosis. The research criteria demonstrated significantly more antisocial personality among the index cases (13%) than among the controls (0%). Unexpectedly, however, there was no trend toward a spectrum of related disorders among the index subjects. Alcoholism was diagnosed in 2% of the index and control subjects, respectively, drug dependency in 2% of each, and alcoholism plus drug dependency in 4% of the controls. Even more striking was the fact that no cases of hysteria were found in either group. It should be noted, however, that one of the antisocial index subjects was strongly suggestive of hysteria as well, but this diagnosis could not be made because she was not located for interview and the diagnosis was based on her records. Since all of the hysteria criterion questions were asked of every subject, it is possible to compare the 17 personally interviewed index females with the 13 personally interviewed female controls, and when this is done the former account for a total of 63 symptoms compared with 53 among the controls. When one corrects for the smaller size of the control group there are actually a few more symptoms among the control subjects, but the difference is hardly appreciable. Likewise, the DSM-II diagnoses failed to provide evidence in support of a spectrum. Excluding antisocial personality, 17% of the index subjects received a diagnosis of alcoholism, drug dependence, or personality disorder, compared with 15% of the control group. Another way of looking for spectrum pathology is by measuring level of psychosocial functioning rather than looking at diagnoses. This was measured by means of the Menninger Health Sickness Rating Scale (MHSRS) (22). The distribution of scores on this scale demonstrates that eight of the index subjects stand apart from the other index subjects as well as from the controls by virtue of their low scores. These eight subjects included the six diagnosed as antisocial personalities, plus another two diagnosed as schizoid personality and inadequate personality, respectively. Thus, once the antisocials are excluded, the MHSRS scores provide no evidence in support of a spectrum of other psychopathology among the index subjects.

Thus, this study supports a genetic factor in the familial nature of antisocial personality but fails to support the spectrum concept. Several explanations are possible. First, it is possible that persons with spectrum diagnoses would be more difficult to locate for interview because of greater geographic mobility, but at the same time, less likely than the antisocials to leave behind records which might have aided in their location. This possibility is supported by the fact that all of the antisocials were known through their records before they were actually located and some may not have been located had it not

[1] Ming T. Tsuang, M.D., Ph.D.

[2] Ming T. Tsuang, M.D., Ph.D., Irving I. Gottesman, Ph.D., and Paul Huston, M.D.

been for their records. Although all of the state mental health facilities were searched for records, alcoholics and hysterics may be less likely than the antisocials to leave behind records early in life. Secondly, it is possible that the psychopathy spectrum disorders reflect an interaction between genetic and environmental factors and would be more likely to develop when the predisposed subjects are reared in the more disruptive environments of their natural homes. This would explain why the family studies and the adoptees family studies would find the spectrum, whereas an adoptees study might not. Finally, there is the possibility of sampling error. The adoptees study invariably deals with small numbers of subjects and it would be easy to miss relatively low frequency occurrences. Nevertheless, from the Cloninger et al. data one would predict a 30% rate of hysteria among the women offspring of female offenders or 5 of the 17 interviewed index women, whereas none were found.

A study by Cadoret et al. (4,5) of 59 adoptees born to psychiatrically disturbed parents is pertinent to this review because 22 of the adoptees had at least one parent diagnosed as antisocial personality from adoption agency records. The majority of adoptees were adolescents at the time of follow-up and interviews were conducted with the adoptive parents. Due to the age of the adoptees, the analyses of symptoms are likely to be more revealing than psychiatric diagnoses. One comparison contrasted the 22 adoptees of antisocial parentage with the 37 others on (a) Thomas-Chess-Birch temperament items, (b) hyperactive behavior items, and (c) antisocial behavior items. Although a significant difference was not found on antisocial behavior items or temperament items, a significant difference was found on the hyperactive behavior items supporting the connection between adult psychopathy and the hyperkinetic child syndrome. Further, it was found that female adoptees of antisocial parentage had significantly more somatic complaints than either the female control adoptees or the remainder of the female adoptees from non-antisocial psychiatrically disturbed parents, further supporting the place of hysteria in the psychopathy spectrum.

The link between antisocial personality and the hyperkinetic child syndrome is further strengthened by two adoptive parents studies by Morrison and Stewart (24) and Cantwell (7). Morrison and Stewart interviewed the parents of 35 hyperkinetic adoptees and compared them with the biologic parents of hyperkinetic children from his previous study. The striking finding was the total absence of antisocial personality and hysteria and the presence of alcoholism in 3% of the fathers. This compared with 5% antisocial fathers, 10% hysteric mothers, and 20% and 5% alcoholic fathers and mothers, respectively, from the previous study. Cantwell reported similar results with no instances of antisocial personality or hysteria among the parents of his 39 hyperkinetic adoptees and alcoholism in only 5% of the adoptive fathers. Although the hyperkinetic child syndrome is likely to be a heterogeneous disorder, these data taken along with the Cadoret material strongly implicate at least some cases of the hyperkinetic child syndrome in the psychopathy spectrum.

Bohman (2,3) studied a large group of children which was composed of 163 adoptees, 205 babies released for adoption but returned to their biological mothers, and 124 children reared in foster homes. The study is germane to the present review because 27%, 34%, and 40% of the three groups, respectively, had biological fathers who appeared on the criminal registry. The children were followed up when they were 10 to 11 years of age by means of interviews with parents and teachers, and their overall adjustment was rated on a five-point scale. The pertinent finding was that having a criminal biological father was not associated with either antisocial juvenile behavior or poor adjustment among the boys. For the girls, there was a trend toward an association between poor adjustment and a criminal biological father in the second and third groups of children but not among the adoptees. Bohman noted that when maladjustment was encountered among the boys it usually took the form of what we consider the hyperkinetic reaction (i.e., psychomotor hyperactivity, poor concentration, disturbed relations with peers, defiance, and aggressiveness), but he did not comment on whether this correlated with a criminal biological father. Thus, the Bohman material contradicts the findings of the adoption studies on adults but could be construed as consistent with the Cadoret material. Neither Cadoret nor Bohman found a greater amount of antisocial behavior among their children, but Cadoret found increased hyperkinetic behavior. It is difficult to compare these two studies with the three involving adult adoptees because it is possible that some of the children (possibly the hyperkinetic ones) will turn out to be antisocial adults.

CONCLUSION

Based on the foregoing review of genetic studies on antisocial personality, two conclusions appear to be justified. First, the evidence points toward a genetic predisposition to the development of this disorder. This is supported by family studies, twin research, and, most importantly, the recent adoption studies. There is a discrepancy between the studies of adults and those which have involved children, in the failure of the latter to find antisocial behavior among the children, but this could relate to their age and to the psychopathology being manifested in other ways at that age. Thus, the genetic research taken as a whole supports the validity of the diagnosis of antisocial personality.

The second conclusion which appears to be justified is that antisocial personality is related in some way to a spectrum of disorders which includes hysteria, alcoholism, drug dependency, and the hyperkinetic child syndrome. The family studies have elegantly demonstrated the familial nature of this spectrum of disorders and the preponderance of the evidence from the adoption studies supports the conclusion. The latter are of particular interest because they indicate that the relationship between these disorders is a genetic one.

In conclusion, how can we explain the association between this group of disorders? It has been suggested that antisocial personality and hysteria represent alternate expressions of the same predisposition in the male and female, respectively (8). This hypothesis is supported by several lines of evidence. In a study of female felons, 40% of the women diagnosed as antisocial personalities also met the criteria for hysteria (8). Similarly, male antisocials have considerably more somatic symptomatology than non-antisocial men (26), and hysterics frequently have histories of antisocial behavior (20). Finally, in addition to the familial clustering of the two disorders already described, family studies of women with hysteria reveal an increased prevalence of antisocial personality among their male relatives (1). Cloninger et al. (10,11) have reviewed the data on these two disorders in light of the multifactorial model of disease transmission (25). Their findings were consistent with the idea that the two disorders are indeed alternate expressions of the same predisposition. In particular, if the liability to develop these diseases can be viewed as continuous and normally distributed, then the disorders behave as threshold traits such that if the liability exceeds a hypothetical threshold the individual is affected, but with liabilities below that threshold he appears normal. The transmission of these disorders behaves in such a way that (a) in the female the threshold for antisocial personality is higher than that of hysteria so that hysteria represents a less severe form of the same condition, and (b) in the male only one threshold exists and that is for antisocial personality. This model is consistent with the finding that the prevalence of spectrum disorders is higher in the relatives of female antisocials than male antisocials and that antisocial personality is more prevalent among male relatives than among female relatives of those with each disorder.

The sociopathy spectrum is a fascinating and puzzling finding to emerge from psychiatric family research. It is tempting to speculate that some forms of the hyperkinetic child syndrome may represent early manifestations of the sociopathy spectrum, which in adult life may lead to antisocial personality as well as some cases of alcoholism and drug dependency in the male and predominantly to hysteria in the female. When these relationships are understood, it will represent a major advance in our understanding of the antisocial personality.

REFERENCES

1. Arkonac, O., and Guze, S. B. (1963): A family study of hysteria. *N. Engl. J. Med.*, 268:239–242.
2. Bohman, M. (1971): A comparative study of adopted children, foster children and

children in their biological environment born after undesired pregnancies. *Acta Paediatr. Scand. [Suppl.]*, 221.

3. Bohman, M. (1972): A study of adopted children, their background, environment, and adjustment. *Acta Paediatr. Scand.*, 61:90–97.
4. Cadoret, R. J., Cunningham, L., Loftus, R., et al. (1975): Studies of adoptees from psychiatrically disturbed biological parents: II. Temperament, hyperactive, antisocial, and developmental variables. *J. Pediatr.*, 87:301–306.
5. Cadoret, R. J., Cunningham, L., Loftus, R., et al. (1976): Studies of adoptees from psychiatrically disturbed biological parents: III. Medical symptoms and illnesses in childhood and adolescence. *Am. J. Psychiatry*, 133:1316–1318.
6. Cantwell, D. P. (1972): Psychiatric illness in the families of hyperactive children. *Arch. Gen. Psychiatry*, 27:414–417.
7. Cantwell, D. P. (1975): Genetic studies of hyperactive children: Psychiatric illness in biologic and adopting parents. In: *Genetic Research in Psychiatry*, edited by R. R. Fieve, D. Rosenthal, and H. Brill. Johns Hopkins University Press, Baltimore.
8. Cloninger, C. R., and Guze, S. B. (1970): Psychiatric illness and female criminality: The role of sociopathy and hysteria in the antisocial woman. *Am. J. Psychiatry*, 127:303–311.
9. Cloninger, C. R., and Guze, S. B. (1973):Psychiatric illness in the families of female criminals: A study of 288 first degree relatives. *Br. J. Psychiatry*, 122:697–703.
10. Cloninger, C. R., Reich, T., and Guze, S. B. (1975): The multifactorial model of disease transmission: II. Sex differences in the familial transmission of sociopathy (antisocial personality). *Br. J. Psychiatry*, 127:11–22.
11. Cloninger, C. R., Reich, T., and Guze, S. B. (1975): The multifactorial model of disease transmission: III. Familial relationship between sociopathy and hysteria (Briquet's syndrome). *Br. J. Psychiatry*, 127:23–32.
12. Crowe, R. R. (1972): The adopted offspring of women criminal offenders: A study of their arrest records. *Arch. Gen. Psychiatry*, 27:600–603.
13. Crowe, R. R. (1974): An adoption study of antisocial personality. *Arch. Gen. Psychiatry*, 31:785–791.
14. Dalgard, O. S., and Kringlen, E. (1976): A Norwegian twin study of criminality. *Br. J. Criminol.*, 16:213–232.
15. Feighner, J. P., Robins, E., Guze, S. B., et al. (1972): Diagnostic criteria for use in psychiatric research. *Arch. Gen. Psychiatry*, 26:57–63.
16. Guze, S. B. (1967): The diagnosis of hysteria: What are we trying to do? *Am. J. Psychiatry*, 124:491–498.
17. Guze, S. B. (1976): *Criminality and Psychiatric Disorders*. Oxford University Press, New York.
18. Guze, S. B., Tuason, V. B., Gatfield, P. D., et al. (1962): Psychiatric illness and crime with particular reference to alcoholism: A study of 223 criminals. *J. Nerv. Ment. Dis.*, 134:512–521.
19. Guze, S. B., Wolfgram, E. D., McKinney, J. K., et al. (1967): Psychiatric illness in the families of convicted criminals: A study of 519 first degree relatives. *Dis. Nerv. Syst.*, 28:651–659.
20. Guze, S. B., Woodruff, R. A., and Clayton, P. J. (1971): Hysteria and antisocial behavior: Further evidence of an association. *Am. J. Psychiatry*, 127:957–960.
21. Hutchings, B., and Mednick, S. A. (1975): Registered criminality in the adoptive and biological parents of registered male criminal adoptees. In: *Genetic Research in Psychiatry*, edited by R. R. Fieve, D. Rosenthal, and H. Brill. Johns Hopkins University Press, Baltimore.
22. Luborsky, L. (1962): Clinicians' judgments of mental health: A proposed scale. *Arch. Gen. Psychiatry*, 7:407–417.
23. Morrison, J. R., and Stewart, M. A. (1971): A family study of the hyperactive child syndrome. *Biol. Psychiatry*, 3:189–195.
24. Morrison, J. R., and Stewart, M. A. (1973): The psychiatric status of the legal families of adopted hyperactive children. *Arch. Gen. Psychiatry*, 28:888–891.
25. Reich, T., Cloninger, C. R., and Guze, S. B. (1975): The multifactorial model of

disease transmission: I. Description of the model and its use in psychiatry. *Br. J. Psychiatry,* 127:1–10.

26. Robins, L. N. (1966): *Deviant Children Grown Up: A Sociological and Psychiatric Study of Sociopathic Personality.* Williams & Wilkins, Baltimore.
27. Rosenthal, D. (1970): *Genetic Theory and Abnormal Behavior.* McGraw-Hill, New York.
28. Schulsinger, F. (1972): Psychopathy: Heredity and environment. *Int. J. Ment. Health,* 1:190–206.

Critical Issues in Psychiatric Diagnosis,
edited by Robert L. Spitzer and Donald F. Klein.
Raven Press, New York © 1978.

Familial Subtyping of Schizophrenia and Affective Disorders

Ming T. Tsuang

Department of Psychiatry, University of Iowa College of Medicine, Iowa City, Iowa 52242

I will present data from the Iowa 500 research project (10), which we have used in an attempt to subtype schizophrenia and affective disorders. First, of course, I should briefly summarize what the Iowa 500 is for those who may not be familiar with this project.

THE IOWA 500 PROJECT

Study Population

This is a study of approximately 500 psychiatric cases, the ultimate goal of which is to identify homogeneous subgroups in schizophrenia and affective disorders by utilizing all available information from long-term follow-up and family studies of these cases. These psychiatric cases were selected from 3,800 admissions to the Iowa Psychiatric Hospital between 1934 and 1944. By reviewing extensively well-documented records, we selected 200 cases of schizophrenia, 100 cases of bipolar and 225 cases of unipolar affective disorder according to specified research criteria (3).

In order to obtain a control sample to use as a base line for comparisons, we selected 160 cases with appendectomy and herniorrhaphy from the surgical department of the same medical center. The controls were selected from about 3,000 admissions with diagnoses of herniorrhaphy and appendectomy from 1938 to 1948. These 160 controls represent a stratified random sample of cases proportionally matched to the psychiatric cases for sex and admission pay status. In the psychiatric cases, 41% were males (27% public pay and 14% private pay) and 59% females (46% public pay and 13% private pay). The stratified random sample of 160 surgical controls was selected on the basis of these proportions. Surgical cases with a record of psychiatric symptoms at admission, or those younger than 14 or older than 61 (the age range of psychiatric cases) were excluded.

The final Iowa 500 index population consists of 525 psychiatric cases and 160 controls for a total of 685. This includes 225 unipolars instead of the 200 as originally planned, due to a miscalculation of one of the original investigators. Strictly speaking, therefore, the study should be called the Iowa 525 rather than the Iowa 500. We intentionally kept these additional 25 unipolar because we think that some of them may eventually become bipolars in the course of the long-term follow-up.

We originally estimated that an average of three family members of each index case could be interviewed, and, therefore, an estimated number of 2,055 family members are to be interviewed. The total study population therefore numbers 2,740, index cases and first-degree relatives.

Field Work

We are now interviewing these cases without knowing their original diagnosis, and also without knowing whether they are index cases or family members. Until now we have been able to trace approximately 98% of the index cases living and dead, and have completed about 1,500 interviews of family members. The interviews were conducted by trained interviewers using the Iowa Structured Psychiatric Interview (ISPI) form (4). This form was specifically designed for this project, after reliability and validity studies were conducted. The data which I am going to present to you are based on 1,331 ISPI forms on which we have completed an initial diagnostic assessment.

Diagnostic Assessment

The diagnostic assessment was done by four staff psychiatrists and conducted in such a fashion that blind, independent, and consensus diagnoses were obtained by reviewing the ISPI forms. Here I have used three qualifiers to describe the diagnostic assessment. First, by "blind" I mean that the diagnosticians were blind to the original diagnosis of the index cases and also blind to whether the form being assessed was that of an index cases or a family member. Second, "independent diagnoses" means that an interview form was sent to the first psychiatrist for assessment according to research criteria (2,9), after which the form was sent to the second psychiatrist for independent diagnostic assessment according to DSM-II criteria (1). Third, "consensus diagnosis" indicates that if the diagnoses of the first and second psychiatrist concurred, that diagnosis became the final diagnosis. However, if there was disagreement between the first and second diagnostician, the form was sent to a third psychiatrist for another independent diagnostic assessment. The final diagnosis was then made by me, taking into consideration all three diagnoses. These final diagnoses were used for the data analysis to be presented here.

There have been many family studies on schizophrenia and affective disorder which have been reviewed previously (5–7). The reasons I have spent some time in describing our material and methods are quite obvious. In designing our study, we have taken into consideration the many criticisms made of family studies. We are not studying schizophrenia or affective disorder separately, we are studying them simultaneously. The index cases were selected according to specified research criteria, and a control group was also included. Blind interview and structured interview techniques were utilized. Rigorous diagnostic assessment procedures were enforced.

Now with this background of materials and methods in mind, let us proceed to discuss the results.

FAMILIAL DIFFERENTIATION OF SCHIZOPHRENIA AND AFFECTIVE DISORDERS

The mean ages of first-degree relatives interviewed were as follows. There were 414 control relatives with a mean age of 49.8 years; 314 schizophrenia relatives with a mean age of 60.6, and 603 relatives of affective disorder cases with a mean age of 57.3.

The schizophrenia index cases were younger than other index cases at the time of admission 35 years ago, and most of them were single. Most of the schizophrenia relatives interviewed, therefore, were siblings, and this helps explain the older mean age in this group. The affective disorder cases were older at the time of index admission and the majority of them were married; therefore, the majority of the first-degree relatives interviewed were represented by children, a fact which accounts for their younger mean age.

Schizophrenia

The rate of schizophrenia among the relatives of each index group is shown in Table 1. Only one case of schizophrenia was diagnosed in the control relatives which represents 0.2%. In schizophrenia relatives 16 cases were found, namely, 5.1%, and in affective disorder relatives 9 cases, namely, 1.5%, were found. In comparison with the control group, the rate of schizophrenia among the schizophrenia relatives is statistically significantly higher, but there is no difference between the affective disorder and control groups. The mean age of the schizophrenia relatives was over 60, meaning most of them have already passed the risk period for schizophrenia. Therefore, their morbidity risk using Weinberg abridged form of age correction results in figures very similar to the crude rates. Comparison of schizophrenia between relatives of those with schizophrenia and affective disorder also showed a very significant difference. Therefore, using the rates of familial schizophrenia from our data, we can say that schizophrenia is quite different from the affective disorder and control groups.

I would like to comment on the lower rate of schizophrenia found in our study compared to other studies (8). These figures are based only on interviews with living relatives who freely agreed to participate in the study. We have no way at this time of assessing the rate of illness among the relatives who have refused. From our own experience of following schizophrenia for a long time, we found that these patients had mortality in excess of that of the general population (11). Therefore, we are also attempting to assess the rate of illness among the deceased relatives, particularly those who had been admitted to the state mental hospitals in Iowa. We expect that after a complete ascertainment of the illness rates in deceased relatives, the rates will increase.

Affective Disorders

Now let us proceed to our results for the affective disorders (Table 1). The rate of 10.1% among the affective disorder relatives was significantly

TABLE 1. *Schizophrenia and affective disorders among 1,331 interviewed first-degree relatives*

Research diagnosis of index case	Relatives		
	N	# Schizophrenia (%)	# Affective disorder (%)
Control (C)	414	1 (0.2)	20 (4.8)
Schizophrenia (S)	314	16 (5.1)	9 (2.9)
Affective disorder (AD)	603	9 (1.5)	61 (10.1)
Pairwise comparisons	C:S	a	NS
for significant	C:AD	NS	a
difference in rates	S:AD	a	a

[a] $p < 0.01$.

higher than those of the control and schizophrenia relatives. There were no significant differences between the rates of affective disorder among control and schizophrenia relatives. Because of the longer period of risk for affective disorders, and also because of the overrepresentation of children among the affective disorder and control relatives, the morbidity risk in these two categories could be expected to increase after age correction.

From our data, it is quite apparent that the significantly different rates of schizophrenia and affective disorder among the relatives demonstrate that schizophrenia and affective disorder are two separate disorders. Having shown this, let us now proceed to a discussion of subtyping.

Subtyping of Schizophrenia

Of course, many subdivisions of schizophrenia have been proposed (6,7). Some are widely recognized and supported by a large body of data. These include the primary division into organic versus idiopathic, and the subdivision of idiopathic schizophrenia into atypical (good prognosis, non-

TABLE 2. *Rate, morbidity risk (MR), and subtype diagnoses of schizophrenia among the interviewed relatives of schizophrenia index cases*

| Subtype diagnosis of index case | Interviewed relatives | | | | | |
	# Schizo-phrenia	N (%)	BZ (MR in %)	# Para-noid	# Nonpara-noid
Paranoid	4	83 (4.8)	81.5 (4.9)	3	1
Nonparanoid	12	231 (5.2)	225.5 (5.3)	1	11

Subtype concordance: p = 0.0269 (Fisher's exact test).

process, reactive, schizophreniform) and typical (poor prognosis, process). Others of the proposed subdivisions of schizophrenia are less well accepted and research to substantiate them continues. These include the division of typical schizophrenia into paranoid and nonparanoid types, and the subdivision of nonparanoid into simple, catatonic, and hebephrenic subtypes.

The schizophrenia cases in our study were subdivided into paranoid and nonparanoid subgroups according to their clinical features at the time of index admission. The data from our family study show no differences between the rates of schizophrenia in the relatives of paranoids and nonparanoids (Table 2). The morbidity risks for schizophrenia in these two groups of relatives were also similar.

The concordance of subtype diagnoses between index cases and relatives is also shown in Table 2. When we divide all schizophrenics among the relatives of paranoid schizophrenics into paranoid and nonparanoid subtypes, there are three paranoids and only one nonparanoid; whereas among the relatives of nonparanoid schizophrenics, out of the total of 12 schizophrenics only 1 was classified as paranoid and the other 11 were classified as nonparanoid. The subtype concordance reaches statistical significance at 0.0269. Therefore, in terms of subtype diagnosis our family data seem to suggest that there are two subtypes of schizophrenia, paranoid and nonparanoid.

Of course, when we complete our study we may be able to rediagnose subtypes of index cases and relatives according to long-term follow-up information, and this may affect the rate of concordance. Also, the number of diagnoses of schizophrenia among the deceased relatives will increase total cases so that further analysis of subtyping could be done, especially with regard to the further subdivision of nonparanoid schizophrenia into hebephrenic, catatonic, and simple subtypes.

Subtyping of Affective Disorders

Several divisions of primary affective disorder have likewise been proposed (7). The major division is into bipolar (manic or manic and depressive episodes) and unipolar (only depressive episodes) affective disorder. The evidence for this division is fairly well established. A further subdivision has been proposed for each of these main divisions: namely, X-linked and non-X-linked for bipolar, and depressive spectrum (early onset females) and pure depressive (late onset males) diseases for unipolar affective disorder. The present study deals with the primary division into unipolar and bipolar subtypes only.

The rates and morbidity risks of affective disorder among relatives of those with bipolar and unipolar affective disorder are shown in Table 3. It can be seen that the rates of affective disorder among the bipolar and unipolar relatives are very similar, 9.7% and 10.3%, respectively. Likewise, after age correction the morbidity risk of 13.4% among bipolar relatives is also very close to the 14.0% among the unipolar relatives.

The subtype diagnoses of affective disorder relatives also appear in Table 3. Out of 19 affective disorder diagnoses in the bipolar relatives, there were 2 bipolars and 17 unipolars. The distribution of the 42 affective disorder diagnoses among the unipolar relatives is 4 bipolars and 38 unipolars. The concordance of subtypes here is obviously not statistically significant. The subtypes of the index cases were based on the records of index admissions of 35 years ago. Of course, it is quite possible that in the course of follow-up some unipolars would become bipolars. In fact, according to follow-up information in the original medical records, 9 out of the total 225 unipolar index cases became bipolar (12).

The diagnoses of relatives as unipolars and bipolars were made blindly without knowing the original diagnosis of the index cases. Several possibilities might account for the deficiency of the diagnosis of bipolars. The diagnoses were made solely on the basis of information obtained directly from the interviewees and recorded on the ISPI forms. There is a possibility that the interviewees tend to respond positively to depressive symptoms, and deny manic symptoms as such, because the manic symptoms are rather pleasurable and give the person a sense of well-being. Therefore, they might not be experienced, and thus not reported, as symptoms.

In fact, when we did a pilot study to test the validity of our interviewing

TABLE 3. Rate, morbidity risk (MR), and subtype diagnoses of affective disorders among the interviewed relatives of affective disorder index cases

Subtype diagnosis of index case	Interviewed relatives				
	# Affective disorder	N (%)	BZ (MR in %)	# Bi-polar	# Uni-polar
Bipolar	19	195 (9.7)	141.5 (13.4)	2	17
Unipolar	42	408 (10.3)	299.5 (14.0)	4	38

Subtype concordance: p = 0.7303 (Fisher's exact test).

instrument, we found that responses to mania screening questions did not differentiate psychiatric and nonpsychiatric cases; whereas depression and schizophrenia screening questions differentiated psychiatric and nonpsychiatric cases very clearly.

We conclude, therefore, that a diagnosis of bipolar affective disorder cannot easily be made solely based on interview data without obtaining information from other sources. This may be the case particularly when the interviewee is of an advanced age, and the manic symptoms were experienced at a much younger age.

At the present time, we view our findings regarding the rate of affective disorder among bipolar relatives as results that need further explanation since they do not agree with the findings of other studies in this matter (5). We hope to find some explanation when we have completed the collection of data from other sources, including medical records of those relatives who have been admitted to any mental hospital in Iowa. This will include not only some of those whom we have already interviewed, but deceased relatives as well.

SUMMARY

To summarize, then, we have applied the preliminary results of our family study to the problem of differentiating and subtyping schizophrenia and affective disorder. Schizophrenia, affective disorder, and control relatives were clearly distinguished according to their rates of schizophrenia and affective disorder, respectively: schizophrenia relatives had a significantly higher rate of schizophrenia than the affective disorder and control relatives, whose rates were not significantly different; affective disorder relatives had a significantly higher rate of affective disorder than either the schizophrenia or control relatives, and the rates for the latter groups were not significantly different from each other.

With regard to subtyping, there is a significant tendency for diagnoses of paranoid and nonparanoid schizophrenia to occur in the relatives of paranoid and nonparanoid index cases, respectively, thus providing support for this subdivision on the basis of subtypes breeding true. Among the affective disorder relatives we found no significant tendency for subtype to be associated with like subtype in the index cases, that is, for unipolar to go with unipolar, bipolar with bipolar. We believe this finding may be explained, among other reasons, by methodological problems, rather than assuming that the unipolar/bipolar subdivision is not a valid one.

I would like to emphasize that the results presented here are preliminary, and based on one source of information, a structured interview; also, the subtype diagnoses of the index cases are based on index admission data, not follow-up information.

We are currently engaged in gathering a more complete set of information on both living and deceased relatives and index cases. We are anxious to see whether our preliminary results will hold up when the data set is more comprehensive. Our larger goal, however, is not merely to provide support for the differentiation and subdivision of schizophrenia and affective disorder. Our goal is to use all available information with regard to symptoms, course, final outcome, and familial illness to provide reliable criteria on which to base any subdivision. We will use computerized diagnostic assessment as well as clinical diagnoses in the process, and when possible, the cluster analysis technique will be applied to the data. This technique would identify clusters of features and take us beyond the boundaries of currently available diagnostic categories.

ACKNOWLEDGMENTS

The following staff psychiatrists, Department of Psychiatry, The University of Iowa College of Medicine, participated in the diagnostic assessment of the relatives: Drs. George Winokur, John Clancy, and Raymond Crowe. The following individuals participated in the collection, management, and analysis of the data for the present study: Thomas Bray, M.S., Jerome Fleming, M.S., and Larry Scriven, B.A. This study has been supported by National Institute of Mental Health Grant MH 24189.

REFERENCES

1. American Psychiatric Association (1968): *Diagnostic and Statistical Manual of Mental Disorders, Ed. 2.* American Psychiatric Association, Washington, D.C.
2. Feighner, J. P., Robins, E., Guze, S. B., Woodruff, R. A., Winokur, G., and Munoz, R. (1972): Diagnostic criteria for use in psychiatric research. *Arch. Gen. Psychiatry,* 26:57–63.
3. Morrison, J., Clancy, J., Crowe, R. R., and Winokur, G. (1972): The Iowa 500: Diagnostic validity in mania, depression, and schizophrenia. *Arch. Gen. Psychiatry,* 27:457–461.
4. Tsuang, M. T., with the assistance of Bray, T. (1974): *The Iowa Structured Psychiatric Interview.* Department of Psychiatry, University of Iowa College of Medicine, Iowa City.
5. Tsuang, M. T. (1975): Genetics of affective disorder. In: *The Psychobiology of Depression,* edited by J. Mendels, pp. 85–1000. Spectrum Publication, New York.
6. Tsuang, M. T. (1975): Heterogeneity of schizophrenia. *Biol. Psychiatry,* 10(4): 465–474.
7. Tsuang, M. T. (1975): Schizophrenia and affective disorders: One illness or many? In: *Biology of the Major Psychoses,* edited by D. X. Freedman, pp. 27–39. Raven Press, New York.
8. Tsuang, M. T. (1976): Genetic factors in schizophrenia. In: *Biological Foundations of Psychiatry,* edited by R. G. Grenell and S. Gabay, pp. 633–644. Raven Press, New York.
9. Tsuang, M. T., and Winokur, G. (1974): Criteria for subtyping schizophrenia: Clinical differentiation of hebephrenic and paranoid schizophrenia. *Arch. Gen. Psychiatry,* 31:43–47.
10. Tsuang, M. T., and Winokur, G. (1975): The Iowa 500: Field work in a 35-year follow-up of depression, mania, and schizophrenia. *Can. Psychiatr. Assoc. J.,* 20:359–365.

11. Tsuang, M. T., and Woolson, R. F. (1977): Mortality in patients with schizophrenia, mania, depression and surgical conditions: A comparison with general population mortality. *Br. J. Psychiatry,* 130:162–166.
12. Winokur, G., and Morrison, J. (1973): The Iowa 500: Follow-up of 225 depressives. *Br. J. Psychiatry,* 123:543–548.

Critical Issues in Psychiatric Diagnosis,
edited by Robert L. Spitzer and Donald F. Klein.
Raven Press, New York © 1978.

Genetic Relationships Within the Schizophrenia Spectrum: Evidence from Adoption Studies

*Seymour S. Kety, **David Rosenthal, and *†Paul H. Wender

*Department of Psychiatry, Harvard Medical School, Cambridge, Massachusetts 02115;
**Laboratory of Psychology, National Institute of Mental Health,
Bethesda, Maryland 20014; and *†Department of Psychiatry, Medical School,
University of Utah, Salt Lake City, Utah 84132*

The diagnostic process in psychiatry suffers from a handicap which beset medical diagnoses a century ago—the absence of objective and pathognomonic criteria by which to characterize its most common and most serious disorders. To a large extent psychiatric diagnosis represents a nosologic convention based on symptom clusters evaluated subjectively. That is not to suggest that these clusters or their evaluation is spurious; in fact, subjective judgments can be extremely sensitive and reliable. There are musicians who can recognize a particular note and distinguish it from another which differs in frequency by one part in several thousand. For this they need no oscilloscope to aid their subjective discrimination. More complex subjective judgments, however, are notoriously corruptible, with the result that psychiatric observation and diagnosis can be biased by preconceived notions and circular validations. In addition, a major source of confusion derives from the tendency to broaden a phenomenological syndrome or nosologically link it to a new syndrome without compelling evidence of their similarity or relatedness.

Criteria do exist and have been used to examine the validity of a newly recognized subgroup of the original syndrome. This has involved longitudinal observation with evidence of symptomatic convergence, response to a particular drug, discovery of an objective and pathognomonic marker such as the spinal fluid Wasserman test in paresis, or the significant association of the new subgroup with the original syndrome in studies of families. It is not necessary that the basis of the association in families be genetic, since a disorder may have a common environmental basis in its etiology but take different forms within a family. The findings of a large number of studies that schizophrenia and manic-depressive illness tend to cluster in different families or are separately concordant in monozygotic twins have been responsible for the generally accepted tenet that these are different syndromes.

Recently, studies of adopted individuals and their families have adduced evidence bearing on the relationship between syndromes. They have the limitation that the number of probands is small and their biological relatives more difficult to identify than has been the case for probands reared in their natural families, but the advantage that mimicry is not likely to account for phenomenological similarities and that with appropriate design, selective and subjective bias can be minimized in ascertainment and diagnosis.

In the several studies of schizophrenia that have been completed using the adoption strategy (2–4,8), there has been a consistent finding that the biological relatives (parents, offspring, siblings, and half-siblings) of schizophrenic individuals show a significant prevalence of schizophrenic illness, even though they have lived apart from them. The adoptive relatives of schizophrenics who have reared or been reared with them without sharing their genetic endowment have no higher prevalence of schizophrenia than is found in the general population. The obvious relevance of these observations to the importance of genetic factors in the transmission of schizophrenia has been pointed out in each of these studies.

Another aspect of some of these studies is the information they may contribute regarding the validity and relationship of various putative subgroups of schizophrenia. In the early stages of the studies in Denmark we were confronted with the problem of the disagreement among schools of psychiatry regarding the syndromes that were or could be regarded as appropriate subdivisions of schizophrenia. There was little difficulty in arriving at agreement on a diagnostic category of "chronic schizophrenia," which included the classic features that had been described by Kraepelin (5) and since that time have been recognized by psychiatrists throughout the world. On the other hand, that is the only syndrome which merits the designation of schizophrenia in Denmark, and in many other countries in Europe, whereas in the United States, a diagnosis of "borderline" or "latent" schizophrenia has been recognized as well as the diagnosis of "acute schizophrenic reaction" (1). Instead of attempting to decide between Danish and American psychiatry on the basis of inadequate evidence, we decided tentatively to retain these two putative subtypes of schizophrenia in the hope that our studies might shed some light on their relationship to chronic schizophrenia. These were the three subgroups which we included as "definite" schizophrenia in our selection of index cases. In the diagnosis of their relatives where we could not select only those with definite diagnoses, we also included a diagnosis of "uncertain" schizophrenia, where schizophrenia appeared to be the best diagnosis but was nevertheless questionable because the symptoms were too few, too mild, or atypical. In diagnosing the relatives, we also included a final hypothetical subgroup "inadequate" or "schizoid" personality, taken from the APA Diagnostic Manual (1), which there was some reason to believe might be a "forme fruste" of schizophrenia. All of these, which we employed along with other diagnoses in the characterization of relatives, we combined into a "schizophrenia spectrum" as a hypothesis or group of hypotheses which could be tested for their relationship to chronic schizophrenia.

We spelled out the characteristics we would use for these diagnoses (3), leaning heavily on the APA Diagnostic Manual (DSM-II):

Chronic schizophrenia (synonyms—chronic undifferentiated schizophrenia, true schizophrenia, process schizophrenia)

Characteristics:

1. Poor prepsychotic adjustment; introverted, schizoid; shut in; few peer contacts; few heterosexual; usually unmarried; poor occupational adjustment.
2. Onset—gradual and without clear-cut psychological precipitant.
3. Presenting picture—presence of primary Bleulerian characteristics; presence of clear rather than confused sensorium.
4. Post-hospital course—failure to reach previous level of adjustment.
5. Tendency to chronicity.

Acute schizophrenic reaction (synonyms—acute undifferentiated schizophrenic reaction, schizoaffective psychosis, schizophreniform psychosis, acute paranoid reaction)

Characteristics:

1. Relatively good premorbid adjustment.
2. Relatively rapid onset of illness with clear-cut psychological precipitants.
3. Presenting picture—presence of secondary symptoms and comparatively lesser evidence of primary ones; presence of affect (manic-depressive symptoms, feeling of guilt); cloudy rather than clear sensorium.
4. Post-hospital course—good.
5. Tendency to relatively brief episode(s) responding to drugs, EST, etc.

Latent or borderline schizophrenia (synonyms—pseudoneurotic schizophrenia, ambulatory schizophrenia, questionable simple schizophrenia, "psychotic character," severe schizoid individual)

Characteristics:

1. Thinking: strange or atypical mentation; thought shows tendency to ignore reality, logic, and experience to an excessive degree resulting in poor adaptation to life experience despite the presence of a normal IQ; fuzzy, murky, vague speech.
2. Experience—brief episodes of cognitive distortion (the patient can and does snap back but during the episode the idea has more the character of a delusion than an ego-alien obsessive thought); feelings of depersonalization or strangeness or unfamiliarity with or toward the familiar; micropsychosis.
3. Affective: anhedonia, never happy, no deep or intense involvement with anyone.
4. Interpersonal behavior—may appear poised but lacking in depth ("as if" personality); sexual adjustment—chaotic fluctuation, mixture of hetero- and homosexuality.
5. Psychopathology—multiple neurotic manifestations which shift

frequently (obsessive concerns, phobias, conversion, psycho-somatic symptoms); severe widespread anxiety.

Uncertain schizophrenia—schizophrenia most likely diagnosis but in-sufficient information available, or symptoms are too mild, too few, or sufficiently atypical to warrant a more definite diagnosis.

Inadequate or schizoid personality
    Characteristics:
    1. A somewhat heterogeneous group consisting of individuals who would be classified as either inadequate or schizoid by the APA Diagnostic Manual; persons so classified often had many of the characteristics of the latent schizophrenic, but to a considerably milder degree.

By making our criteria for schizophrenia broad enough to include chronic, acute, and latent types as are more conventionally used by American psychi-atrists, we could examine the syndrome as a whole; by defining and classify-ing the subjects into one or another of the three subtypes, we would be able to examine the relationship of the putative forms "acute" or "latent" to classic schizophrenia. Similarly, the remaining syndromes in the "schizo-phrenia spectrum," including uncertain schizophrenia, schizoid and inade-quate personality, could be examined for their relationship to schizophrenia.

Using institutional records that were abstracted, translated into English, and edited to remove biasing information, we selected 34 index adoptees whom we diagnosed as chronic, borderline, or acute schizophrenia from the nearly 5,500 adult adoptees in the Greater Copenhagen sample. More recently, the number of index adoptees was increased to 74 in the total sample of more than 14,000 adult adoptees in all of Denmark. Having chosen suitably matched control adoptees with no known history of mental illness, we identified the biological and adoptive relatives. Where any of these had been seen in a mental institution in Denmark, the information obtainable became the basis for blind, independent, and consensual diagnoses by four raters. The finding of a highly significant concentration of schizophrenia spectrum disorders in the biological relatives of the schizophrenic index cases in the Greater Copenhagen Sample, which was confirmed in the remainder of Denmark, was compatible with the hypothesis that genetic factors operated significantly in the transmission of schizophrenia.

Examining the pattern of schizophrenia-related disorder in the biological relatives of index cases with chronic, latent, and acute schizophrenia indi-cated even in the first study (3) that we were not dealing with homogeneous entities. Whereas the biological relatives of chronic and latent schizophrenic adoptees showed both chronic and latent schizophrenia, none were diagnosed as acute schizophrenia. Moreover, none of the biological relatives of the acute schizophrenic adoptees fell within the schizophrenia spectrum. This suggested that whereas latent schizophrenia was related to chronic schizo-

TABLE 1. *Prevalence of schizophrenia spectrum disorders in biological relatives of schizophrenic adoptees according to diagnosis in adoptee (total national sample—institutional records)*

Index adoptees		Biological index relatives							
N	Diagnosis	N	Dx:	Chronic sz.	Latent sz.	Acute sz.	Uncertain sz.	Schizoid	Total spectrum
37	Chronic sz.	217		6	6	1	4	1	18
24	Latent sz.	128		1	3	0	1	0	5
13	Acute sz.	61		0	0	0	0	0	0

phrenia, acute schizophrenia was not. The results obtained in the total Danish sample (Table 1) confirm that finding. In the 217 biological relatives of the 37 index adoptees with chronic schizophrenia, we found chronic schizophrenia, latent schizophrenia, and uncertain schizophrenia significantly represented, suggesting that the two latter groups are genetically related to classic schizophrenia. The 61 biological relatives of 13 index adoptees with acute schizophrenia yielded none who were hospitalized with a mental illness in the schizophrenia spectrum. The failure of these results to associate acute schizophrenic reaction with chronic schizophrenia is compatible with accumulating evidence from family studies, outcome observations, and pharmacological response (6) that most of the acute psychoses which in America have been labeled "acute schizophrenic reaction" are not subtypes of schizophrenia.

The results summarized thus far have been based entirely on institutional records. Schizoid or inadequate personality is usually not a basis for hospitalization with the result that such diagnoses were made too rarely to constitute any test of their relationship to chronic schizophrenia. Recognizing that there might be more mental illness in a population than appeared in mental hospital records, and to obtain more systematic information, we decided to seek psychiatric interviews with the relatives in a large subsample.

From 1970 to 1973 Dr. Bjørn Jacobsen conducted extensive interviews with more than 90% of the biological and adoptive relatives of the 34 schizophrenic adoptees and their matched controls in the Greater Copenhagen Sample. Of 512 parents, siblings, and half-siblings identified, 119 had died, 26 had emigrated beyond Scandinavia, and 3 had disappeared. Of the 364 alive and accessible, 329 (90%) participated in an interview which obtained a large amount of information on environmental variables, medical history, and a complete mental status examination. Information adequate for a presumptive psychiatric diagnosis was obtained in an additional 12 subjects. The 6% in whom inadequate information was obtained were randomly distributed between the biological and adoptive relatives of index and control probands. The typescripts of the 35-page interviews were edited to remove extraneous information and were read by three raters who made independent and consensual psychiatric diagnoses while remaining ignorant regarding the relationship of the subject to an index or control proband. About 30% of the relatives were found to be normal or to have no psychiatric diagnosis, and nearly 45% received a consensus diagnosis outside of the schizophrenia spectrum. These, as well as the diagnosis of normal, were randomly distributed among the relatives. Nor was there a concentration of organic, neurotic, affective, or personality disorder in the individuals genetically related to a schizophrenic adoptee. This study therefore failed to find any overlap between schizophrenia and other psychiatric diagnoses.

Schizophrenic illness, on the other hand, was highly significantly concentrated in the individuals genetically related to the schizophrenic adoptees with whom they had not lived. There were 115 interviews among the biological relatives of the schizophrenic adoptees and 250 interviews among individuals not genetically related to the index adoptees (their adoptive relatives, relatives of control probands, and control adoptees). A consensus diagnosis of chronic schizophrenia was made in 4.3% of the biological relatives of the schizophrenic adoptees, and in 0.8% of the remaining relatives ($p = 0.03$). Each rater independently found a significantly greater number of chronic schizophrenics among the biological index relatives ($p = 0.03$, 0.01, 0.04). A consensus diagnosis of latent schizophrenia was made in 5.2% of the biological index relatives and in 1.6% of the others, a difference that fell short of statistical significance ($p = 0.06$). The independent diagnoses of latent schizophrenia were each higher in the biological index relatives, but not significantly so.

Our diagnosis of "uncertain schizophrenia" had been left vague and implied merely that the manifestations were closer to schizophrenia than to any other psychiatric diagnosis but were milder, fewer, or not entirely typical of those required for a definite diagnosis of schizophrenia. A consensus diagnosis of uncertain schizophrenia was made in 11.3% of those genetically related to the schizophrenic adoptees and in 2.8% of those not so related ($p = 0.002$). Each independent rater found a similarly highly significant concentration of uncertain schizophrenia in the biological index relatives ($p = 0.003, 0.01, 0.009$).

The results for schizoid or inadequate personality are less clear-cut. These personality disorders were not found more frequently in the biological index relatives by our consensus diagnosis, nor by two of the raters in their independent diagnoses, although one rater made these diagnoses in 13% of those genetically related to a schizophrenic adoptee and in 3.6% of the others ($p = 0.001$).

These results were compatible with the significant influence of genetic factors in the transmission of classic chronic schizophrenia. They also suggested that less severe syndromes, designated by us as latent schizophrenia and uncertain schizophrenia, were genetically related to more typical schizophrenia. The findings in this study were equivocal regarding the relationship of schizoid or inadequate personality to schizophrenia. Rosenthal (7) has pointed out, however, the results of another study where there is a greater risk for schizophrenia in the offspring of a schizophrenic parent if the other parent is schizoid.

In the diagnoses based on the interviews of the Copenhagen subsample, and in those based on the institutional records of the national sample, we had individually and collectively identified a significant number of individuals with classic chronic schizophrenia among the biological relatives of the schizophrenic adoptees, almost entirely confined to the relatives of the adoptees who in turn had been diagnosed as chronic schizophrenic. Moreover, the biological relatives of the chronic schizophrenic adoptees showed, in addition to chronic schizophrenia, a significant number of individuals with less severe but chronic schizophrenia-like syndromes, which we had designated "latent schizophrenia" or "uncertain schizophrenia." Although our characterizations of these syndromes were somewhat vague and hardly explicit, the diagnoses were blind and the vagueness of the characterization could only have operated to diminish the possibility that they would be concentrated in one group of relatives by chance. It appeared to be a tenable conclusion that there were milder disorders of cognition and affect genetically related to classic schizophrenia.

There was thus sufficient validity in our possibly idiosyncratic diagnoses of latent and uncertain schizophrenia to warrant an independent appraisal by more objective and rigorous criteria. It was fortunate that Robert Spitzer and Jean Endicott, in discussions with Paul Wender, became sufficiently interested in these data and their possible implications for an external validation of syndromes presumably related to schizophrenia, that they were willing to undertake an independent review of pertinent interviews to learn how well or poorly our diagnostic categories could be characterized.

Spitzer, Endicott, and their colleagues received 86 of Jacobsen's edited interviews from the Greater Copenhagen Study including all of those in whom we had reached a diagnosis of chronic schizophrenia, latent schizophrenia, or uncertain schizophrenia, 6 with our consensus diagnosis of schizoid or inadequate personality, and 43 to whom we had given no psychiatric diagnosis or diagnoses outside of the schizophrenia spectrum. In addition, they received 34 extensive summaries by Jacobsen of the institutional records available for the schizophrenic index cases, prepared in the format of the interviews. The latter batch was given to their staff without knowledge of our diagnoses, who applied the RDC criteria (9) for schizophrenia and other psychiatric diagnoses. In the remainder, they compared those to whom we had given a "schizophrenia spectrum" diagnosis with those outside the spectrum. By an iterative process that began with a large number of manifestations that we used in arriving at our global judgment, and through successive refinements, they found that they were able, to a satisfactory degree of specificity, to characterize those whom we had diagnosed as latent or uncertain schizophrenia or schizoid personality by the presence of at least three out of

TABLE 2. Comparison of original global consensus diagnosis (WRK) with diagnosis based on explicit symptom check list (Spitzer, Endicott, et al.) (Greater Copenhagen Sample—psychiatric interviews)

	Agreements			Disagreements	
N	WRK consensus	Spitzer, Endicott, et al.	N	WRK consensus	Spitzer, Endicott, et al.
20	Chronic sz.	Chronic sz.			
2	Chronic sz.	Probable Chronic sz.			
1	Chronic sz.	Probable Acute sz.			
1	Chronic sz.	STP[a]			
11	Latent sz.	STP			
4	Latent sz.	Chronic sz.	5	Latent sz.	Not sz. spectrum
4	Acute sz.	STP			
1	Acute sz.	Chronic sz.	2	Acute sz.	Not sz. spectrum
15	Uncertain sz.	STP	5	Uncertain sz.	Not sz. spectrum
5	Schizoid	STP	1	Schizoid	Not sz. spectrum
40	Not sz. Spectrum	Not sz. Spectrum	3	Not sz. Spectrum	STP

[a] Schizotypal personality.

eight particular symptoms, each of which was related to a cardinal feature of classic schizophrenia but less severe in intensity. These criteria and a more extensive presentation of their procedure and results will be published elsewhere by Spitzer et al.

Table 2 presents a summary of these results as they pertain to the present discussion. In the 24 subjects in whom we had arrived at a consensus diagnosis of "chronic schizophrenia," there was excellent agreement with the diagnoses by Spitzer et al. based on RDC criteria: 20 were classed as chronic schizophrenia, 2 as probable chronic schizophrenia, and 1 as probable acute schizophrenia. One subject they designated as not schizophrenic, and eventually as "schizotypal personality."

Spitzer and Endicott did not attempt to differentiate between our diagnoses of latent schizophrenia, uncertain schizophrenia, schizoid or inadequate personality; indeed, it is doubtful that we could demonstrate a significant differentiation between these categories. They therefore lumped them together under a new diagnostic category—schizotypal personality—which will be included in DSM-III. Of the 53 subjects whom we had included in the schizophrenia spectrum outside of chronic schizophrenia, Spitzer and Endicott diagnosed 5 as chronic schizophrenia, 35 as schizotypal personality, and 13 as outside the schizophrenia spectrum. Of the 43 individuals whom we had characterized as outside the schizophrenia spectrum, Spitzer and Endicott agreed in 40, diagnosing the remaining 3 as schizotypal personality. The remarkable agreement between us on classic chronic schizophrenia is diminished, as would be expected, in the case of the vaguer categories.

TABLE 3. *Schizophrenia spectrum diagnosis by two groups independently in the 102 biological relatives of 16 adoptees with agreed diagnoses of chronic schizophrenia (Greater Copenhagen Sample—psychiatric interviews)*

Subjects	WRK consensus	N	Spitzer, Endicott, et al.
Adoptees:	Chronic sz.	7	Chronic sz., undifferentiated
	Chronic sz.	5	Chronic sz., disorganized
	Chronic sz.	3	Chronic sz., paranoid
	Chronic sz.	1	Probable chronic sz.
Biological relatives:	Chronic sz.	5	Chronic sz.
	Latent sz.	5	Schizotypal personality
	Uncertain sz.	6	Schizotypal personality
	Schizoid	1	Schizotypal personality

In 16 of the 17 adoptees in whom we had made a consensus diagnosis of chronic schizophrenia, Spitzer and Endicott made the same diagnosis independently. It is interesting to examine the schizophrenia spectrum diagnoses made by both groups in their biological relatives. The agreement (Table 3) is quite remarkable giving independent support for our previously tentative inference that in addition to chronic schizophrenia, there is a similar but milder syndrome (designated latent or uncertain schizophrenia by us, schizotypal personality by Spitzer et al.) that is genetically related to classic schizophrenia.

SUMMARY

1. The study of adopted individuals and their families permits the independent psychiatric evaluation of adoptees and their biological relatives who have lived apart from them, while minimizing ascertainment, subjective diagnostic bias, and the sharing of symptoms by association or mimicry, which may confound the usual studies of the association of mental illnesses in families. This strategy has been employed to examine the possible relationship of several syndromes that have been presumed to be subtypes of schizophrenia or schizophrenia-related disorders.

2. Blind, global, independent, and consensual diagnoses by three raters, based on hospital records or psychiatric interviews of the biological and adoptive relatives of adoptees who had become schizophrenic, found a spectrum of schizophrenia or schizophrenia-like disorders with a highly significant increased prevalence in the biological relatives as compared to appropriate control populations. The adoptive relatives showed a low prevalence of these disorders which did not differ from the prevalence in their controls.

3. In addition to classic chronic schizophrenia, global diagnoses of a less severe, chronic, schizophrenia-like syndrome that included "latent" and "uncertain" schizophrenia were found, by each rater independently and in

consensus, significantly concentrated in the population genetically related to the schizophrenic adoptees in comparison with the adoptive and control populations of relatives.

4. Both the classic chronic schizophrenia syndrome and the less severe syndromes were found especially prevalent in the biological relatives of adoptees diagnosed as chronic schizophrenia, suggesting that there may be one or more milder syndromes with schizophrenic features genetically related to classic schizophrenia.

5. Schizophrenia and schizophrenia-related disorders were not found to be significantly elevated in the biological relatives of adoptees diagnosed as "acute schizophrenic reaction," which adds to accumulating evidence that such acute psychoses are not necessarily forms of schizophrenia.

6. Exhaustive summaries of interviews or hospital records on which the global diagnoses of "chronic," "latent," or "uncertain" schizophrenia had been based were independently examined by another group of raters, using the RDC criteria and a specific symptom check-list. This confirmed the global diagnosis of "chronic schizophrenia" in 22 of 24 instances, as well as the existence of a milder syndrome ("latent" or "uncertain" schizophrenia, now combined as "schizotypal personality") in the biological relatives of chronic schizophrenics.

ACKNOWLEDGMENTS

This work was supported in part by grants from the National Institute of Mental Health (MH15602, MH30511, MH20712), the Intramural Research Program, NIMH, the Schizophrenia Research Foundation of the Scottish Rite, and the Foundations' Fund for Research in Psychiatry.

REFERENCES

1. American Psychiatric Association (1968): *Diagnostic and Statistical Manual of Mental Disorders, Ed. 2.* American Psychiatric Association, Washington, D.C.
2. Heston, L. L. (1966): Psychiatric disorders in foster home reared children of schizophrenic mothers. *Br. J. Psychiatry,* 112:819–825.
3. Kety, S. S., Rosenthal, D., Wender, P. H., and Schulsinger, F. (1968): The types and prevalence of mental illness in the biological and adoptive families of adopted schizophrenics. In: *The Transmission of Schizophrenia,* edited by D. Rosenthal and S. S. Kety, pp. 345–362. Pergamon Press, Oxford.
4. Kety, S. S., Rosenthal, D., Wender, P. H., Schulsinger, F., and Jacobsen, B. (1975): Mental illness in the biological and adoptive families of adopted individuals who have become schizophrenic: A preliminary report based upon psychiatric interviews. In: *Genetic Research in Psychiatry,* edited by R. Fieve, D. Rosenthal, and H. Brill, pp. 147–165. The Johns Hopkins University Press, Baltimore.
5. Kraepelin, E. (1919): *Dementia Praecox and Paraphrenia,* translated by R. M. Barclay. E. S. Livingstone, Edinburgh.
6. Pope, H., and Lipinski, J. (1978): Differential diagnosis of schizophrenia and manic-depressive illness: A reassessment of the specificity of "schizophrenic" symptoms in the light of current research. *Arch. Gen. Psychiat.* (in press).

7. Rosenthal, D. (1975): The concept of schizophrenic disorders. In: *Genetic Research in Psychiatry*, edited by R. Fieve, D. Rosenthal, and H. Brill, pp. 199–208. Johns Hopkins University Press, Baltimore.
8. Rosenthal, D., Wender, P. H., Kety, S. S., Schulsinger, F., Welner, J., and Oster-gaard, L. (1968): Schizophrenics' offspring reared in adoptive homes. In: *The Transmission of Schizophrenia,* edited by D. Rosenthal and S. S. Kety, pp. 377–391. Pergamon Press, Oxford.
9. Spitzer, R. L., Endicott, J., and Robins, E. (1975): *Research Diagnostic Criteria (RDC) for a Selected Group of Functional Disorders, Ed. 2.* Biometrics Research, New York State Psychiatric Institute, New York.

Critical Issues in Psychiatric Diagnosis,
edited by Robert L. Spitzer and Donald F. Klein.
Raven Press, New York © 1978.

Familial Alcoholism: A Diagnostic Entity?

Donald W. Goodwin

Department of Psychiatry, University of Kansas Medical Center, Kansas City, Kansas 66103

Alcoholics beget alcoholics
—Plutarch

This chapter has two parts. The first consists of a historical review tracing notions about a possible hereditary factor in alcoholism from biblical times to the present. The second presents the results of recent attempts to identify hereditary factors in alcoholism by studying children of alcoholics separated from their alcoholic biological parents early in life and raised by nonalcoholic foster parents.

HISTORICAL BACKGROUND

The idea that alcoholism is a familial disorder is very old. Aristotle, among others, agreed with Plutarch. "Drunken women," he wrote (3), "bring forth children like unto themselves."

Thousands of years ago women were warned against drinking during pregnancy. Often it is uncertain what the warners were concerned about.

The mother of Samson, for example, was warned against drinking wine or "strong drink" during her pregnancy (Judges 13:3–4). In the past several years there has been interest in possible deleterious effects on the fetus produced by maternal drinking, resulting in the term "fetal alcohol syndrome." The latter refers to congenital malformations sometimes observed in the offspring of alcoholic women. It is not clear yet whether alcohol is responsible for these abnormalities. At any rate, Samson's mother was not told why she should abstain. Assuming she took the advice, clearly she did not have a child with the fetal alcohol syndrome. By all accounts, Samson was a strapping lad of normal proportions. (He had poor judgment about women, but this is not considered a feature of the fetal alcohol syndrome.)

In fact, based on other writings of the period, the angelic admonition may have had no connection with fetal abnormalities; rather, it may have arisen from a fear that if she drank Samson would also drink.

The medical and religious literature of the eighteenth and nineteenth centuries is replete with warnings against either parent drinking at time of conception or the mother drinking during pregnancy (20). Two parallel themes are sounded. One is based on a concern, reminiscent of concern about the fetal alcohol syndrome, that alcohol is a teratogen and produces small, mentally defective, or malformed offspring. The other fear was that if the mother drank the child would become an alcoholic.

Benjamin Rush (17), early in the nineteenth century, held the latter view, warning women not to drink "ardent spirits" during pregnancy because the offspring might become alcoholic. Distinguished psychiatrists such as Forel and Morel had similar views. Innumerable religious tracts repeated the theme, often with references to "sins of the father being visited upon the sons."

One popular idea in the nineteenth century, held by many medical men and the clergy, was that a heavy drinking mother (or father) would produce whole generations of defective individuals, some of whom were idiots, others alcoholic, and others simply "depraved." All of this was based on the Lamarckian notion of the inheritance of acquired characteristics.

Late in the nineteenth century, as Lamarckianism was gradually replaced by Darwinianism, the first crude but systematic studies of the effect of maternal drinking on offspring were conducted. Several investigators reported that mentally retarded children had unusually large numbers of alcoholic progenitors (20). One reported that, invariably, the birth rate dropped and more idiots were born exactly 9 months after wine festivals, reflecting a popular view that maternal drinking produced abortions and idiots (1). Then, in 1908, a physician named Crothers (5) reported one of the earliest (if not the earliest) series indicating that alcoholism ran in families. His study population was impressive. Of 4,000 alcoholics whom he had treated over 35 years, 70% had predecessors who drank in excess.

During the second and third decades of the twentieth century many studies appeared on the effects of maternal drinking on fetus and offspring. At least one human study and several animal studies indicated that offspring of heavy drinking animals or humans were as normal as controls or even superior to controls (11,19). The latter was ascribed to "natural selection" and was a good example of the application of Darwinian theory to the eugenics movement. Bathing the egg or sperm in alcohol at time of conception would eliminate the "weaklings" and the same would happen if the mother drank during pregnancy. True, she would have fewer children but they would be hardier because of elimination of the "unfit." There were actually some data to support this concept, but the idea was fairly short-lived, and was not heard of again after the early thirties.

Also, as the century progressed, the notion that alcoholism was inherited lost favor. Jellinek (12), in a 1945 survey of 15 scholars in the field, concluded that heredity was not a factor in alcoholism, and this seemed borne out by a mid-1940 adoption study by Roe (16), which will be discussed later.

At the same time, investigators continued to report an unusually high prevalence of alcoholism among the male relatives of alcoholics. In almost every study, at least 25% of male relatives of alcoholics were alcoholic (6). But what had been attributed in earlier times to "poor stock" or mutagenic or teratogenic effects of alcohol on the germ plasm now was almost universally laid to environmental factors: poor parenting, slums, "society." Haggard and Jellinek (10) in 1942 stated flatly that there was no acceptable evidence to show that alcohol ingestion by one or either parent has "any effect whatsoever on the human germ, or has any influence in altering heredity, or is the cause of any abnormality in the child." They attributed damaged offspring to poor nutrition of the alcoholic mother and the bad influence of the alcoholic home. As for correlations between alcoholic parentage and feeble-minded children, they commented, "While alcohol does not make bad stock, many alcoholics come from bad stock." This was a novel idea for the times, namely, that perhaps the same conditions (environmental, biological, or both) that produced a heavy drinking mother or father also contributed to a higher incidence of fetal abnormalities and excessive drinking in the adult offspring. At least one recent study (14), mentioned later, supports this idea.

At the same time Jellinek dismissed heredity as a factor in alcoholism he acknowledged the overwhelming evidence for the high prevalence of alcoholism in the families of alcoholics (11). This came from his knowledge of family studies and many contacts with alcoholics (particularly in Alcoholics Anonymous). In 1945, indeed, he proposed that "familial alcoholism" might be a real phenomenon, distinguishable from nonfamilial alcoholism. Familial alcoholism, he believed, was characterized not only by having family members who were alcoholic but also by early onset and a particularly malignant form of the disease.

The 1960s saw a renewed interest in investigating possible genetic factors in alcoholism. Twin studies were conducted, one in Sweden and one in Finland. (There subsequently have been two others, of more limited value.) The first by Kaij (14) reported that monozygotic twins were significantly more concordant for alcoholism than were dizygotic twins. Moreover, the more severe the form of alcoholism, the greater the concordance in monozygotic twins.

Kaij also produced a finding reminiscent of Jellinek's speculation that common factors produced both alcoholism in the mother and abnormalities in the children, including excessive drinking. He reported that "deteriorated" alcoholics had deteriorated identical twin brothers, whether the twin brothers drank or not. The implication was that deterioration either was not associated with heavy drinking or might even explain heavy drinking.

The Finnish study (15) had less clear-cut results. Identical twins were more concordant for patterns of drinking, but there was no difference in "loss of control" or adverse consequences of drinking (the usual grounds for diagnosing alcoholism). Among younger twins there was a trend for consequences to distinguish the two groups, but the numbers were too small to draw conclusions.

There also has been a host of "genetic marker" studies, reviewed extensively elsewhere (6). The premise behind the studies is that if a known inherited trait is significantly correlated with the presence or absence of alcoholism, either in single families (pedigree studies) or in populations (association studies), this would suggest a genetic factor in alcoholism. Of the 20 or more genetic marker studies published so far, some have reported positive correlations, others negative, and most show no correlation at all. The most that can be said for this line of research is that the results are inconclusive.

The remainder of this chapter is about adoption studies where offspring of alcoholics are compared with offspring of nonalcoholics with neither group having contact with their biological parents soon after birth.

ADOPTION STUDIES

One approach to separating "nature" from "nurture" is to study individuals separated from their alcoholic biological relatives soon after birth and raised by nonalcoholic, unrelated foster parents. The first study of this type was by Roe (16) in 1944. In 1970 the author and a group of American and Danish investigators started a series of adoption studies in Denmark to study further the possibility that alcoholism in part has genetic roots (7,8). Within the last year two more adoption studies of alcoholism have been completed, and in 1972 Schuckit et al. (18) reported the results of a "half sibling" study, which closely resembles adoption studies.

Danish Studies

The Danish studies have gone through three phases; the most recent was completed in 1976. I will summarize the results, followed by a review of the other adoption studies.

Phase One (7)

Because men are more likely to develop drinking problems than are women, the first phase of the study involved studying a sample of Danish males who had a biological parent with a hospital diagnosis of alcoholism and who had been adopted in the first few weeks of life to nonrelatives. The control group, consisting of age-matched men without, as far as was known, alcoholism in their biological parents, was selected from a large pool of adoptees. A psychiatrist interviewed the total sample of 133 men (average age 30), 55 of whom had a biological parent who was alcoholic, matched with

78 controls with no known alcoholism in their parents (it was possible some did have alcoholic parents, but there was no record of this in the central registries maintained in Denmark). The interviewer did not know whether the interviewees were sons of alcoholics or sons of presumed nonalcoholics and the study was "blind" from its inception until the data were analyzed. Experimenter bias therefore could not have been a factor in the study. The results of the study can be summarized as follows:

1. Of the 55 probands (sons of alcoholics), 10 were alcoholic, using both specific criteria and a history of treatment for alcoholism. Of the 78 controls, 4 met the criteria for alcoholism but none had received treatment. The difference was significant at the 0.02 level.

2. The probands were no more likely to be heavy drinkers or drinkers with occasional problems from drinking than were the controls. About 40% of each group were heavy drinkers, defined as daily drinkers who drank six or more drinks at least several times a month. Having a biological parent who was alcoholic increased the likelihood of the son being alcoholic but did not increase the chance of his being classified as a heavy drinker.

3. The interviewer, a trained psychiatrist, obtained a complete psychiatric history and performed a mental status examination. The probands were no more likely to receive a diagnosis of depression, sociopathy, drug abuse, or other diagnosable psychiatric conditions than were the controls. Both groups had sizable numbers of individuals diagnosed as having various personality disturbances, but these vaguely described traits were as common in the control group as in the probands.

From these data it could be concluded that sons of alcoholics were about four times more likely to be alcoholic as were sons of nonalcoholics, despite having no exposure to the alcoholic biological parent after the first few weeks of life. Moreover, they were likely to be alcoholic at a relatively early age (in their twenties) and have a form of alcoholism serious enough to warrant treatment. Having a biological parent who was alcoholic apparently did not increase their risk of developing psychiatric disorders other than alcoholism and did not predispose to heavy drinking in the absence of alcoholism. The familial predisposition to alcoholism in this group was specific for alcoholism and not on a continuum with heavy drinking.

Phase Two (9)

Some of the probands had brothers who had been raised by their alcoholic biological parents (most of the alcoholic parents, by the way, were fathers). The sons of alcoholics raised by their alcoholic biological parents also had a high rate of alcoholism, compared to controls consisting of nonadopted men raised by nonalcoholic parents. Their rate of alcoholism, however, was no greater than was the rate observed in their brothers raised by nonalcoholic foster parents (about 18% in both groups).

The conclusion from the first two phases was that alcoholism was transmitted in families and that the increased susceptibility to alcoholism in men occurred about equally in men raised by their alcoholic biological parents and men raised by nonalcoholic foster parents. In other words, if indeed there was a genetic predisposition to alcoholism, exposure to the alcoholic parent did not appear to augment this increased susceptibility.

Phase Three (8)

The final phase of the study involved studying the daughters of alcoholics, both those raised by foster parents and those raised by their alcoholic biological parents. The sample consisted of 49 proband women (adopted-out daughters of alcoholics) and 48 controls (adopted-out daughters of presumed nonalcoholics). As was the case of the former studies, the interviews were conducted blindly, with no chance of biased results. The subjects were between the ages of 30 and 41, with a mean age of 35. The major findings were as follows:

1. One of the probands was clearly alcoholic and another was a serious problem drinker who failed to meet the criteria completely for alcoholism. Two of the controls were alcoholic. The three women diagnosed as being alcoholic had all received treatment for their alcoholism. Hence 4% of the women in both groups were either alcoholic or serious problem drinkers. The sample was too small to draw definite conclusions from this, but since there is an estimated prevalence of alcoholism among Danish women of about 0.1 to 1%, the data suggest that there may indeed be an increased prevalence of alcoholism in the two groups. Since nothing is known about the parents of the control women, other than that none had a biological parent with a hospital diagnosis of alcoholism, possibly the two alcoholic controls had parents who had alcohol problems. The parents could not be located and there was no way of determining whether this was the case. However, it was interesting that both of the alcoholic controls had foster parents who were described as alcoholic, suggesting environmental exposure to alcoholism may contribute to alcoholism in women but not to alcoholism in men.

2. More than 90% of the women in both groups were abstainers or very light drinkers. This contrasted with the Danish male adoptees; about 40% of the latter were heavy drinkers.

3. Family history studies have suggested that alcoholics often have male relatives who are alcoholic or sociopathic and female relatives who are depressed (21). In this study, complete psychiatric histories were obtained and mental status examinations performed. Among the adopted women,

there was a low rate of depression in both groups, with no more depression in the daughters of the alcoholics than in the controls. Among daughters of alcoholics raised by their alcoholic parents, depression was significantly more present than in controls. There was no evidence of increased susceptibility to other psychiatric disorders in the daughters of alcoholics, whether raised by foster parents or their own alcoholic biological parents.

It appears, therefore, that alcoholism in women may have a partial genetic basis, but that sample size in the present study precluded any definitive conclusion. Since the great majority of the women were very mild drinkers, it is possible that social factors discouraging heavy drinking may suppress a genetic tendency, if one exists. There was no evidence of a genetic predisposition to depression in the daughters of alcoholics. At any rate, if such a predisposition exists, apparently environmental factors are required to make the depression clinically manifest. Regarding the daughters raised by their alcoholic parents, it is not possible to determine whether their increased rate of depression was due to environmental factors precipitating a genetic predisposition or due to environmental factors.

It should be noted that some evidence indicates that women develop alcoholism at a later age than do men, and possibly these 35-year-old women had not all entered the age of risk for alcoholism. Further follow-up studies are needed to explore this possibility.

Other Adoption Studies

In 1944 Roe (16) obtained information about 49 foster children in the 20- to 40-year age group, 22 of normal parentage and 27 with a biological parent described as a "heavy drinker." Among children with heavy-drinking parents, 70% were users of alcohol, compared to 64% in the control parentage group. In adolescence, two children of alcohol parentage got into trouble because of drinking too much as compared to one in the "normal-parentage" group. The author found that adopted children of heavy drinkers had more adjustment problems in adolescence and adulthood than did adopted children of nonalcoholics, but the differences were not significant and neither group had adult drinking problems. She concluded there was no evidence of hereditary influences on drinking.

This conclusion, however, can be questioned on several grounds. First, the sample was small. There were only 21 men of "alcoholic" parentage and 11 of normal parentage. Since women, particularly at the time of the study, were at very low risk for alcoholism, discovering they had no problem with alcohol was not unexpected. Second, although the biological parents of the proband group were described as "heavy drinkers," it is unclear how many would justify a diagnosis of alcoholism. Most had a history of antisocial behavior, and apparently none had been treated for a drinking problem. All of the biological parents of the proband group in the Danish study received a hospital diagnosis of alcoholism and at a time when this diagnosis was rarely employed in the country where the study took place.

Schuckit et al. (18) also studied a group of individuals reared apart from their biological parents where either a biological parent or a "surrogate" parent had a drinking problem. The subjects were significantly more likely to have a drinking problem if their biological parent was considered alcoholic than if their surrogate parent was alcoholic. Studying 32 alcoholics and 132 nonalcoholics, most of whom came from broken homes, it was found that 62% of the alcoholics had an alcoholic biological parent compared to 20% of the nonalcoholics. This association occurred irrespective of personal contact with the alcoholic biological parent. Simply living with an alcoholic parent appeared to have no relationship to the development of alcoholism.

Two very recent studies (neither published at time of this writing) support the findings of the Danish studies. Both studied adoptees who had presumed alcoholic parents and were raised by nonalcoholic foster parents. One study in Sweden by Professor Michael Bohman at Umea University (2), using Temperance Board records, found that registrations for alcohol abuse among biological parents and registration for alcohol abuse among their adopted sons were positively correlated.

Moreover, when the biological parent had multiple registrations for alcohol abuse (suggesting definite alcoholism), the registration rate in the adopted sons rose proportionately. For the latter group the rate of alcohol abuse was similar to that found in the Danish study of sons of alcoholics. In both cases the adopted-out sons of alcoholics were about four times more likely to be alcoholic than were controls.

The Bohman study did not show a correlation between registered criminality in the biological parents and registered criminality in their adopted children. Nor did criminality in the biological parents predict alcohol problems in the adopted children. This also parallels the finding of the Danish studies that alcoholism in the biological parent predicted alcoholism in their adopted children, but did not predict other psychopathology, including criminality.

Cadoret and Gath (4), in a study in Iowa, also found that children separated at birth from their alcoholic biological parents were significantly more likely to have alcohol problems than were adoptees of nonalcoholic parentage. The sample size was small, but the differences were statistically significant and, again, consistent with those found in the Schuckit et al. study, the Danish studies, and the Bohman study.

DISCUSSION

Of five adoption studies of alcoholism, four report findings compatible with a hereditary factor in alcoholism and one found no indication of hereditary influence. The last study, by Roe (16), differs from the Danish studies in one crucial regard. As mentioned, the alcoholic biological parents in the Danish study were severely and classically alcoholic. The diagnosis of alcoholism, at least until recently, was rarely made in Danish psychiatric hospitals, apparently not because of a low incidence of alcoholism but because of diagnostic fashion. Of the alcoholic biological parents given a hospital diagnosis of alcoholism, many were suffering delirium tremens and had such severe alcoholism the diagnosis was inescapable. In the Roe study it was unclear whether the biological parents were truly "alcoholic." Most had a history of antisocial behavior as well as heavy drinking and there was no record of treatment, withdrawal symptoms, or other indications of definite alcoholism. In other words, severity of parental alcoholism may be a crucial factor in explaining the differences between the Roe study and the results of the other adoption studies.

As mentioned, Jellinek (12) 30 years ago proposed a diagnostic category called "familial alcoholism." The Danish studies, in particular, seem to support this concept. Familial alcoholism, as described by Jellinek and supported by the Danish data, consists of the following features:

1. A family history of severe, unequivocal alcoholism.
2. Early onset.
3. Bender-type alcoholism requiring treatment at a relatively young age.
4. No increased susceptibility to other types of substance abuse or diagnosable psychiatric illness.

A recent study (13) found that if an alcoholic had one family member who was alcoholic, 90% of them reported having two or more family members who were alcoholic, further strengthening the concept of familial alcoholism.

From a research standpoint, separating "familial" from "nonfamilial" alcoholism may reveal some interesting and useful correlations. About half of alcoholic patients on many alcoholism wards give a family history of alcoholism. Hence, separating alcoholic patients into these groups would yield similarly sized cells for comparison purposes.

In conclusion, evidence available at present indicates that alcoholism develops in some people independently of exposure to alcoholism or other gross psychopathology in the family-of-upbringing. Whether this is due, strictly speaking, to genetic factors is unknown. From the moment of fertilization, when the egg cytoplasm exerts environmental influences on the developing organism, through the vicissitudes of intrauterine life and often through the first few weeks or months of life when the infant is still cared for by the biological mother, gene-environmental interaction are inseparable.

If genes do contribute to alcoholism, what are they? There has been speculation that alcoholism is transmitted by a sex-linked recessive gene, but the evidence for this is contradictory and not compatible with the male-to-male transmission commonly seen in alcoholism. Inherited factors in alcoholism presumably are polygenic, assuming they exist.

In any case, there is now sufficient evidence for a genetic factor to encourage investigators to look for mechanisms of transmission. The burgeoning field of pharmacogenetics is steadily producing information bearing on genetic control of drug metabolism and drug effects, and an inquiry into a possible genetic basis for some forms of alcoholism comes at a time when new technology for conducting such research is steadily advancing.

ACKNOWLEDGMENTS

This work was supported in part by Public Health Service grants MH-18484, MH-09247, and a Research Scientist Developmental Award AA-47325 from the National Institute of Alcohol Abuse and Alcoholism (Dr. Goodwin). The cohort of adoptees in the Danish studies was originally identified for a study of schizophrenia sponsored by the National Institute of Mental Health and carried out under the auspices of the Psykologisk Institut at the Kommunehospitalet in Copenhagen. The investigators in this study were Drs. David Rosenthal, Seymour Kety, Paul H. Wender, and Fini Schulsinger. Their cooperation made this material available for our study. Other investigators in the Danish alcoholism studies were Drs. Fini Schulsinger, Sarnoff Mednick, Joachim Knop, Lief Hermansen, Samuel B. Guze, and George Winokur. We are grateful to Drs. Erik Strömgren and Annalise Dupont of the Institute of Psychiatric Demography in Aarhus for the use of the national psychiatric register in Denmark.

REFERENCES

1. Bezzola, D. (1901): A statistical investigation into the role of alcohol in the origin of innate imbecility. *Q. J. Inebr.*, 23:346–354.
2. Bohman, M. (1977): Genetic aspects of alcoholism and criminality—seen through a material of adoptions. Preprint.
3. Burton, R. (1906) (Orig. 1621): ("Democritus Junior"). Causes of melancholy. In: *The Anatomy of Melancholy*, Vol. 1. William Tegg, London.
4. Cadoret, R., and Gath, A. (1977): Inheritance of alcoholism in adoptees. Preprint.
5. Crothers, R. D. (1909): Heredity in the causation of inebriety. *Br. Med. J.*, 2:659–661.
6. Goodwin, D. W. (1976): *Is Alcoholism Hereditary?* Oxford University Press, New York.
7. Goodwin, D. W., Schulsinger, F., Hermansen, L., Guze, S. B., and Winokur, G. (1973): Alcohol problems in adoptees raised apart from alcoholic biological parents. *Arch. Gen. Psychiatry,* 28:238–243.
8. Goodwin, D. W., Schulsinger, F., Knop, J., Mednick, S., and Guze, S. B. (1977): Alcoholism and depression in adopted-out daughters of alcoholics. *Arch. Gen. Psychiatry (in press)*.
9. Goodwin, D. W., Schulsinger, F., Moller, N., Hermansen, L., Winokur, G., and

Guze, S. B. (1974): Drinking problems in adopted and nonadopted sons of alcoholics. *Arch. Gen. Psychiatry*, 31:164–169.

10. Haggard, H. W., and Jellinek, E. M. (1942): *Alcohol Explored*. Doubleday and Co., Garden City, New York.
11. Jellinek, E. M. (1945): Heredity of the alcoholic. Alcohol, science and society. *Q. J. Stud. Alc.*, 5:105–114.
12. Jellinek, E. M., and Jolliffe, N. (1940): Effect of alcohol on the individual; review of the literature of 1939. *Q. J. Stud. Alc.*, 1:110–181.
13. Jones, R. (1972): Alcoholics among relatives of patients. *Q. J. Stud. Alc.*, 33:810.
14. Kaij, L. (1960): Studies on the etiology and sequels of abuse of alcohol. Department of Psychiatry, University of Lund, Lund, Sweden.
15. Partanen, J., Bruun, K., and Markkanen, T. (1966): Inheritance of drinking behavior. Rutgers University Center of Alcohol Studies, New Brunswick, New Jersey.
16. Roe, A. (1944): The adult adjustment of children of alcoholic parents raised in foster homes. *Q. J. Stud. Alc.*, 5:378–393.
17. Rush, B. (1787): *An Enquiry into the Effects of Spirituous Liquors upon the Human Body and Their Influence upon the Happiness of Society*. Thomas Dobson, Philadelphia.
18. Schuckit, M. A., Goodwin, D. W., and Winokur, G. (1972): A half-sibling study of alcoholism. *Am. J. Psychiatry*, 128:1132–1136.
19. Stockard, C. R. (1923): Experimental modifications of the germ-plasm and its bearing on the inheritance of acquired characters. *Proc. Am. Phil. Soc.*, 62:311–325.
20. Warner, R. H., and Rosett, H. L. (1975): The effects of drinking on offspring. An historical survey of the American and British literature. *J. Stud. Alc.*, 36:(11) 1395–1420.
21. Winokur, G., Reich, T., Rimmer, J., and Pitts, F. (1970): Alcoholism: III. Diagnoisis and familial psychiatric illness in 259 alocholic probands. *Arch. Gen. Psychiatry*, 23:104.

Critical Issues in Psychiatric Diagnosis,
edited by Robert L. Spitzer and Donald F. Klein.
Raven Press, New York © 1978.

Exploring Psychiatric Taxa and Their Validity with Genetic Family Studies

*Irving I. Gottesman and **Robert R. Golden

*Department of Psychology, University of Minnesota; and **Department of Psychiatry, University of Minnesota School of Medicine, Minneapolis, Minnesota 55455*

The molar-molecular, macro-micro, holistic-reductionist, and clinical-laboratory kinds of continua are paralleled in the fields of genetics by population genetics-molecular genetics. As might be expected, the ends of the continua represent distant and distinctive kinds of data acquisition techniques; a complete understanding of the nature of human psychopathology requires both ends and the middle of the continuum of techniques. The studies reported or reviewed in this section of the book dealing with genetics as a tool in the validation of psychiatric diagnoses fall under the umbrella of population (psychiatric) genetics. That is, to the extent that the data are of present or future interest to geneticists, they are studies of molar, macro, holistic, or clinical phenomena that require integration into a gene-to-behavior-pathway perspective of psychopathology (11,12). Like clinical research in other areas of medicine or biology, most research in psychiatric genetics represents "prescientific" first steps on the long road to the understanding of pathogenesis, pathophysiology, and treatment of diseases or disorders. Some of the steps will necessarily need retracing and restarting in more valid or fruitful directions, but use of clinical human genetic methods as tools in the armamentarium of psychopathologists concerned with the validity of psychiatric diagnoses will hasten the day when rational treatments and prevention are possible.

Advances in medical genetics (2,9,14), other than psychiatric genetics, have been made possible by relatively unambiguous diagnostic categories under single gene locus "control" (e.g., phenylketonuria) or by quantification of unambiguous dimensions relevant to a disease under polygenic control (e.g., blood pressure/heart disease or serum insulin/diabetes). The very content of this book documents that the diagnostic categories in psychiatry are still arguable, as are posited personality dimensions that may index a predisposition to psychopathology. A large part of this uncertainty is dictated by the fact that our categories and dimensions represent "open concepts" (17,18) in need of what Cronbach and Meehl (5) have called "construct validity." Additional uncertainty is contributed by the fact that classic Mendelian single-locus control over such posited entities as sociopathy, schizophrenia, affective psychosis, and alcoholism has been ruled out by the empirical data reported here and elsewhere (8,13,25). Slater and Cowie (25) describe the use of the concept of incomplete expression of a gene that is needed to retain classic Mendelian techniques in a modified form for psychiatric research. Curnow and Smith (6,27), Gottesman and Shields (11, 12), and Reich et al. (20) describe the application of techniques from quantitative genetics for traits that appear to depend on a continuum of gene effects but which manifest themselves in a quasi-continuous or threshold fashion at the phenotypic level. The latter kinds of traits are common by the standards of medical genetics, with lifetime risks in the general population of 1% and higher; whereas such diseases as PKU (a recessive condition) or Huntington's disease (a dominant) occur with a frequency close to 1 in 10,000, and, unlike the conditions discussed in this section, occur in 25% or 50% of the siblings of probands, respectively.

Questions about the validity of diagnoses of psychiatric conditions logically precede questions about the degree to which these conditions are under genetic control (their heritabilities) and their modes of genetic transmission (monogenic with a certain gene frequency and penetrance, multifactorial with a certain heritability and n thresholds, etc.). Questions dealing with the subclinical or premorbid manifestations of various conditions (X-spectrum disorder) and the manner and extent that phenotypically different conditions may be related to each other genetically, logically precede questions about heritabilities and modes of transmission since they determine the answers to the latter questions. Shields et al. (24) and Rosenthal (22) have discussed some of these issues as they relate to schizophrenia and schizoidia. As witnessed by the chapters in this section, we often find ourselves working on many of these questions simultaneously. If we do this without awareness, we stand exposed to the dangers of circular reasoning. With awareness, the dangers are lessened and we may profit from self-corrective feedback. For example, Shields and Gottesman (23) asked which of their blind judges and which of their combinations of consensus diagnoses yielded a concept of schizophrenia that made the most sense biologically as indexed by the ratio of identical twin to fraternal twin concordance rates (see below).

THE CONCEPT OF GENETIC HETEROGENEITY

One useful orientation to the use of genetics as a tool in validating diagnoses comes from a familiarity with the concepts of etiological and phenotypical heterogeneity. A classic example of the latter is the wide range of symptom patterns associated with the one disease, general paresis. Etiological heterogeneity refers to patently one syndrome that has many different causes, both environmental and genetic. Mental retardation, for example, has many environmental causes including CNS traumas, prenatal viral infections, anoxia, and sensory deprivations. It also has many genetic causes including chromosomal abnormalities, dominant gene loci, autosomal and sex-linked recessive loci, and polygenic combinations leading to low intelligence. Table 1, derived from an analysis of the entries in McKusick (14), illustrates just a portion of the genetic heterogeneity that can be documented by restricting ourselves to the simple mendelizing conditions that have mental retardation or cognitive deficits that markedly diminish intelligence as part of the phenotypic picture. Although it is clear from the data presented that about 11% of the more than 2,000 known Mendelian phenotypes are associated with one or another distinct kind of retardation, it needs to be emphasized that the 263 phenotypes all together account for only a small proportion of all cases diagnosable as retarded because each is rare. Even Down's syndrome, the most common chromosomal abnormality associated with retardation, occurs with an incidence of 1/660 newborns. The vast majority of retardation, using IQ test scores under 70 in West European environments as a criterion, appears to be causally related to the polygenic system that underlies the genetic contribution to variation in normal intellectual ability (9,21,25).

One important conclusion to be reached from the example of heterogeneity in mental retardation is that it would be foolish to use the diagnosis of retardation as a sufficient category in research into the etiology of retardation. The combination of the various kinds of probands into one sample with a subsequent look at the prevalence of retardation in their relatives would permit the conclusion that we were dealing with something familial, but it would not permit the various signals to be discerned among the noise. We could not find out about the various specific etiologies (14) (i.e., the different inborn errors of metabolism) and their different but specific treatments. It is quite difficult to determine on present evidence whether the clinical variations seen among the schizophrenias, the affective disorders, the alcoholisms, and the sociopathies are associated with specific genetic etiologies or with simpler phenotypical heterogeneity. Both kinds of arguments have their merits. Davison and Bagley (7), for example, have docu-

TABLE 1. *Percentage of known Mendelian phenotypes[a] associated with mental retardation/ cognitive deficits*

Category	No. definite (+ probable)	Phenotypes associated with MR	
		N	%
Autosomal dominant	583 (+ 635) = 1,218	42	3.4
Autosomal recessive	466 (+ 481) = 947	187	19.7
X-linked	93 (+ 78) = 171	34	19.9
Total	1,141 (+1,194) = 2,336	263	11.3

[a] McKusick, 1975 (14).

mented the various kinds of organic brain insults that may mimic a genuine schizophrenia, but such "symptomatic phenocopies" are likely to account for a tiny proportion of all schizophrenic phenotypes (13,25).

Multiple heterogeneity implies that the bulk of cases of some disorder can be accounted for by pooling a number of rare and sufficient causes. To the extent that one of the causes, a major gene, is found in the majority or a large plurality of cases, an etiological theory will be a monogenic theory. To the extent that the different causal factors are common, insufficient, and variable across cases, etiology will depend on the combination of the several contributors. In such a situation heterogeneity theories overlap with polygenic and other multifactorial theories. An extension of the concept of heterogeneity for polygenic theories, not necessarily an obfuscating one, implies that the kinds of disease seen in the relatives of probands in genetic family or twin studies involve different weights for genetic and environmental contributors from those seen in isolated or sporadic instances of the disease. For example, it might be that the schizophrenias observed in the adopted-away children of schizophrenics or in the co-twins of schizophrenics are especially genetically loaded variations, whereas the schizophrenias in sporadic, nonfamilial cases (the vast majority indeed) involve especially environmentally loaded variations. Both variations are compatible with the current emphasis on diathesis-stressor models in psychiatric genetics (12, 25), where genes are necessary but not sufficient.

THE TAXONOMIC USE OF TWIN STUDIES

The adoption and family studies presented in this volume by Crowe, Tsuang, Kety et al., and Goodwin provide good illustrations of those methodologies and their exploratory use in the problem of validating diagnostic concepts. We shall return to the Tsuang data from the Iowa 500 below to illustrate another strategy. Some illustrations of the use of twin data from psychiatric genetic studies to supplement that from other kinds of methods follow. Pairs of identical twins who are discordant for a disorder and who remain that way to the end of the risk period provide an opportunity for maximizing the detection of environmental phenocopies. Identical pairs initially discordant who become concordant provide the chance to detect and characterize the premorbid states and any "spectrum" associated with a disorder. Twins, both fraternal and identical, who have been independently diagnosed or characterized provide a chance, in the context of discovery, for choosing the breadth (wide to narrow) of diagnostic orientation that may yield the most lawful and biologically meaningful results (23,24).

If we were dealing with simple Mendelian conditions in twins, the concordance rates in MZ (identical) pairs would be 100% whereas in DZ (fraternal) pairs the concordance rates would be 50% for dominant gene diseases and 25% for recessive conditions, and the MZ:DZ concordance rate

TABLE 2. *Effects of different diagnostic criteria on twin concordance rates for schizophrenia and affective psychoses*

Criterion of concordance[a]		Concordance rate (b/a)		Ratio of rates	
(a) Pair with index case:	and (b) Co-twin:	MZ (%)	DZ (%)	MZ:DZ	Reference
1. S or ?S	S or ?S	11/22 (50)	3/33 (9)	5.5	23
2. S	S	8/20 (40)	3/31 (10)	4.1	23
3. S or ?S	S, ?S, or O	17/22 (77)	12/33 (36)	2.1	23
4. Narrow S	S, ?S, or schizoid	9/9 (100)	2/18 (11)	9.0	12
5. Broad S	Broad S	14/24 (58)	8/33 (24)	2.4	12
6. S or ?S	Loose spectrum	20/22 (91)	15/33 (45)	2.0	24
7. MD	MD	32/55 (58)	9/52 (17)	3.4	1
8. UP	UP	11/28 (39)	2/16 (12)	3.2	1
9. BP	BP	14/27 (52)	2/36 (6)	8.7	1
10. BP	Affective disorder	26/27 (96)	13/36 (36)	2.7	1

[a] See text for abbreviations.

ratios would be 2.0 and 4.0, respectively. Once simple Mendelian inheritance has been ruled out on other grounds, the ratios can be used, clinically at least, to get a feeling for the specificity of a diagnostic concept that is highly heritable. If liability to a trait were entirely environmentally determined, intra- or interfamilially, we would expect equal concordance rates and a ratio of 1.0 as we find for measles and for juvenile delinquency (4,25). Although we must be wary of numerology, the ratios *within* a sample diagnosed with differing orientations to wide versus narrow concepts of a disorder suggest specificity if they are relatively high. The first six lines in Table 2 are from diagnoses of the Maudsley Hospital Schizophrenic Twin Study (12,23,24). The first three lines show the concordance rates and ratios obtained from the consensus diagnoses of six blind judges for each of 114 twins (24 starting pairs of MZ and 33 of DZ wherein one member of each pair, at least, had a hospital diagnosis of schizophrenia). S refers to a consensus diagnosis of schizophrenia; ?S, to one of probable schizophrenia; and 0, to some other psychiatric diagnosis. From the ratios of MZ:DZ concordance rates formed by these varying concepts about schizophrenia (5.5, 4.1, and 2.1), we entertained the conclusion that a "middle-of-the-road" orientation might yield the most biologically meaningful and specific results; that is, using definite and probable diagnoses from our panel of six judges for both the proband and the co-twin gave a ratio of 5.5 even though other concepts (e.g., line 3) gave higher MZ and DZ concordance rates. Line 4 shows the results from a seventh judge, Erik Essen-Möller from Sweden; his narrow conception of schizophrenia in probands combined with a somewhat broader criterion in co-twins yielded a very high ratio, but it was at the expense of greatly reducing the sample size. Line 5 shows the diagnoses of P. E. Meehl (the most inclusive consensus judge) who works within a Radovian framework emphasizing pseudoneurotic and borderline schizo-phrenia and schizotypal personality organization; the lowered ratio of 2.4 suggests a loss of specificity from too inclusive a view of the disorder. Line 6 reveals what happens with a consensus diagnosis in the proband and a loose definition of a schizophrenia spectrum that included normal histories but schizoid personality test results or interview impressions; we get almost a "dominant gene picture" with a ratio of 2.0. Such a finding needs to be considered in the light of results of twin studies of diabetes (3,11); diabetes in the proband and diabetes or an abnormal glucose tolerance test gave re-sulting concordance rates like those in line 6.

Lines 7 through 10 in Table 2 show data taken from the study of Bertelsen et al. (1) using the Danish Twin Register to examine the affective psychoses from traditional manic-depressive (MD) and contemporary unipolar (UP) and bipolar (BP) affective disorder viewpoints. They used a definition of UP that did not require more than one attack of depression. The ratios shown suggest, again only clinically, that traditional manic-depressive unipolar categories as defined here are much less specific diagnoses than bipolar af-fective disorder with its ratio of 8.7. Using BP in the proband and any kind of affective disorder in the co-twin including cycloid personalities or suicide leads to results like those in line 6 for schizophrenia and a loose spectrum. The data in Table 2 are presented as food for thought and as "prescientific." All the concordance rates are from simple pairwise calculations with no twin counted more than once. Similar approaches have been taken to explore the neuroses by Slater and Shields (26), somatic and psychiatric disorders by Pollin et al. (19), and criminality by Christiansen (4).

A BRIEF DESCRIPTION OF THE MULTIFACTORIAL
MODEL FOR TWO DISEASE FORMS

The model [after Smith (27), but see Reich et al. (20)] is intended to explain the four frequencies given in Table 3 in relation to those that would correspond to general population prevalence rates. These frequencies are directly observable (as given in the Iowa 500 data), and can be compared with model-based estimates of the same, as is described below. Let S = schizophrenia and A = affective psychoses. Besides the four frequencies, the model also requires the total number of first-degree relatives of probands who have disease S, and that of probands who have disease A. The required data can also be given in the form of prevalence rates of each disease for the general population and for the first-degree relatives of probands with each disease, ideally using lifetime risks.

The basic assumptions of the model concern the concepts of "liability" and "threshold." The term "liability" does not refer here only to an innate predisposition, but rather to the degree that an individual is affected or to the likelihood of becoming affected. An increase in the liability is generally

TABLE 3. *The frequencies explained by the multifactorial model*

			First-degree relatives Disease form	
			S	A
		S	f_{SS}	f_{SA}
Probands	Disease form			
		A	f_{AS}	f_{AA}

regarded as a result of both genetic and environmental contributors (12). It is assumed that when the liability is greater than a certain point, the threshold, the individual is then and only then affected and is correctly diagnosed as such. That is, the diagnosis is evidently assumed to be a perfect criterion or an infallible indicator of the disease. Another basic assumption of the model is that the liabilities of two first-degree relatives have a bivariate normal distribution. Each liability distribution will indeed be a quasi-normal one if, for example, it is approximately the sum of a large number of quasi-independent environmental and genetic sources.

In short, it is hypothesized that each of the four frequencies in the 2×2 table (above) results from a two-way dichotomization at the two threshold points of the latent bivariate normal distribution for the appropriate liability variates. It can be shown that the prevalence rates which result from these dichotomizations are sufficient to determine the latent correlation between the liabilities of pairs of first-degree relatives. Conversely, if the correlation between liabilities to diseases S and A, and the population and first-degree relative prevalence rates are known, then the model provides an estimate of the prevalence rate of, for example, disease A in first-degree relatives of probands with disease S. Such a procedure can be used with the roles of S and A reversed and with S the same as A. The formula for the tetrachoric correlation coefficient or a variety of easier-to-use approximations can be used for this purpose.

The correlation between the liabilities of first-degree relatives to the same disease can thus be estimated, yielding, say, r_{SS} for disease S and r_{AA} for disease A. The correlation between the liabilities of two first-degree relatives to the two different diseases, r_{SA}, could also be estimated in a similar fashion. We already know something about the relationships of these correlations, since it has been shown that $r_{SS} = \frac{1}{2}h^2_S$, $r_{AA} = \frac{1}{2}h^2_A$, and $r_{SA} = \frac{1}{2}h_S h_A r_G$ where h denotes "heritability." The term r_G is a measure of "genetic" correlation (27) between the two disease forms; it has the value of 1 when the two disease forms are genetically identical, and has the value 0 when the two disease forms are genetically independent.

Under the hypothesis $r_G = 1$, we have $r_{SS} = r_{AA} = r_{SA} = r$. Here we combine the data for the two disease forms, as if these were only one disease, to obtain an estimate of r. With the value of r and the population prevalence rate for the single disease we can then obtain model-based estimates of the four frequencies in the table above. A chi-square goodness of fit test can be used to make a preliminary assessment of the validity of the model. Similarly, under the hypothesis $r_G = 0$, we have $r_{SS} = \frac{1}{2}h^2_S$, $r_{AA} = \frac{1}{2}h^2_A$, and $r_{SA} = 0$. In this case we estimate r_{SS} and r_{AA} separately from the data of each of the two diseases. The goodness-of-fit of the model is tested in a manner similar to that used in the previous case. Finally, if r_G is hypothesized to have some intermediate value, then r_{SS} and r_{AA} are first determined as in the case of two genetically independent diseases. Then the value of r_G can be found which minimizes the chi-square value (with the degrees of freedom reduced accordingly). Presumably, the model fit will be superior for one of the three hypothesized situations regarding the genetic relation between the two disease forms (identical, independent, correlated). The model thereby provides one with a rational basis for making such a choice especially in the context of discovery. It remains to develop internal validity tests (15) of the model assumptions so it can be determined if the main consequence of the model, the estimate of r_G, is likely to be of sufficient accuracy.

CONSISTENCY TESTING

One purpose of quantitative models is that of testing substantive theories. Diagnoses used in clinical psychiatric genetic research can be seen in this context. Naturally, it is necessary to have sufficient faith in the model if we are to have a useful test of the substantive theory. Most importantly, we hope that the model will not give us "spurious" results. Results are spurious if they are both deceptive to the investigator and totally wrong. For example, we would not want the multifactorial model to tell us that two diseases are highly genetically related when, in fact, they are genetically independent.

When a quantitative model is used for testing a substantive theory, the results of the analysis will approximate the actual but unknown situation to the extent that the assumptions of the model approximate the truth. It follows that checking the truth of the assumptions is a matter of critical importance. In the multifactorial model we are concerned with the assumptions regarding normality of distribution, existence of threshold points, and validity of diagnosis.

What is needed then is a rational means of evaluating the model with regard to its estimation accuracy, likelihood of producing spurious results, disease detection power, and the like, for the actual but unknown latent situation under study. That is, when using the multifactorial model we need to obtain an accurate estimate of r_G, for example, but it is probably even more important to somehow know that such estimates are likely to be accurate enough or not.

Currently model fit is usually evaluated by a goodness-of-fit null hypothesis test (27). In this approach, the values of various manifest parameters (i.e., frequencies of various affected relatives) are derived from the assumptions of the model. These "expected" values are compared with the observed sample values in terms of a chi-square which has a known distribution when the assumptions of the model are perfectly satisfied; that is, the distribution is known when the only source of discrepancy between model-based or derived values and the observed values is sampling error. If a statistically significant discrepancy is found then the model is rejected; if not, it is accepted. The problem is that since we know that this model and all models are literally false, the multifactorial model will be rejected or not solely on the basis of the power of chi-square test used. Unless we have some means of properly controlling the power of this test, it will not tell us if the results are likely to be spurious or if the parameter estimates are likely to be accurate enough. When using the model in its present form we have to decide if we should accept the assumptions or not on *a priori* grounds, not if observable consequences of the assumptions are adequately satisfied by the data.

The parameter estimation procedures of a quantitative model can normally be complemented by "consistency tests" (15,16), the results of which describe how well the assumptions of the model can be trusted. The major purposes of consistency tests are to avoid spurious findings and to detect when parameter estimates are too erroneous for the particular purposes of the study. In the multifactorial model there is at least one obvious candidate for a consistency test. There are two ways to derive r_G if it is conjectured that the two diseases are genetically related but not identical. One can use probands with the disease S and relatives with the disease A and vice versa. For example, in the Iowa data reported by Tsuang (*this volume*), if the probands have disease S we find r_G is approximately 0; whereas if the probands have disease A, we find r_G is nearly 0.9. It would appear that the two values are so discrepant that the model must be rejected, but it may be that the pooled r_G estimate of 0.24 is still quite accurate. Presumably, the difference in the two separate estimates is due in part to sampling error, to invalidity and unreliability of diagnoses, and to violations of the other assumptions. It is of interest to note that if 6 of the 25 relatives diagnosed as schizophrenic had, rather, been diagnosed as affective, then the model would nearly fit perfectly according to the chi-square test, and resulting r_G value is very close to 0. Knowing how much unreliability exists in such psychiatric diagnoses does not make it difficult to fear that the r_G estimate could easily be highly erroneous. We conclude that the model can not be safely used to estimate or test the degree of genetic relationship between schizophrenia and affective psychosis with the present data. The model may, in fact, yield an accurate r_G result but we do not know that.

The assumptions of the model are probably never perfectly true; but, of course, it is necessary only that the assumptions be approximately true, or, to put it another way, that the assumptions be adequately "robust," so that parameter estimates are accurate enough. The assumptions can be checked by the use of statistical tests which are derived in part by analytical study, and in part from Monte Carlo and empirical trials of the model. This approach, very briefly, consists of studying the effects of various kinds and degrees of assumption violation on the consistency test statistic. By so doing, the latter can eventually serve as an indicator of flaws in the model (10).

CONCLUSIONS

We confidently expect to look back with fondness at the ferment of activity in psychiatric genetics in the post-World War II period to the present as a "prescientific" era of useful trial and error that led to the final melding of biochemistry, molecular genetics, psychometrics, and careful descriptive clinical psychopathology into a structure for valid psychiatric diagnosis. Neither DSM-III nor PSE (28) and its variants will bring about a cosmological revolution wherein medicine and biology would permit psychiatry to be numbered among their fraternities without prejudice; such guarantors of reliability will, however, move us rapidly in the direction of valid diagnoses if they are accompanied by psychiatric genetics and the tools listed above. We are still awaiting the invention of a "telescope" that will protect psychopathologists from their favorite myths. In the interim we must beware of the seductive powers of the richness of clinical phenomena as well as of the elegance of mathematical models.

REFERENCES

1. Bertelsen, A., Harvald, B., and Hauge, M. (1977): A Danish twin study of manic-depressive disorders. *Br. J. Psychiatry,* 130:330–351.
2. Carter, C. O. (1969): The genetics of common disorders. *Br. Med. Bull.,* 25:52–57.
3. Cerasi, E., and Luft, R. (1967): Insulin response to glucose infusion in diabetic and non-diabetic monozygotic twin pairs. Genetic control of insulin response? *Acta Endocrinol. (Kbh.),* 55:330–345.
4. Christiansen, K. O. (1974): The genesis of aggressive criminality: Implications of a study of crime in a Danish twin study. In: *Determinants and Origins of Aggressive Behavior,* edited by J. de Wit and W. Hartup, pp. 233–253. North Holland, Amsterdam.
5. Cronbach, L. J., and Meehl, P. E. (1955): Construct validity in psychological tests. *Psychol. Bull.,* 52:281–302.
6. Curnow, R. N., and Smith, C. (1975): Multifactorial models for familial diseases in man. *J. R. Stat. Soc. A,* 138:131–156.
7. Davison, K., and Bagley, C. R. (1969): Schizophrenia-like psychoses associated with organic disorders of the central nervous system: A review of the literature. *Br. J. Psychiatry,* Special Publication No. 4:113–184.
8. Fieve, R. R., Rosenthal, D., and Brill, H. (Eds.) (1975): *Genetic Research in Psychiatry.* Johns Hopkins University Press, Baltimore.
9. Fraser Roberts, J. A. (1973): *An Introduction to Medical Genetics, Ed. 6.* Oxford University Press, London.
10. Golden, R. R., and Meehl, P. E. (1977): *Contributions to Taxometrics.* Academic Press, New York (*in press*).
11. Gottesman, I. I., and Shields, J. (1968): In pursuit of the schizophrenic genotype. In: *Progress in Human Behavior Genetics,* edited by S. Vandenberg, pp. 67–103. Johns Hopkins University Press, Baltimore.

12. Gottesman, I. I., and Shields, J. (1972): *Schizophrenia and Genetics: A Twin Study Vantage Point.* Academic Press, New York.

13. Gottesman, I. I., and Shields, J. (1976): A critical review of recent adoption, twin, and family studies of schizophrenia: Behavioral genetics perspectives. *Schiz. Bull.,* 2:360–401.

14. McKusick, V. A. (1975): *Mendelian Inheritance in Man: Catalogs of Autosomal Dominant, Autosomal Recessive, and X-linked Phenotypes, Ed. 4.* Johns Hopkins University Press, Baltimore.

15. Meehl, P. E. (1965): Detecting latent clinical taxa by fallible quantitative indicators lacking an accepted criterion. *Reports from the Research Laboratories of the Department of Psychiatry,* University of Minnesota, Minneapolis, Report No. PR-65-2.

16. Meehl, P. E. (1973): MAXCOV-HITMAX: A taxonomic search method for loose genetic syndromes. In: *Psychodiagnosis: Selected Papers.* University of Minnesota Press, Minneapolis.

17. Meehl, P. E. (1977): Specific etiology and other forms of strong influence: Some quantitative meanings. *J. Med. Philos.,* 2(1):33–53.

18. Pap, A. (1953): Reduction-sentences and open concepts. *Methodos,* 5(17):3–30.

19. Pollin, W., Allen, M. G., Hoffer, A., Stabenau, J. R., and Hrubec, Z. (1969): Psychopathology in 15,909 pairs of veteran twins. *Am. J. Psychiatry,* 126:597–609.

20. Reich, T., Cloninger, C. R., and Guze, S. B. (1975): The multifactorial model of disease transmission: I. Description of the model and its use in psychiatry. *Br. J. Psychiatry,* 127:1–10.

21. Roberts, G. E. (1973): The relevance of biochemistry to the problem of mental retardation. In: *Biochemistry and Mental Illness,* edited by L. L. Iversen and S. P. Rose, pp. 7–17. The Biochemical Society, London.

22. Rosenthal, D. (1975): Discussion: The concept of schizophrenic disorders. In: *Genetic Research in Psychiatry,* edited by R. R. Fieve and D. Rosenthal, pp. 199–208. Johns Hopkins University Press, Baltimore.

23. Shields, J., and Gottesman, I. I. (1972): Cross-national diagnosis of schizophrenia in twins. *Arch. Gen. Psychiatry,* 27:725–730.

24. Shields, J., Heston, L. L., and Gottesman, I. I. (1975): Schizophrenia and the schizoid: The problem for genetic analysis. In: *Genetic Research in Psychiatry,* edited by R. R. Fieve, D. Rosenthal, and H. Brill, pp. 167–197. Johns Hopkins University Press, Baltimore.

25. Slater, E., and Cowie, V. (1971): *The Genetics of Mental Disorders.* Oxford University Press, London.

26. Slater, E., and Shields, J. (1969): Genetical aspects of anxiety. In: *Studies of Anxiety,* edited by M. H. Lader, pp. 62–71. *Br. J. Psychiatry,* Special Publication No. 3.

27. Smith, C. (1976): Statistical resolution of genetic heterogeneity in familial disease. *Ann. Hum. Genet.,* 39:281–291.

28. Wing, J. K., Cooper, J. E., and Sartorius, N. (1974): *The Measurement and Classification of Psychiatric Symptoms.* Cambridge University Press, London.

Discussion

Dr. Kety: I have very little to say because Dr. Gottesman was rather easy with me this time. That may be partly because of my own negligence in that I did not write the paper and have the data analyzed early enough to send it to him in time for him to read it very carefully. But, then, Dr. Gottesman has not always depended upon careful reading of our work in order to criticize it. (Laughter)

It is true that if chronic schizophrenia, latent schizophrenia, and uncertain schizophrenia, as we define it, are combined in our interviewed population, the prevalence is 6.9%. Dr. Gottesman appropriately raised the question as to what that means, are 7% of the Danes and Americans walking around with these horrible, unlabeled illnesses?

Actually, I think that there are ways of dissecting that compound figure that would provide a more realistic understanding of the situation. For example, if you would simply list those that we diagnosed as chronic schizophrenia you would find that in this interviewed population the incidence of this disorder in people that are not genetically related to an index case is about 1.8%. That is still high, but we must remember that this is an interviewed population. When one interviews people, whether or not they have ever been in a mental hospital—and most of these people have not—you inevitably find the possibility of making more diagnoses than you might expect.

As far as the rest of the spectrum—at least my spectrum—and, by the way, Rosenthal and Wender and I do not always agree on what is in the spectrum—as far as borderline schizophrenia and uncertain schizophrenia are concerned, this would account for about 4% out of the 6.9% in the people not genetically related to schizophrenics.

We are throwing a very wide net, and are including as uncertain schizophrenia anybody that we think might have schizophrenia, smells like a schizophrenic, and by all of our subjective supersensitive and possibly erroneous techniques that we can muster, might have something related to schizophrenia. That does not mean that we are ready to say that everybody ought to be labeled schizophrenia who comes into this category. This is a research study, and the people in Denmark do not even know that we have labeled them with these diagnoses. What we are doing is testing a hypothesis, which is: suppose we open our minds to the possibility that somebody might be schizophrenic. If we throw out as wide a net as we can, isn't it interesting that with this vague, uncertain kind of thing, we still find a very significant concentration of it, whatever "it" is, in the people who are genetically related to schizophrenics as opposed to people who are not genetically related. There is a lot of noise in the system, and that noise is adding to the total figure of 6.9%, but in that noise there still is a signal, and the signal has, as always observed by Spitzer and Endicott, using other criteria, something that is suggestive of schizophrenic traits. We do not claim to have a hard and fast diagnosis ready to be put into the literature.

Dr. Zubin: I have a brief comment to make about that 6.8% of schizophrenics that Dr. Kety did not expect to occur in his data.

Just as you have concordant twins, both of whom are phenotypic schizophrenics, you probably also have concordance for the schizophrenic genotype in twins, neither of whom expresses himself phenotypically.

When you take siblings where you expect a genotypic concordance of 50%, according to some genetic hypotheses, and phenotypically you get only about 12%, you have a 4 to 1 ratio of people who carry the genotype that never expresses itself to those in whom it is expressed phenotypically.

I wonder what that does to our control group. It is possible that the presence of a 4 to 1 ratio of genotypic carriers who do not express themselves phenotypically brought about your unexpected finding?

Until we develop markers that will identify the genotype carriers, there will always be a danger of getting into our control group people who do not belong there.

Dr. Klein: I think one thing that we come away from this discussion with is the need for the most exquisite methodology in doing diagnosis. I would like to raise one small question about Dr. Crowe's report on hyperkinetic children. In those two particular studies the criteria for being considered a hyperkinetic child were not firm.

In the Cantwell study, some 28 traits were considered markers of hyperkinesis, and a child needed only 6 of them to qualify, in addition to hyperactivity and distractibility. Many of those criteria were simply elements of conduct disorders; not necessarily related to hyperkinesis.

In our own studies, I think we have fair evidence that children who have conduct disorders will tend to be rated by teachers as hyperkinetic, even if not factually hyperkinetic.

Therefore, it is possible that those studies show that antisociality is related to antisociality rather than that hyperkinesis is related to antisociality.

Dr. Kety: Dr. Spitzer wants to talk, but I want to give him something to talk about. I want to ask a question which I thought might have come up in the discussion, but did not. That is the question of acute schizophrenia, not so much from our own data, which is too small to rule really out the possibility that acute schizophrenia is related genetically to chronic schizophrenia. I am concerned about the thousands of papers which have found that acute and chronic schizophrenia do not seem to be related, and the many papers that now show that the so-called acute schizophrenic responds well to lithium. In view of all this, why will acute schizophrenia continue to be perpetuated in DSM-III?

Dr. Spitzer: There are several problems here. One problem is that even if it is true that acute schizophrenia seems to be genetically different from chronic schizophrenia, one could argue, as Dr. Zubin has, that the difference may not be in the illness as much as in the host factor which protects one against the illness. Maybe the host factor has a genetic component that accounts for some individuals developing a chronic course, and others only an acute course, in schizophrenia.

The other problem is more a practical one in that we do have to have some correspondence between DSM-III and the *International Classification of Diseases.* We have made a compromise and have said that if the acute psychosis is of less than 2 weeks' duration, one should reserve judgment as to whether or not that is schizophrenia, and we have therefore provided another category, brief reactive psychosis. Many of the cases which in DSM-I and II would have been called acute schizophrenia will now no longer be called schizophrenia, but would receive that diagnosis. It seems to us that in this time of history, it would be premature for us to tell our European colleagues that we know where schizophrenia begins and where it ends. We have a similar problem with schizoaffective schizophrenia. We have been asked why we have not separated schizoaffective disorders from schizophrenia, as we have done in developing the Research Diagnostic Criteria. We felt that in a similar fashion we did not believe that there was sufficient evidence to remove schizoaffective disorder from schizophrenia. There will be a DSM-IV, a DSM-V, and a DSM-VI. At least we will have provided clear criteria in DSM-III so that some of these questions will be answered.

(*Editor's Note:* At the May, 1977, meeting of the American Psychiatric Association's Task Force on Nomenclature, it was decided to exclude acute schizophrenia from schizophrenia and to list schizoaffective disorder outside of the category of Schizophrenia in the next draft of DSM-III.)

Critical Issues in Psychiatric Diagnosis,
edited by Robert L. Spitzer and Donald F. Klein.
Raven Press, New York © 1978.

EEG Response Strategies in Psychiatric Diagnosis

Max Fink

*Department of Psychiatry and Behavioral Sciences Health Sciences Center,
S.U.N.Y. at Stony Brook, Stony Brook, New York 11794*

The lesson of the history of psychiatry is that progress is inevitable and irrev-ocable from psychology to neurology, from mind to brain, never the other way round. Every medical advance adds to the list of diseases which may cause men mental derangement. The abnormal mental state is not the disease, nor its essence or determinant, but an epiphenomenon. This is why psycho-logical theories and therapies, which held out such promise at the turn of the century when so much less was known of localisation of function in the brain, have added so little to the understanding and treatment of mental ill-ness, despite all the time and effort devoted to them.

—Macalpine and Hunter (37)

Classification provides structure for observations and reduces the chaos of sensory stimuli to meaningful clusters. In the biological and physical sciences, classification schemes begin with an implicit assumption that there is order and differentiation in the structures under study. The basis for the order is sought in verifiable and measurable phenomena. The ability of in-dividuals to produce like offspring is an example of a particularly useful classification device in biology. Classifications are derived from heuristic or theoretic models, serving science best when they provide a framework not only for the initial data on which they are based, but when they allow the incorporation of new data and new classes (35).

Modern psychiatric classifications lack a common theoretic model, there being at least three triangulating ("polar") schemata that are derived from prevailing models of madness—the organic, the psychotherapeutic, and the sociotherapeutic. Despite heroic attempts by eclecticists to integrate these models, their views are so different as to make an integration virtually im-possible within the limits of our present knowledge (1). Yet classification schemes seek to accommodate these positions. Perhaps they attempt too much, encompassing in one classification disorders that may be rooted in neurophysiology and neurochemistry, in educational lack, in social and economic deprivation, in genetic predispositions, as well as in the uneven application of often illogical laws.

One approach may be to use a single view of mental illness as the basis for a classification scheme, thereby maximizing the benefits that may accrue from a unitary view and hazarding the loss of those benefits that may have accrued on the selection of another model of mental illness. The organic model of mental illness is considered here as a basis for a classification strategy.

In 1929 Hans Berger published his records of rhythmic, patterned electrical activity from the intact human scalp, establishing the science of electroencephalography (16). His interest in brain function derived from the same roots in pathology that stimulated Kraepelin's classification; the same roots from which fever, insulin coma, Metrazol, and electroseizure therapies developed. Berger, and many of the early electroencephalographers, sought diagnostic validity in the EEG patterns. They were highly successful, in some ways beyond their hopes and expectations. Four examples readily come to mind (24,65).

1. Patients with epileptic seizures and episodic behavior disturbances were found to have identifiable diffuse or focal, spike and/or burst EEG abnormalities. Therapies were developed and soon this large population was wrested from the multitude of undiagnosed and untreated mentally ill.

2. Children with learning difficulty, headaches, and mood and motor disturbances were shown to have characteristic 3-Hz spike and wave patterns. These were related in time to "absences" and to automatic behaviors. Treatments for this population were soon found and these patients are no longer a significant diagnostic (or therapeutic) problem.

3. EEG slow waves accompanied severe dementias, whether post-traumatic, senile degenerative, arteriosclerotic, or toxic. The amount of EEG slowing was related to the severity of the organic mental syndrome, and changes in the frequency patterns were predictive of outcome in the reversible dementias (postinfectious, traumatic, or toxic, especially alcoholic). Although these patients are still of concern to psychiatrists, their classification is eased by EEG methods.

4. Slow waves observed on one side of the scalp or in a well-defined area were related to focal brain pathology, as following brain hemorrhages or tumors. With this pathologic identification, the accompanying abnormal language, mood, and mental states were no longer defined as "psychiatric syndromes," and the patients became the charge of practitioners other than psychiatrists.

These successes of diagnosis, reflecting abnormalities in cerebral pathophysiology and pathology, are now an integral part of medical assessment. When similar identifiable EEG patterns were not readily forthcoming in the "functional" mentally ill, disappointment led to an abandonment of EEG methodology in psychiatry; and with it, an implicit rejection of disordered cerebral pathophysiology as the basis for the "functional" abnormal mental states. Greater emphasis was placed on psychodynamic, psychosocial, and environmental theories of mental illness, and symptoms assumed primacy in classification systems.

Three questions relate to the focus of this volume:

1. Was the rejection of cerebral pathophysiology as a mechanism for "functional" mental states justified?
2. Is there merit in reassessing brain electrophysiology for nosologic purposes?
3. Would it be useful to include quantitative EEG measures in proposed nosologic schemes?

TECHNICAL CHANGES IN EEG ANALYSIS

Before answering these questions, it is necessary to note that modern brain electrophysiology has undergone, and is undergoing, rapid change. Since the first reports by Berger in 1929, the methods used to record and to measure EEG activity have changed. From single electrode pairs and primitive galvanometers, modern EEG methods record from multiple lead pairs, with stable and sensitive solid-state amplifiers. Recordings are made with subjects alert and asleep as well as after activation procedures such as hyperventilation, drugs, or repetitive sensory stimuli. Brain responses to sensory stimuli are averaged and the evoked response pattern measured; and in a special activation paradigm, the subject's electrophysiologic response to an anticipated sensory stimulus is measured (the CNV).[1]

Analytic systems also differ. To supplement the visual holistic analysis commonly used in reading clinical EEG records, digital computer programs now provide quantitative temporal and spatial analyses of brain rhythms.[2] But these developments are very recent, the greatest progress being made in this decade, and the methods have been applied only occasionally to the diagnostic problems that interest us. We must answer our questions using data collected in an earlier period, with methods that are less sensitive and less reliable than more recent techniques.

EEG AS A DIAGNOSTIC STRATEGY

Two tactics are used to relate EEG measures to behavioral and clinical variables. In resting, alert EEG recordings, EEG samples are usually recorded with eyes closed. After EEG parameters are described or measured, the

---

[1] These aspects of cerebral activity are discussed by others. Useful reviews are those of Shagass (53), Regan (42), Itil (26), and Saletu (45).

[2] New computer analytic methods have been developed to identify organic brain dysfunctions and the epilepsies, and to classify psychotropic drugs. For details see the volumes edited by Schenk (47), Itil (26), Dolce and Künkel (6), Matecjek and Schenk (38), Kellaway and Petersen (34), and Saletu (45).

scores are related to a psychologic test score, to a clinical diagnostic label, or to a value on a behavioral scale.

An alternate method is to use the activated EEG, in which a subject's behavioral, linguistic, and EEG responses to a test substance are the basis for classification. This method is similar to the use of the therapeutic response to establish a clinical diagnosis, as in the relabeling of lithium responders as cases of "mania," and EST responders as cases of "depressive psychosis."

Clinical EEG and Diagnosis

It has been difficult to determine characteristic EEG patterns in cases of "schizophrenia," "depression," or the "neuroses," perhaps because of the unreliability of clinical classifications.[3] Some reports suggest that patients with schizophrenia have choppy rhythms, greater variability in amplitude measures, greater amounts of fast activity, or greater amounts of theta activity than normal or depressed subjects (27). Others contrast different regions of the scalp and find that schizophrenic patients have low interareal correlations of frequencies (19). Schizophrenic patients who fail to respond to treatment are found to have hyperstabile records (4). Changes in EEG patterns with treatment are prognostic of outcome with better results occurring in patients with EEG records showing characteristic changes (29). In studies of depressives, the depth of depression is related to the EEG mean integrated amplitude and to hemispheric differences (5,41).

These findings are made in group data and do not provide information regarding the individual case. The studies are often poorly controlled for age and sex differences among the subjects, and even when controls are studied, their suitability in terms of diet, hospitalization, and prior treatment makes conclusions difficult.

Some studies relate EEG aspects to changes in the behavior of individual patients. Stevens (57) found episodic disturbances in perception or in the stream of thought of patients to accompany low-voltage EEG fast activity, posteriorly localized monophasic sharp waves, or paroxysmal discharges with or without photic stimulation. Depth electrode recordings in chronic schizophrenic patients elicit abnormal spike activity in the midline septal area (22); a finding recently corroborated by Hanley (21) in a single case.

Others ask whether a common electrophysiologic pattern can be defined in patients who are homogeneous for a pattern of symptoms, a genetic trait, or a clinical response to treatment. Volavka et al. (64) found a significantly lower average frequency of occipital alpha activity in noninstitutionalized men with an XYY sex chromosome pattern compared to men with an XXY chromosome pattern. In a carefully selected group of children defined as

---

[3] Citations in this review will be selective. They are culled from an extensive literature; see Wilson (65), Fink (7,8), Shagass (52,54,55), Vianna (62), Itil (27), and Kietzman et al. (36).

"high risk for schizophrenia" because of their birth to schizophrenic mothers, Itil et al. (28) reported more high-frequency beta activity, less alpha activity, and more very slow waves than in controls whose mothers were not schizophrenic, and who were matched for demographic characteristics. A third example is the separation of hyperkinetic children into responders or nonresponders by the degree of episodic EEG activity in their resting EEGs (46).

> *Comment:* Abnormal EEG patterns have often been defined in population samples of the functional mentally ill. But the differences are poorly established, and controls are often inadequate. Some recent studies, however, using larger sample sizes, objective selection criteria, and controls suggest that abnormal behaviors may have reflections in abnormal EEG patterns. Most critical, none of the suggested relations of EEG variables and behavior are valid for the individual.

Activated EEG and Diagnosis

Activated EEG presents some promising findings, not only for group data, but also for individual subjects. Early studies were focused on the response of blood pressure to cholinergic and adrenergic drugs, pupillary response, and the galvanic skin response (7). The first stressors in EEG studies were hyperventilation, a technique which served to define a group of epileptics, and visual flicker, useful in defining epilepsy and to measure the intensity of anxiety (30,31). For psychiatric purposes, studies of barbiturates led to the development of the sedation threshold, a response to amobarbital (49–51,54) and the pentothal response (17,18,25). Roth and his co-workers (43,44) used pentothal to define responders and nonresponders to EST. Sleep was often used and is the most widely used activation procedure in clinical studies today (7,26,45).

With the development of computer techniques for EEG response averaging, many studies used the response to visual, tactile, and auditory stimuli. This voluminous literature[4] will not be reviewed here, except to note that the power of the associations resides in response characteristics, and not in any stable, resting patterns of behavior or electrophysiology.

Activated EEG has been extensively studied. Two types of studies are models for a diagnostic strategy—the sedation threshold and sleep activation of specific EEG patterns.

Sedation Threshold

The physiologic responses to an intravenous barbiturate include slurred and slowed speech, errors in simple mathematical tasks, nystagmus, ataxia,

---

[4] See footnote 1 for reviews, and the report by Sutton (*this volume*).

and increased EEG beta activity, usually in 18 to 25 Hz in a characteristic spindling pattern. Shagass and his co-workers (49–51,54) found that the intravenous administration of amobarbital at a set rate (1 cc/40 sec), delivering a set amount by body weight (0.5 mg/kg), elicited EEG beta spindling at different doses. They related the amount necessary for a statistical endpoint (inflection point in the EEG beta activity curve) to clinical diagnosis; finding that anxious neurotics and active schizophrenic patients required greater amounts of amobarbital than psychotic depressed or patients with an organic mental syndrome (56). Their findings were confirmed by some authors, often using other endpoints (39,40), and criticized by others (2). Claridge (3), reviewing his studies, reported significant differences in sedation thresholds for dysthymics (high threshold, average $= 9.3$) and hystericopsychopaths (low threshold, average $= 6.7$). Much of the criticism of the sedation threshold is related to technical problems, and to problems in defining homogeneous samples according to behavioral criteria.[5]

Sleep Activation

Subjects passing from waking to light sleep may exhibit identifiable EEG patterns as slow-wave bursts and spikes, 14 and 6 positive spikes, and B-mitten patterns. Slow-wave bursts and spikes are characteristic of seizure disorders (24). The significance of the other patterns is still obscure. In an extensive series of studies, 14 and 6 positive spikes were found in epileptics (9,11–13) and in children with behavior disorders (32,33). The patterns have been described by many authors (23,48), but their significance remains undeveloped (66).

The B-mitten is uncommon in the normal population, occurring in less than 3% of controls (10,14,15). Its occurrence is high in epileptics with psychosis and schizophrenia. Halasz and Nagy (20), and more recently Struve and Becka (58), suggest that B-mittens are associated with psychotic decompensation as seen in "reactive schizophrenia." The latter observation was replicated in a carefully studied sample of 85 schizophrenics (59). These authors first thought B-mitten patterns were characteristic of reactive adult schizophrenic patients, but lately they associate these EEG signs with "dysphoric affective dysregulation" (60). Interestingly, they noted that this type of cerebral dysfunction "cuts across broad diagnostic boundaries."

In another diagnostic study, Struve, Klein, and Saraf (61) found that

---

[5] The rate of development of beta activity is influenced not only by the subject's clinical state but also by the characteristics of the resting electroencephalogram and especially the amount of alpha activity. When tests are repeated on different occasions, the results show considerable variability. The criteria of the measurement are selected because of technical simplicity rather than theoretical grounds. For example, in the sedation threshold, nystagmus, onset of sleep, cessation of verbalization, and the maximum amount of beta activity have each been used as endpoints (7).

patients reporting suicidal ideation and suicidal attempts often exhibited paroxysmal EEG activity.

Comment: These activation techniques elicit identifiable EEG patterns of slow-wave bursts, B-mittens, 14 and 6 positive spikes, and beta spindling. Most scientists have sought to relate these phenomena to clinical diagnoses. When correlations between EEG phenomena and clinical diagnosis were low, criticism was leveled at the EEG measure. Is it possible that these EEG criteria provide an independent means to identify homogeneous populations for therapeutic or prognostic studies, and that the criticism for the failure of the relationships to clinical diagnosis should more properly be leveled at weaknesses in the diagnostic scheme and not the physiologic index?

DISCUSSION

The need for a defined and reliable nosology in clinical psychiatry is great. A nosology rooted in pathophysiology or in objective pathologic data would do much to improve our understanding of etiology, develop new therapies, and provide clues to prevention. Present and proposed schemes rely on an eclectic amalgam of incompatible views of madness, relying on clinical descriptions and on subjective assessments of mood, thought process, and psychomotor functions as criteria—criteria that are difficult to define and even more difficult to quantify.

An alternative may be to seek a classification based on a single physiologic or biochemical view of mental illness. Studies rooted in cerebral pathophysiology during this century have parcelled out populations of the mentally ill: the adult and childhood epilepsies, toxic and post-traumatic psychoses, and temporal lobe disorders are examples. Some parcelling devices have yet to by systematically explored: separation of high- and low-anxiety psychoses by the sedation threshold; disorders accompanying 14 and 6 positive spikes and B-mitten patterns; abnormal patterns in genetic subpopulations, as XYY and XXY males; frequency spectral differences in children of schizophrenic mothers; and hyperactive children with epileptic EEG representing a therapeutic responsive group to stimulant drug therapy.

It is probable that these patterns can be expanded by studies of phobics responsive to imipramine and young male schizophrenics worsened by imipramine. These clinical subgroups defined by drug response patterns (partially independent of specific symptoms) provide an interesting starting point for careful electrophysiologic analysis.

Electrophysiologic measures provide a noninvasive, safe, repeatable, behaviorally sensitive way to define a common basis for the symptom clusters now under study. Instead of approaching clinical diagnosis as the independent measure and electrophysiology as the dependent measure—the conventional wisdom—this survey suggests that EEG measures be viewed as the independent classification device with the usual clinical, phenotypic symptom clustering as the dependent measure. Electrophysiology is not the only basis to examine a theory of disordered brain function in mental illness, for as others suggest, biochemical, hormonal, and genetic models also provide interesting theories for understanding the clustering of symptoms and subjects (63).

An EEG response strategy should be considered in any nosologic scheme. Despite the problems of selecting a useful stressor or appropriate response measure, the inclusion of EEG measures in a proposed classification will encourage an operational view of mental illness.

SUMMARY

Classificatory schemes for the mentally ill usually include the results of dysfunctions in brain pathophysiology as well as disorders related to social regulations, interpersonal difficulties, sexual object choices, and social deviancy accompanying poverty and inadequate education. These patterns have diverse etiologies and it has been difficult to encompass them in a single classification scheme.

Cerebral electrophysiology provides measures which reflect normal and abnormal brain functioning. Resting EEG measures have parcelled out four major types of mental illness associated with cerebral dysfunction. The brain response to drug stressors and sensory stimuli provides sensitive, noninvasive, and relevant ways to classify groups of the so-called functional mentally ill.

The inclusion of an EEG response strategy in proposed diagnostic schemes is recommended.

ACKNOWLEDGMENTS

This study was aided, in part, by the International Association for Psychiatric Research, Inc., and NIMH Grants MH 24020 and 28471.

REFERENCES

1. Clare, A. (1976): *Psychiatry in Dissent.* Tavistock Publications, London.
2. Claridge, G. S. (1967): *Personality and Arousal.* Pergamon Press, Oxford.
3. Claridge, G. S. (1975): Psychophysiological indicators of neurosis and early psychosis. In: *Experimental Approaches in Psychopathology,* edited by M. Kietzman, S. Sutton, and J. Zubin, pp. 89–107. Academic Press, New York.
4. Dasberg, H., and Robinson, S. (1969): Correlation between electroencephalographic deviations following anti-psychotic drug treatment and the course of mental illness. *Isr. Ann. Psychiatry,* 7:185–200.
5. d'Elia, G., and Perris, C. (1973): Cerebral functional dominance and depression. An analyses of EEG amplitude in depressed patients. *Acta Psychiatr. Scand.,* 49: 191–197.
6. Dolce, G., and Künkel, H. (Eds.) (1975): *CEAN: Computerized EEG Analyses.* G. Fischer Verlag, Stuttgart.
7. Fink, M. (1968): Neurophysiological response strategies in the classification of

mental illness. In: *The Role of Methodology of Classification in Psychiatry and Psychopathology,* edited by M. M. Katz, J. O. Cole, and W. E. Barton, pp. 535–540. U.S. Government Printing Office, Washington, D.C.

8. Fink, M. (1973): The electroencephalogram in clinical psychiatry. In: *Biological Psychiatry,* edited by J. Mendels, pp. 331–344. J. B. Lippincott, New York.
9. Gibbs, E. L., and Gibbs, F. A. (1951): Electroencephalographic evidence of thalamic and hypothalamic epilepsy. *Neurology (Minneap.),* 1:136–144.
10. Gibbs, F. A., and Gibbs, E. L. (1963): The mitten pattern—An electroencephalographic abnormality correlating with psychosis. *J. Neuropsychiatry,* 5:6–13.
11. Gibbs, F. A., and Gibbs, E. L. (1963): Fourteen and six per second positive spikes. *Electroencephalogr. Clin. Neurophysiol.,* 15:553–558.
12. Gibbs, F. A., and Gibbs, E. L. (1971): Anti-epileptic treatment of patients with 14 and 16 per second positive spikes in electronencephalogram. *Clin. Electroencephalogr.,* 2:52–55.
13. Gibbs, E. L., and Gibbs, F. A. (1973): Clinical significance of 14 and 6 per second positive spikes in the electroencephalograms of patients over 29 years of age. *Clin. Electroencephalogr.,* 4:140–144.
14. Gibbs, F. A., and Gibbs, E. L. (1973): Tumor sites in cases of brain tumor with mitten patterns in the electroencephalogram. *Clin. Electroencephalogr.,* 4:206–208.
15. Gibbs, E. L., Gibbs, F. A., Tasher, D., and Adams, C. (1960): An electroencephalographic abnormality correlating with psychosis. *Electroencephalogr. Clin. Neurophysiol.,* 12:265.
16. Gloor, P. (1969): Hans Berger on the electroencephalogram of man. *Electroencephalogr. Clin. Neurophysiol. [Suppl.],* 28.
17. Goldman, D. (1959): Specific electroencephalographic changes with pentothal activation in psychotic states. *Electroencephalogr. Clin. Neurophysiol.,* 11:657–667.
18. Goldman, D. (1960): Differential response to drugs useful in treatment of psychoses revealed by pentothal-activated EEG. In: *Recent Advances in Biological Psychiatry,* edited by J. Wortis, pp. 250–267. Grune & Stratton, New York.
19. Goldstein, L., and Sugerman, A. A. (1969): EEG correlates of psychopathology. In: *Neurobiological Aspects of Psychopathology,* edited by J. Zubin, pp. 1–19. Grune & Stratton, New York.
20. Halasz, P., and Nagy, T. A. (1965): The mitten pattern—An EEG abnormality in sleep. *Acta Med. Acad. Sci. Hung.,* 21:311–318.
21. Hanley, J. (1972): Automatic recognition of EEG correlates of behavior in a chronic schizophrenic patient. *Am. J. Psychiatry,* 128:1524–1528.
22. Heath, R. G. (1954): *Studies in Schizophrenia.* Harvard University Press, Cambridge, Mass.
23. Henry, C. E. (1963): Positive spike discharges in the EEG and behavior abnormality. In: *EEG and Behavior,* edited by G. H. Glaser, pp. 315–344. Basic Books, New York.
24. Hill, D., and Parr, G. (1963): *Electroencephalography.* Macmillan, New York.
25. Itil, T. (1964): *Elecktroencephalographische Studien bei Psychosen und psychotropen Medikamenten.* Ahmet Sait Matbaasi, Istanbul.
26. Itil, T. M. (Ed.) (1974): *Psychotropic Drugs and the Human EEG.* S. Karger, Basel.
27. Itil, T. M. (1975): Electroencephalography in psychiatry. In: *Psychopharmacologic Treatment: Theory and Practice,* edited by H. Denber, pp. 241–262. Marcel Dekker, New York.
28. Itil, T. M., Hsu, W., Saletu, B., and Mednick, S. (1974): Computer EEG and auditory evoked potential investigations in children at high risk for schizophrenia. *Am. J. Psychiatry,* 131:892–900.
29. Itil, T. M., Marasa, J., Saletu, B., Davis, S., and Mucciardi, A. (1975): Computerized EEG: Predictor of outcome in schizophrenia. *J. Nerv. Ment. Dis.,* 160:188–203.
30. Johnson, L. C., and Ulett, G. A. (1959): Quantitative study of pattern and sta-

bility of resting electroencephalographic activity in a young adult group. *EEG Clin. Neurophysiol.*, 11:233–249.

31. Johnson, L. C., and Ulett, G. A. (1959): Stability of EEG activity and manifest anxiety. *J. Comp. Physiol. Psychol.*, 52:284–288.

32. Kellaway, P., Crawley, J. W., and Kagawa, N. (1959): A specific electroencephalographic correlate of convulsive equivalent disorders in children. *J. Pediatr.*, 55: 582–592.

33. Kellaway, P., Crawley, J. W., and Kagawa, N. (1960): Paroxysmal pain and autonomic disturbances of cerebral origin: A specific electro-clinical syndrome. *Epilepsia*, 1:466–483.

34. Kellaway, P., and Petersen, I. (Eds.) (1976): *Quantitative Analytic Studies in Epilepsy.* Raven Press, New York.

35. Kety, S. (1968): Problems in psychiatric nosology from the viewpoint of the biological sciences. In: *Role and Methodology of Classification in Psychiatry and Psychopathology,* edited by M. M. Katz, J. O. Cole, and W. E. Barton, pp. 190–196. U.S. Government Printing Office, Washington, D.C.

36. Kietzman, M. L., Sutton, S., and Zubin, J. (Eds.) (1975): *Experimental Approaches to Psychopathology.* Academic Press, New York.

37. Macalpine, I., and Hunter, R. (1974): The pathography of the past. *Times Literary Supplement,* March 15.

38. Matecjek, M., and Schenk, G. K. (eds.) (1975): *Quantitative Analysis of the EEG: Methods and Applications.* AEG Telefunken, Konstanz, Switzerland.

39. Perez-Reyes, M. (1972): Differences in sedative susceptibility between types of depression: Clinical and neurophysiologic significance. In: *Recent Advances in the Psychobiology of the Depressive Illnesses,* edited by T. A. Williams, M. Katz, and J. A. Shields, pp. 119–130. U.S. Government Printing Office, Washington, D.C.

40. Perez-Reyes, M., Shands, H. C., and Johnson, G. (1962): Galvanic skin reflex inhibition threshold: A new psychophysiologic technique. *Psychosom. Med.*, 24: 274–277.

41. Perris, C. (1975): EEG techniques in the measurement of the severity of depressive syndromes. *Neuropsychobiology*, 1:16–25.

42. Regan, D. (1972): *Evoked Potentials in Psychology.* Chapman and Hall, London.

43. Roth, M. (1951): Changes in the EEG under barbiturate anaesthesia produced by electro-convulsive treatment and their significance for the theory of ECT action. *Electroencephalogr. Clin. Neurophysiol.*, 3:261–280.

44. Roth, M., Kay, D. W. K., Shaw, J., and Green, J. (1957): Prognosis and pentothal induced electroencephalographic changes in electro-convulsive treatment. *Electroencephalogr. Clin. Neurophysiol.*, 9:225–237.

45. Saletu, B. (1976): *Psychopharmaka, Gehirtätigkeit und Schlaf.* S. Karger, Basel.

46. Satterfield, J. H., Lesser, L. I., Saul, R. E., and Cantwell, D. P. (1973): EEG aspects in the diagnosis and treatment of minimal brain dysfunction. *Ann. N.Y. Acad. Sci.*, 205:274–282.

47. Schenk, G. K. (Ed.) (1973): *Die Quantifizieruug des Elektroencephalogramms.* AEG Telefunken, Konstanz, Switzerland.

48. Schwade, E. D., and Geiger, S. G. (1960): Severe behavior disorders with abnormal electroencephalograms. *Dis. Nerv. Syst.*, 21:616–620.

49. Shagass, C. (1954): The sedation threshold. A method for estimating tension in psychiatric patients. *Electroencephalogr. Clin. Neurophysiol.*, 6:221–233.

50. Shagass, C. (1956): Sedation threshold. A neurophysiological tool for psychosomatic research. *Psychosom. Med.*, 18:410–419.

51. Shagass, C. (1957): A measurable neurophysiological factor of psychiatric significance. *Electroencephalogr. Clin. Neurophysiol.*, 9:101–108.

52. Shagass, C. (1969): Neurophysiological studies. In: *The Schizophrenic Syndrome,* edited by L. Bellak and L. Loeb. Grune & Stratton, New York.

53. Shagass, C. (1972): *Evoked Brain Potentials in Psychiatry.* Plenum Press, New York.

54. Shagass, C. (1972): Electrophysiological studies of psychiatric problems. *Rev. Can. Biol. [Suppl.]*, 31:77–95.

55. Shagass, C. (1975): EEG and evoked potentials in the psychoses. In: *Biology of the Major Psychoses,* edited by D. X. Freedman, pp. 101–128. Raven Press, New York.

56. Shagass, C., and Jones, A. L. (1958): A neurophysiological test for psychiatric diagnosis: Results in 750 patients. *Am. J. Psychiatry,* 114:1002–1010.

57. Stevens, J. (1973): An anatomy of schizophrenia? *Arch. Gen. Psychiatry,* 29:177–189.

58. Struve, F. A., and Becka, D. R. (1968): The relative incidence of the B-mitten EEG pattern in process and reactive schizophrenia. *Electroencephalogr. Clin. Neurophysiol.,* 24:80–82.

59. Struve, F., Becka, D., and Klein, D. F. (1972): B-mitten EEG pattern and process and reactive schizophrenia. *Arch. Gen. Psychiatry,* 26:189–192.

60. Struve, F. A., and Klein, D. F. (1976): Diagnostic implications of the B-mitten EEG pattern: Relationship to primary and secondary affective dysregulation. *Biol. Psychiatry,* 11:599–611.

61. Struve, F., Klein, D. F., and Saraf, K. R. (1972): EEG correlates of suicide ideation and attempts. *Arch. Gen. Psychiatry,* 27:363–365.

62. Vianna, U. (1975): The electroencephalogram in schizophrenia. In: *Studies of Schizophrenia,* edited by M. H. Lader. *Br. J. Psychiatry [Suppl.],* 10:54–58.

63. Vogel, W., Broverman, D. M., Klaiber, E. L., Kobayashi, Y., and Clarkson, F. E. (1976): A model for the integration of hormonal, behavioral, EEG, and pharmacological data in psychopathology. In: *Psychotropic Action of Hormones,* edited by T. Itil, G. Laudahn, and W. H. Hermann, pp. 121–134. Spectrum, New York.

64. Volavka, J., Mednick, S. A., Sergeant, J., and Rasmussen, L. (1977): Electroencephalograms of XYY and XXY men. *Br. J. Psychiatry,* 130:43–47.

65. Wilson, W. P. (Ed.) (1965): *Applications of Electroencephalography in Psychiatry.* Duke University Press, Durham, N.C.

66. Woerner, M. G., and Klein, D. F. (1974): Fourteen and six per second positive spiking. *J. Nerv. Ment. Dis.,* 159:356–361.

Critical Issues in Psychiatric Diagnosis,
edited by Robert L. Spitzer and Donald F. Klein.
Raven Press, New York © 1978.

Evoked Potentials and Diagnosis

Samuel Sutton and Patricia Tueting

New York State Psychiatric Institute, New York, New York 10032

Whatever our hypotheses about the sources or nature of mental illness, an important manifestation is often some deviation in thought process. Evoked potential recording constitutes a tool for observing the time-locked activity of the brain associated with specific conscious processes in human subjects. Of course, these evoked potential recordings are made with the physical barriers of the cerebrospinal fluids, the meninges, the skull, and the scalp. There is also the difficulty that many repetitions of the same stimuli are required. But with experimental and technical ingenuity, these problems have not proven a barrier to rather impressive findings in normal subjects. The average evoked potential has been shown to be sensitive to a wide variety of variables ranging from sensory differences among stimuli such as intensity, color, and acuity; to perceptual differences such as geometrical form, contour sharpness, and perceptual grouping. It has also been found to reflect cognitive variables such as the influence of stimulus salience or significance, the degree to which a stimulus reduces prior uncertainty or matches a template stored in memory, and the relation of the stimulus to the task required of the subject. In addition, attentional and motivational states of the subject influence the shape and amplitude of various components of the evoked potential. We have even been able to demonstrate emitted potentials—these are totally endogenous responses of the brain to significant stimuli which are expected at specific points in time, but do not actually occur. If you like, it is as if we can record the brain saying, "I distinctly heard that clock not strike!"

Although a fairly large body of evoked potential work addressed at issues of interest to psychiatry has already been done, the greatest promise of evoked potential work for the area of psychopathology lies largely in the future. The aim of this chapter is to discuss evoked potential research in psychopathology from a methodological standpoint, that is, from the standpoint of basic research where rigorousness of methodology is a primary goal. The reason for this stance is the hope that by analyzing the nature of the difficulties that lie in our path, we can move forward at a more rapid pace. For the most part, therefore, this chapter is addressed to evoked potential researchers. However, it is also addressed to those whose primary focus is the area of psychopathology to aid them in putting current evoked potential findings in perspective. Charles Shagass, who was one of the first pioneers in evoked potential research, and in evoked potential research in psychopathology, rarely misses an opportunity to remark, "The best way to diagnose the patient is to talk to him!" The analysis provided in this chapter of the current state of evoked potential work in psychopathology does not provide any basis for a fundamental disagreement with this point of view.

TRIAL-TO-TRIAL VARIABILITY OF EVOKED POTENTIALS IN PATIENTS

A key difficulty in evoked potential research in psychopathology may be summarized as follows:

> In comparing patient groups with each other and with normal subjects, the very sensitivity of evoked potentials to so many psychological variables alluded to above—the sensitivity of the evoked potential to every passing thought and every fluctuation of attention—is an embarrassment of riches. Given this high degree of sensitivity of the evoked potential, many of the symptoms of psychosis—delusions, hallucinations, affective states, poor attention, distractibility—create barriers to good experimental methodology. Consider the following example:

Some years ago, Callaway et al. (6) had the ingenious notion of using evoked potentials to verify Shakow's segmental set hypothesis. This hypothesis argued that schizophrenic patients do not hold on to larger sets, but rather get involved with minor sets. For example, schizophrenic patients rather than maintaining the required set for a whole experimental session might change set much more often, even from one trial to the next. In Callaway's design, two tones of different pitches, 600 Hz and 1,000 Hz, were presented in random order. Subjects were instructed to ignore the differences between the tones. The hypothesis was that the average waveforms for the 600-Hz and 1,000-Hz tones for the normal subjects—who were following the major set—would be very much alike. On the other hand, the schizophrenic patients—who could less easily hang on to the major set—would show larger differences between the two average waveforms. This would be so because they would attend to the difference they should be ignoring. This prediction was verified.

However, in a subsequent analysis the evoked potentials for each trial were considered (9). It was found that there was considerably greater trial-to-trial variability in the evoked potentials of the patients than in the evoked potentials of the normal subjects. Therefore, the average waveforms of the patients to the two tones were more different, not because they were attending to a difference they should have been ignoring, but because the individual trials of which the two average waveforms were composed were more varied.

The whole issue of variability is one of the fundamental problems in evoked potential research in general and perhaps an even large one in evoked potentials in psychopathology. The implications of variability for evoked potential research in psychopathology can only be touched on lightly here. We are dealing with something much broader than the usual finding that variability among subjects for almost any measure will be larger for a patient group than for a normal group, although we have that problem too, many times over.

In the evoked potential situation, each trial in each individual consists of several hundred sequential time points, a series of correlated measures. We take the average over many such trials within an experimental condition for each individual to increase the signal-to-noise ratio. This maneuver will serve if the events, or components, in the individual trials occur more or less at the same point in time. When components do not occur at the same point in time, the average waveform will be artificially flattened because peaks from some trials and troughs from other trials will cancel each other out. Procedures have been worked out for coping with the problem (29,51). One such procedure deals with the inconstant latency of the brain's response to the absence of an expected event. Although the brain will generally signal the absence, the brain is not a perfect clock and the timing of the signal will vary from trial to trial (29). The procedures for dealing with trial variability in latency become infinitely more complicated if the different components of the evoked potential do not maintain the same latency with respect to each other across trials.

Against the background of these problems involved in evoked potential measurement, the increased variability of patient waveforms from trial to trial and from subject to subject provides an additional source of difficulty. One ray of light in this morass of variability has been reported by Shagass (38). He found that trial-to-trial variability is lower in chronic schizophrenic patients than in normal controls or in other patient groups in the first 100 msec of the average evoked response to somatosensory stimulation. The importance of the finding is that it is difficult to see how it could be produced as an artifact or through carelessness in experimental design. It is not at all clear what interpretation can be put on this apparent lack of plasticity for chronic schizophrenic patients in the portion of the evoked response most related to input processing.

Shagass' data are not in conflict with the more general finding (Shagass included) that the later portions of the evoked potential, beyond 100 msec, are more variable in schizophrenic patients than in normal subjects (17,19, 22,32,38). These later components are the components thought to be involved in the perceptual-cognitive aspects of information processing (48).

Our use of the phrase "the sensitivity of the evoked potential to every passing thought" is perhaps not just rhetoric. This is suggested by the fact that trial-to-trial variability of the later components of the evoked potential is more highly correlated with thought disorder than with any other symptom category (17,19,32). Average waveforms are more aberrant in schizophrenic patients with thought disorder than in schizophrenic patients without thought disorder. Inderbitzen et al. (15) have shown that nonparanoid process schizophrenic patients who were more variable in performance on perceptual tasks had high evoked potential variability, whereas paranoid reactive patients who were less variable in performance on perceptual tasks had lower evoked potential variablity. What such data seem to suggest is that the trial-to-trial variability of evoked potentials stems, if you will permit the leap, from the variable "state of mind" of the patients.

APPROACHES TO CONTROLLING
THE EXPERIMENTAL SITUATION

In the Callaway et al. design (6), it was assumed that because the normal subjects were instructed to ignore the difference between the tones, the instruction was followed. In fact, however, ignoring or not ignoring the difference between the tones was an option for the normal subjects and not under the control of the experimenter. For some subjects the instruction may have operated like the instruction "Don't think of pink elephants!" If, as hypothesized, the patients could not ignore the differences between the tones, then for the patient sample the lack of experimenter control inherent in the design was not consequential. However, if ignoring or not ignoring the tones was an option available to the patients (or at least to some of them), depending, for example, on their level of effort or motivation, then the lack of experimenter control becomes a serious fault. Because of the high sensitivity of the evoked potential to psychological variables, control of subject option is a key problem in research design (46). Our own solution to the problem in evoked potential studies of cognitive variables with normal subjects has been to create what we call *full demand* situations. These are experimental situations in which the task is difficult and/or absorbing and the rewards, often monetary, are large enough to engage the subject. For example, we have used guessing situations in which the subject must guess which of two stimuli will be presented. The occurrence of the stimulus to which the evoked potential is recorded informs the subject that the guess was right or wrong, and that money was won or lost on that trial.

In the guessing situation just described, correct guesses and incorrect guesses can be segregated for separate averaging. In a variety of performance tasks, discrimination, target identification, or learning paradigms, different categories of performance such as hits or misses can also be segregated for separate averaging. All of these procedures also provide approaches to quantification in that evoked potentials can be compared for blocks of trials at different levels of performance. For example, blocks of trials in which accuracy of discrimination is relatively low can be compared with blocks of trials in which accuracy of discrimination is relatively high (16). More direct approaches to quantification are provided by procedures like reaction time for each trial which can provide evidence of the subject's degree of attention or motivation. Unfortunately, reaction time involves movement which tends to contaminate the evoked potential (48). A procedure with useful possibilities is one in which a quantitative rating of the degree of confidence in the decision or judgment is made by the subject in each trial (44). Evoked potentials have been shown to vary systematically in amplitude as a function of confidence, being larger the more confident the subject is of the correctness of the response. The relevance of these methods to this discussion is that they all provide ways of obtaining, for the same trials, information about the relationship of the subject to the stimuli to which the evoked potentials are recorded.

To determine whether the use of any one of these approaches introduces sufficient experimenter control into the situation requires empirical evaluation. Recently, we have obtained evidence that our guessing situation was not under adequate experimenter control. We discovered this when we instituted the apparently cumbersome and unnecessary procedure of having the patient report after every trial whether his guess had turned out to be right or wrong. We found that a disturbing number of patients could not make this report accurately. For example, patients who guessed that a low tone would occur, and who received a low tone, might nevertheless report that they had guessed incorrectly.

The need for such control arises from the need to know what the data represent precisely in the context of testing patients who often appear confused or who have difficulty in maintaining attention and in following instructions. In this context, one wonders what it is that careful training to maintain fixation, not to blink, and not to move—yet not to be tense, may be doing to the data. On the one hand, we are trying to focus the subject's attention on the experimental task; on the other hand, we have an additional and possibly interfering task, that of controlling muscular reactions. The task of maintaining ocular and muscular control may be more difficult and hence more distracting for patients than for normal subjects. A better strategy might be to relax rigid muscular requirements and live with more eye blinks and movements. Since such trials are in any case segregated from the record, the major disadvantage would be that the sequence of usable trials would be under less experimental control. This would only create serious problems in experiments in which the sequence of usable trials is important, e.g., in habituation studies.

In one study, we found that the evoked potentials of schizophrenic and depressive patients were dramatically different from the evoked potentials of normal controls (23,49). In contrast, the differences we found between the waveforms of schizophrenic and depressive patients were relatively marginal.

We reported that the difference between the waveforms of patients and normal controls was in the P$\overline{300}$ component.[1] This is the component of the evoked potential which is more sensitive to the cognitive variables mentioned earlier. But it should be noted that P$\overline{300}$ is the largest component of the evoked potential under the experimental conditions we used, and therefore could be measured with some degree of reliability in the patient waveforms. Even to the casual observer, the patient waveforms, particularly those of the schizophrenic patients, were smaller and were grossly aberrant throughout. Smaller amplitude for waveforms of schizophrenic patients has been widely reported (7,19,28,32,42,47), and Saletu et al. (32) have found that evoked potential waveforms are most aberrant in those schizophrenic patients with thought disorder. In view of the overall differences between the waveforms of schizophrenic patients and normal subjects, and in view of the unusual features of the waveforms of the schizophrenic patients which made identification of components difficult, we were, in fact, not able to tell whether the differences were limited to the P$\overline{300}$ component. The variability problem made it impossible to discover which of the other components of the evoked potential were deviant, and which were perhaps normal. This component identification problem in patients is unfortunate because there is a fair amount of information about how various components are involved in different psychological processes.

NO INSTRUCTION PROCEDURES

In contrast to the full-demand approach, most other investigators working with patients have used relatively uninstructed subjects except for the usual injunctions to fixate the eyes and avoid movement. Not requiring a behavioral task has the important advantage of decreasing the length of experimental sessions and therefore of decreasing fatigue. A typical session might consist of the presentation of stimuli 1 sec apart in groups of 60. Even with rests, 20 min would suffice to collect several hundred responses. These studies, in common with full-demand studies, have used own-control procedures, i.e., they have compared different experimental conditions within the subject. Within-subject design reduces the influence of sampling variables such as age and sex. The further control of randomization of experimental conditions by trial reduces other sources of experimental error.

To clarify these last points let us review briefly the work of Buchsbaum, Silverman, and their colleagues. They based their conceptualization on a proposal by Petrie that individuals differ along a personality dimension—the augmenter who tends to increase and the reducer who tends to decrease the perceived intensity of stimuli. Petrie had used a behavioral procedure, a

---

[1] The finding of smaller P$\overline{300}$s in psychotic patients has been reported by three other laboratories (28,42,47).

measure of a kinesthetic figural aftereffect. She found that reducers were more tolerant of pain (26). However, the kinesthetic figural aftereffect procedure has poor repeat reliability in the same subjects, and although a search for a measure with greater reliability was not the original motivation for designing an evoked potential analogue, the evoked potential procedure did serve to tie the concept to a more reliable paradigm (4).

In Buchsbaum's evoked potential procedure, four different intensities of light are presented and a measurement is made of several components of the average evoked potential at each intensity. In the earlier studies, the different intensities were presented in blocks of trials. This procedure left the question of the source of the group differences ambiguous, since after the first trial of a block the subject might make a peripheral adjustment, such as the diameter of the pupil, or an attitudinal or attentional adjustment. Although in one study a control was instituted by reanalyzing the data of only the first trial of each block, a much more satisfactory control was introduced in later studies by making all intensities random by trial.

To summarize the findings of the Buchsbaum group briefly, acute non-paranoid schizophrenic patients tend to be reducers. They speculate that reducing serves to protect these individuals from flooding by sensory stimuli, presumably because such patients are particularly vulnerable to flooding (37). Paranoid patients tend to be augmenters, presumably because they are involved in vigilant scanning of their environment. Chronic schizophrenic patients reduce less than acute schizophrenic patients although why this might be so is not clear. Finally, patients with bipolar affective disorders are extreme augmenters, in the sense that they augment more than normal subjects do (21). In an earlier paper, Buchsbaum et al. (2) suggest that augmenting in patients with bipolar depression may be interpreted as related to the fact that the manic patient is "caught up in seeking ever-increasing amounts of stimulation" (p. 24). In this 1971 study, patients with unipolar depression had shown less augmenting than patients with bipolar depression or even had shown reducing slopes, but a more recent study found no differences between unipolar and bipolar depressive patients (10). Augmenting-reducing has also been shown to be related to biochemical factors. Amplitude /intensity slope and monoamine oxidase activity in platelets were found to be negatively correlated in unipolar depressive patients (3) and L-DOPA tended to normalize the amplitude/intensity slopes of patients with unipolar and bipolar depression (14).

Somewhat disturbing for the interpretation of the augmenting-reducing findings are studies of normal subjects from Buchsbaum's group that indicate that muscle tension and attention may be variables which affect the augmenting-reducing slope. Experimentally inducing muscle tension by having subjects hold weights tended to shift slopes in the reducing direction (20). Obviously the problem which is presented by these data is that different diagnostic groups may differ from each other and from normal controls in their level of muscle tension. Therefore, the differences between patient groups in augmenting-reducing slopes could be interpreted in terms of muscle tension.

In their attention study, Schechter and Buchsbaum (36) found that slopes of normal subjects were shifted by various instructions which manipulated the attention of the subject. The authors took comfort from the fact that in these normal subjects slopes were particularly stable in the no instruction condition. This is the condition under which normal-patient comparisons are usually made. However, under a condition of no instructions patients are more likely than normals to self-instruct or to be involved in internal processes which alter their attention. The disturbance of attention in schizophrenia is a well-known phenomenon both phenomenologically and experimentally. Therefore, the important and disturbing finding of the study is that augmenting-reducing slopes are affected by attentional factors.

Nevertheless, these and several other efforts of the Buchsbaum group illustrate another important methodological point—one perhaps so general that we do not think of it as methodology in the narrow sense. That is, the importance of staying with an idea and continually working it through and trying to improve it.

Perhaps no one has been more systematic in this way than Shagass. He began by examining the evoked potential to a second stimulus after various short intervals (from 2.5 to 200 msec) following a first stimulus. The procedure is based on the model for measuring the recovery cycle of peripheral nerve, but here it was addressed to the question of obtaining a measure of cortical excitability. In pursuing a paradigm which might yield more stable, more diagnostically specific, and more interpretable results, he has investigated the effect of varying the intensity of the first (or conditioning) stimulus, and also the effect of varying the number of conditioning stimuli. The effects on his recovery paradigm of age, sex, drugs, sensory modality, and a number of psychological variables have been studied (38). More recently, he has been investigating habituation within an experimental session (C. Shagass, *personal communication*).

Shagass' major finding with the recovery function was that psychotic patients in general have reduced recovery, but there is little difference as a function of diagnosis (39). However, when using conditioning stimuli of different intensity and number, he found that nondepressed floridly psychotic schizophrenic patients showed less recovery than more depressed, less overtly psychotic schizophrenic patients (41). The reduced recovery was more marked for male than for female schizophrenic patients.

CONTROL OF DRUG EFFECTS

A consideration of all of the variables which must be routinely dealt with in good experimental design would be out of place in a discussion of this kind. It should be noted in passing though that evoked potentials do alter with age, and show some differences between males and females. Drugs clearly cannot be ignored as a potential confounding variable when making comparisons among different patient groups and between patient groups and normal controls. There is really no adequate solution to the drug problem and it must ultimately be dealt with by a series of converging operations. Perhaps closest to an optimal procedure is to use patients who have not yet been medicated, but these are rare and would probably constitute a selected population. Patients who have had a drug washout period are highly desirable, but such patients are not available to many investigators. There is also some evidence that drug effects on the EEG may persist through rather long washout periods (50). In a study conducted at a hospital which was not addicted to diagnostic precision, we were able to match schizophrenic and depressive patients for type of phenothiazine, dosage, and total drug intake since hospital admission (23). All patients had been classified as schizophrenic by the hospital psychiatrists, but they were reclassified for our study using the Spitzer and Endicott CAPPS structured interview (43). Of course, this control is not perfect since it does not eliminate the possibility that the same drug could have different effects on the evoked potentials of the two different diagnostic groups.

Studies of the effects of drugs on the evoked potential are increasing in number and may in time help us part of the way out of our dilemma to the extent that they indicate which component or components of the evoked potential are most vulnerable to the effects of a given drug (22,28,30,33). Saletu has, in fact, claimed that he can predict the clinical classification of some drugs on the basis of their effects on the evoked potential and EEG (30).

In general, evoked potentials have tended to become more normal with clinical improvement (2,13,18,27,40). Saletu et al. (34) have reported that for patients whose clinical course deteriorated while on therapeutic drugs, evoked potentials became more abnormal instead of normalizing. It would balance out our information if there were parallel data on the evoked potentials of remitted patients who were off drugs, i.e., evoked potentials are normal when the patients are well and become abnormal if the patients relapse. To our knowledge, no such study has been done, but Levit et al. (23) in our laboratory had the opportunity to retest and reinterview two of his schizophrenic patients several months after discharge from the hospital when they were no longer under phenothiazine. One patient was symptom free and his evoked potentials were more normal. The other patient was symtomatic and showed evoked potential waveforms which were quite similar to the abnormal waveforms recorded on the initial testing. The general thrust of these and other data suggests that the major aspects of the evoked potential differences between patients and normals observed so far are more related to the sick versus well dimension than to the drug versus off-drug dimension.

LONGITUDINAL STUDIES

Studies of the effects of drugs on evoked potentials and studies of the evoked potentials during therapy are steps along the way to more long-range longitudinal studies. Shagass (39) has recently argued that longitudinal studies would permit a better evaluation of the more permanent electrophysiological traits of the individual. Longitudinal studies, he feels, could make a more valuable contribution to studies of the genetic basis of psychotic illness. Another argument for longitudinal studies can be made from the common observation that even in normal subjects evoked response waveforms, although highly variable from individual to individual, are quite stable within the individual *under carefully controlled experimental conditions.* It would seem, therefore, highly worthwhile to study a few patients over a long period, during different phases of symptomatology, over the course of therapy, or over the course of different therapies, when the patient is well, and perhaps if the patient relapses. This approach would eliminate one of the largest sources of variance. It is the kind of study with a low publication yield which understandably few have undertaken.

Some recent data of Buchsbaum et al. (5) do suggest that evoked potentials may differentially reflect state versus trait variables. They studied a manic-depressive patient for 113 days and found that late evoked potential components (vertex and occipital $P\overline{200}$ to light stimuli) changed synchronously with a mood switch while amplitude/intensity slope measures for $P\overline{100}$ decreased about 8 to 10 days prior to a switch from depression to mania. These data, if replicated in other subjects, would indicate that P200 is more state dependent than $P\overline{100}$.

To return for a moment to the idea of using longitudinal studies as a way of looking for a genetic marker in the evoked potential, it should be clear that even if one were found it might not be the same characteristic which most distinguished the evoked potential of the patient when sick. In fact, ideally evoked potential correlates of *state* variables would be different from evoked potential correlates of *trait* variables. We have often used one variant of the longitudinal technique to advantage in our studies with normal subjects. We try out a number of different versions of a new experimental procedure in two or three subjects who we know from experience produce reliable data and whose evoked potential components are easy to identify. We have generally found that once we discover the experimental variant that works reliably, running a full sample of subjects is a routine operation because we know exactly what we are doing.

Our position on the importance of adequate methodology may seem to imply that we are engaged in a hunt for the single best experimental procedure or even more outlandishly the best evoked potential component to measure. This, of course, is not the case, and not what one would expect from any robust tool. Different experimental procedures and different aspects of the evoked potential may turn out to be useful for different purposes. Thus, as has already been indicated, Shagass (38) showed that it was in the first 100 msec of the average evoked potential that chronic schizophrenic patients showed less variability than any other group of subjects. In our study comparing hyperkinetic children and normal children, we found that differences emerged only in components in the 200- to 300-msec range of latencies and only when subjects were tested in an attention demanding task (27). Saletu (31) has used a complex set of measures of latencies, involving different portions of the evoked potential for different drugs, in his battery approach to predicting response to treatment. Finally, as indicated earlier, the general finding has been that with clinical improvement there has been normalization of the evoked potential.

THE ITERATIVE APPROACH

It is useful to consider some of the ways that, at least in principle, evoked potentials might contribute to questions of diagnosis. A good objective methodology could potentially contribute in one or both of two ways. Where there are disease entities whose nosological definition is satisfactory, a routine objective method might serve as a useful adjunct, reducing the pressures on the high-level skills of the trained clinician. In addition, an objective method might contribute to the identification of borderline cases. Evoked potentials are being developed for these purposes in the case of neurological diseases of the sensory pathways of the nervous system (see 1,11,12,25,45). For example, subclinical lesions of the visual pathways can be detected, and this has been shown to assist in establishing the diagnosis of multiple sclerosis (12,24).

The situation is more complex where we are dealing with disease entities which the clinician may well classify under some set of diagnostic labels, but which for a variety of reasons can be considered ad hoc. Although symptomatology may be sharply different and may be a source of differential grouping, one knows from the history of physical medicine that reliance on symptomatology alone can be misleading. One is therefore left with many questions such as: Are good premorbid schizophrenic patients quantitatively or qualitatively different from poor premorbid schizophrenic patients? Where do schizoaffective patients fit in? What about the distinction between unipolar and bipolar depressive patients? And what about distinctions that are made within the bipolar classification such as bipolar I and bipolar II?

It would therefore be useful if a technique like the evoked potential which does not rely on symptomatology could indicate a direction for answering such questions. Pushing this approach a step further, one could conceivably, on the basis of evoked potential findings, segregate some subgroup of patients and then turn to the clinician, to the biochemist, to the geneticist, and to other disciplines and ask what other characteristics do these patients share?

But it should be clear that this is a logical turnabout. Our normal approach is to take the diagnosis, usually as provided by structured interviews, as the independent variable, and the evoked potential findings as the dependent variable. Yet in what is proposed here as possibly the most useful contribution, the evoked potential researcher would turn this around and take evoked potentials as the independent variable and the structured interview as the dependent variable.

This apparent paradox has to be raised because the independent variable, the diagnosis, is difficult to define unambiguously. Therefore, although research into the problem normally begins with diagnosis as the independent variable, if an interesting finding begins to emerge the experimenter may consider reversing the procedure. For example, some years ago Satterfield (35) studied the rate of recovery of evoked potentials as a function of the rate of click presentation. He found, among his depressive patients, some whose evoked potentials showed less recovery than normal subjects, and others whose evoked potentials showed greater recovery than normal subjects. On further investigation of these two patient groups, it turned out that although the two groups did not differ in depressive symptoms, those patients with less recovery had a history of depressive illness in a first-degree relative, whereas none of the patients with greater recovery had a similar family history. In addition, the two groups responded differently to electroshock therapy. Unfortunately, the samples were quite small and there has been no follow-up of this study. It provides, however, an illustration of the logic of the methodology. The logical next step in such a bootstrap, or iterative, operation would be to bring family history into the picture as an independent variable.

The value of such post hoc approaches is not that they generate statistically acceptable findings. In all cases, they require replication before they can be accepted. What they do is generate interesting leads. For example, in our work on visual temporal integration—this was not an evoked potential study—we found by a post hoc analysis that it was schizophrenic patients with thought disorder who most deviated from other psychotic patients and normal controls (8). It was noted above that schizophrenic patients with thought disorder had more aberrant evoked potentials than other schizophrenic patients (15,17,32). The convergence of the findings from these two kinds of studies points to thought disorder as a key symptom and suggests a potentially productive line of further research.

In summary, in this chapter we have tried to place evoked potential research in psychopathology within the context of available research strategies. In general, the stance has been critical in the sense that the field has not sufficiently come to grips with the special problem presented by testing patients with such a highly sensitive tool. The importance of obtaining behavioral responses for the same trials in which evoked potential recordings are obtained has been emphasized as one approach to coping with the problem. In a final section, we presented an argument for iterative methodology, which while apparently violating experimental rules, can be shored up by replication, and can provide the bonus of important research leads.

ACKNOWLEDGMENTS

The authors are indebted to Dr. Susan Makiesky-Barrow for a critical reading of the chapter and to Ms. Marion Hartung for assistance with the preparation of the manuscript. Supported in part by Grant MH19812 from the National Institute of Mental Health, United States Public Health Service.

REFERENCES

1. Abraham, F. A., Melamed, E., and Lavy, S. (1975): Prognostic value of visual evoked potentials following basilar artery occlusion. *Appl. Neurophysiol.*, 38:126–135.
2. Buchsbaum, M., Goodwin, F., Murphy, D., and Borge, G. (1971): AER in affective disorders. *Am. J. Psychiatry*, 128:19–25.
3. Buchsbaum, M., Landau, S., Murphy, D., and Goodwin, F. (1973): Average evoked response in bipolar and unipolar affective disorders: Relationship to sex, age of onset, and monoamine oxidase. *Biol. Psychiatry*, 7:199–212.
4. Buchsbaum, M., and Pfefferbaum, A. (1971): Individual differences in stimulus intensity response. *Psychophysiology*, 8:600–611.
5. Buchsbaum, M. S., Post, R. M., and Bunney, W. E., Jr. (1977): Average evoked responses in a rapidly cycling manic-depressive patient. *Biol. Psychiatry*, 12:83–99.
6. Callaway, E., III, Jones, R. T., and Layne, R. S. (1965): Evoked responses and segmental set of schizophrenia. *Arch. Gen. Psychiatry*, 12:83–89.
7. Cohen, R. (1973): The influence of task-irrelevant stimulus variations on the reliability of auditory evoked responses in schizophrenia. In: *Average Evoked Responses and Their Conditioning in Normal Subjects and Psychiatric Patients*, edited by A. Fessard and G. Lelord, pp. 373–388. INSERM, Paris.
8. Collins, P. J., Kietzman, M. L., Sutton, S., and Shapiro, E. (1977): Visual temporal integration in psychiatric patients. In: *Nature of Schizophrenia: New Findings and Future Strategies*, edited by L. Wynne, R. Cromwell, and S. Matthysse. John Wiley & Sons, New York (*in press*).
9. Donchin, E., Callaway, E., III, and Jones, R. T. (1970): Auditory evoked potential variability in schizophrenia. *Electroencephalogr. Clin. Neurophysiol.*, 29:421–428.
10. Gershon, E. S., and Buchsbaum, M. S. (1976): A genetic study of average evoked response augmenting/reducing in affective disorders. Paper presented at American Psychopathological Association, New York, March.
11. Halliday, A. M., McDonald, W. I., and Mushin, J. (1972): Delayed visual evoked response in optic neuritis. *Lancet*, 1:982–985.
12. Halliday, A. M., McDonald, W. I., and Mushin, J. (1973): Visual evoked response in diagnosis of multiple sclerosis. *Br. Med. J.*, 4:661–664.
13. Heninger, G., and Speck, L. (1966): Visual evoked responses and the mental status of schizophrenics. *Arch. Gen. Psychiatry*, 15:419–426.
14. Henry, G. M., Buchsbaum, M., and Murphy, D. L. (1976): Intravenous L-DOPA plus carbidopa in depressed patients: Average evoked response, learning, and behavioral changes. *Psychosom. Med.*, 38:95–105.
15. Inderbitzen, L. B., Buchsbaum, M., and Silverman, J. (1970): EEG-averaged evoked

response and perceptual variability in schizophrenics. *Arch. Gen. Psychiatry,* 23: 438–444.

16. Jenness, D. (1972): Auditory evoked-response differentiation with discrimination learning in humans. *J. Comp. Physiol. Psychol.,* 80:75–90.
17. Jones, R. T., Blacker, K. H., and Callaway, E. (1966): Perceptual dysfunction in schizophrenia: Clinical and auditory evoked response findings. *Am. J. Psychiatry,* 123:639–645.
18. Jones, R. T., Blacker, K. H., Callaway, E., and Layne, R. S. (1965): The auditory evoked response as a diagnostic and prognostic measure in schizophrenia. *Am. J. Psychiatry,* 122:33–41.
19. Jones, R. T., and Callaway, E. (1970): Auditory evoked responses in schizophrenia—a reassessment. *Biol. Psychiatry,* 2:291–298.
20. Landau, S. G., and Buchsbaum, M. (1973): Average evoked response and muscle tension. *Physiol. Psychol.,* 1:56–60.
21. Landau, S. G., Buchsbaum, M. S., Carpenter, W., Strauss, J., and Sacks, M. (1975): Schizophrenia and stimulus intensity control. *Arch. Gen. Psychiatry,* 32:1239–1245.
22. Levit, R. A. (1972): Averaged evoked potential correlates of information processing in schizophrenics, psychotic depressives and normals. Unpublished doctoral dissertation, Columbia University.
23. Levit, R. A., Sutton, S., and Zubin, J. (1973): Evoked potential correlates of information processing in psychiatric patients. *Psychol. Med.,* 3:487–494.
24. Mastaglia, F. L., Black, J. L., and Collins, D. W. K. (1976): Visual and spinal evoked potentials in diagnosis of multiple sclerosis. *Br. Med. J.,* 2:732–733.
25. Noël, P., and Desmedt, J. E. (1975): Somatosensory cerebral evoked potentials after vascular lesions of the brain-stem and diencephalon. *Brain,* 98:113–128.
26. Petrie, A. (1967): *Individuality in Pain and Suffering.* University of Chicago Press, Chicago.
27. Prichep, L. S., Sutton, S., and Hakerem, G. (1976): Evoked potentials in hyperkinetic and normal children under certainty and uncertainty: A placebo and methylphenidate study. *Psychophysiology,* 13:419–428.
28. Roth, W. T., and Cannon, E. H. (1972): Some features of the auditory evoked response in schizophrenics. *Arch. Gen. Psychiatry,* 27:466–471.
29. Ruchkin, D. S., and Sutton, S. (1977): Latency characteristics and trial by trial variation of emitted potentials. In: *Brussels International Symposium on Cerebral Evoked Potentials in Man,* edited by J. E. Desmedt. S. Karger, Basel (*in press*).
30. Saletu, B. (1974): Classification of psychotropic drugs based on human evoked potentials. In: *Modern Problems of Pharmacopsychiatry,* Vol. 8, edited by T. M. Itil, pp. 258–285. S. Karger, Basel.
31. Saletu, B. (1976): *Psychopharmaka, Gehirntätigkeit und Schlaf: Neurophysiologische Aspekte der Psychopharmakologie und Pharmakopsychiatrie.* S. Karger, Basel.
32. Saletu, B., Itil, T. M., and Saletu, M. (1971): Auditory evoked response, EEG, and thought disorder in schizophrenics. *Am. J. Psychiatry,* 128:336–344.
33. Saletu, B., Saletu, M., and Itil, T. M. (1973): Effect of tricyclic antidepressants on the somatosensory evoked potential in man. *Psychopharmacologia,* 29:1–12.
34. Saletu, B., Saletu, M., and Itil, T. M. (1973): The relationships between psychopathology and evoked responses before, during, and after psychotropic drug treatment. *Biol. Psychiatry,* 6:45–74.
35. Satterfield, J. H. (1972): Auditory evoked cortical response studies in depressed patients and normal control subjects. In: *Recent Advances in the Psychobiology of the Depressive Illnesses,* edited by T. A. Williams, M. M. Katz, and J. A. Shields, Jr., pp. 87–98. Government Printing Office, Washington, D.C.
36. Schechter, G., and Buchsbaum, M. (1973): The effect of attention, stimulus intensity and individual differences on the average evoked response. *Psychophysiology,* 10:392–400.
37. Schooler, C., Buchsbaum, M. S., and Carpenter, W. T. (1976): Evoked response

and kinesthetic measures of augmenting-reducing in schizophrenics: Replications and extensions. *J. Nerv. Ment. Dis.*, 163:221–232.

38. Shagass, C. (1973): Evoked response studies of central excitability in psychiatric disorders. In: *Average Evoked Responses and Their Conditioning in Normal Subjects and Psychiatric Patients,* edited by A. Fessard and G. Lelord, pp. 223–252. INSERM, Paris.

39. Shagass, C. (1976): An electrophysiological view of schizophrenia. *Biol. Psychiatry,* 2:3–30.

40. Shagass, C., Schwartz, M., and Amadeo, M. (1962): Some drug effects on evoked cerebral potentials in man. *J. Neuropsychiatry,* 3:549–558.

41. Shagass, C., Soskis, D. A., Straumanis, J. J., and Overton, D. A. (1974): Symptom patterns related to somatosensory evoked response differences within a schizophrenic population. *Biol. Psychiatry,* 9:25–43.

42. Shagass, C., Straumanis, J. J., Roemer, R. A., and Amadeo, M. (1976): Evoked potentials of schizophrenics in several sensory modalities. Paper presented at the Annual Meeting of the Society of Biological Psychiatry, San Francisco, June.

43. Spitzer, R. L., and Endicott, J. (1968): *Current and Past Psychobiology Scales—CAPPS.* Interview schedule. Biometrics Research, New York State Department of Mental Hygiene, New York, New York.

44. Squires, K. C., Hillyard, S. A., and Lindsay, P. H. (1973): Vertex potentials evoked during auditory signal detection: Relation to decision criteria. *Percept. Psychophys.,* 14:265–272.

45. Starr, A. (1975): Auditory brain stem responses in neurological disease. *Arch. Neurol.,* 32:761–768.

46. Sutton, S. (1969): The specification of psychological variables in an average evoked potential experiment. In: *Average Evoked Potentials—Methods, Results and Evaluations,* edited by E. Donchin and D. B. Lindsley, pp. 237–262. NASA, Washington, D.C.

47. Timsit-Berthier, M., and Gerono, A. (1977): P$\overline{300}$ in psychotic patients. In: *Multidisciplinary Perspectives in Event-Related Brain Potential Research,* edited by D. Otto. U.S. Government Printing Office, Washington, D.C. (*in press*).

48. Tueting, P. (1977): Event-related potentials, cognitive events, and information processing. In: *Multidisciplinary Perspectives in Event-Related Brain Potential Research,* edited by D. Otto. U.S. Government Printing Office, Washington, D.C. (*in press*).

49. Tueting, P., and Levit, R. A. (1977): Long-term changes in evoked potentials of normals, psychotic depressives and schizophrenics. In: *Brussels International Symposium on Cerebral Evoked Potentials in Man,* edited by J. E. Desmedt. S. Karger, Basel (*in press*).

50. Ulett, G. A., Heusler, A. F., and Word, T. J. (1965): The effect of psychotropic drugs on the EEG of the chronic psychotic patient. In: *Applications of Electroencephalography to Psychiatry,* edited by W. P. Wilson, pp. 241–257. Duke University Press, Durham, N.C.

51. Woody, C. D. (1967): Characterization of an adaptive filter for the analysis of variable latency neuroelectric signals. *Med. Biol. Eng.,* 5:539–553.

Critical Issues in Psychiatric Diagnosis,
edited by Robert L. Spitzer and Donald F. Klein.
Raven Press, New York © 1978.

Amine Neurotransmitter Studies and Psychiatric Illness: Toward More Meaningful Diagnostic Concepts

Rex W. Cowdry and Frederick K. Goodwin

Clinical Psychobiology Branch, National Institute of Mental Health, Bethesda, Maryland 20014

Psychiatric diagnoses have always been the subject of lively and sometimes acrimonious debate, since they imply disturbances in man's reason, affect, or social behavior—precisely those qualities which are central to our concepts of humankind. Yet these disturbances in reason, affect, and behavior have proven difficult to classify in a meaningful and reliable way. The uncertainties of psychiatric diagnosis have been a source of dissatisfaction to clinicians and researchers striving for a better understanding of these disorders. The uncertainties have also given comfort to those who criticize psychiatry as primarily a social mechanism for labeling and treating deviant individuals rather than a medical specialty treating defined illnesses.

In psychiatry it is still true that clinical phenomena (including present signs and symptoms, past history, family history, course, and prognoses) provide virtually the entire basis for our diagnoses. The majority of this volume reviews the state of the art in these areas. Clearly, considerable progress has been made particularly in the recent past with the development of the Research Diagnostic Criteria and similar systems with demonstrated reliability. It is equally clear, however, that controversy and confusion are still with us and the answers to some fundamental questions are still elusive.

In this chapter we address the following question: Can the introduction of biological measures be of any value in psychiatric diagnoses, or rather will that further confuse the picture? Although sound psychobiological underpinnings would seem to be necessary if psychiatric diagnosis is to be considered firmly in the medical realm, the critical question is whether the biological hypotheses and data are sufficiently developed to allow a meaningful assessment of their potential usefulness to diagnosis, either by defining meaningful subgroups within existing diagnostic groups, or, more radically, by defining biological groups cutting across the more traditional clinical diagnoses.

In order to provide a clear and comprehensive framework in which to discuss these issues, we have focused on the monoamine neurotransmitters, particularly as they relate to affective illness. The amine neurotransmitters, particularly the catecholamines, norepinephrine and dopamine, and the indoleamine, serotonin, are central to the most extensively developed and researched biological hypotheses of psychiatric disorders. The affective disorders in particular provide a rich set of interactions between these hypotheses on the one hand and current states, enduring traits, genetics, and drug responses on the other.

AMINE NEUROTRANSMITTERS IN PSYCHIATRIC ILLNESS

The Hypotheses

It would seem reasonable to assume that the biologic substrates of syndromes as complex as psychiatric illnesses, with their interrelated cognitive, emotional, psychomotor, appetitive, and autonomic manifestations, are not likely to be found in highly localized specialized systems, but rather in systems that are complex, widely distributed throughout the brain, and essentially integrative in function. The proposed biological substrate would also have to be affected by drugs which have long been known to produce changes in mood or cognition. The monoamine neurotransmitter systems meet both these qualifications.

As is well known, the amine hypotheses of affective illness suggest that clinical depression is associated with a functional deficit of one or more monoamines in the central nervous system, whereas mania is seen as being related to a functional excess of amine(s). Most formulations of these hypotheses focus on a single amine (either norepinephrine, dopamine, or serotonin) and involve the implicit assumption that in some way the amine abnormality causes the clinical condition. [The reader is referred to comprehensive reviews (9,22,46,48) for a more detailed discussion of these hypotheses.] Prominent support for the amine hypotheses comes from a series of studies of reserpine, monoamine oxidase inhibitors, tricyclic antidepressants, and lithium whereby biochemical effects of these drugs on *in vivo* or *in vitro* animal systems (and to some extent also in man) can be correlated with their clinical effects on mood and behavior. Because the tricyclic antidepressants have only a weak effect on blocking the presynaptic reuptake of dopamine compared to their effect on norepinephrine and serotonin [reviewed in (35)], these latter two amines have played a central role in clinical hypotheses and investigations; recent studies, however, suggest that dopaminergic mechanisms may also be involved in at least some of the symptomatology involved in depression or mania (27).

The major neurological hypothesis of schizophrenia focuses on dopamine, a focus primarily motivated by the observation that virtually all of the major antipsychotic medications block central dopamine receptors, and the relative effectiveness of blockade seems to parallel clinical potency to an impressive degree. These data have been the subject of excellent reviews by Snyder et al. (50), Matthysse (38), and others.

Direct Assessment of Amine Function in Patients

Most efforts to study the functional state of neurotransmitter systems in the central nervous system (CNS) of human subjects have involved the measurement of amine neurotransmitter metabolites in urine and cerebrospinal fluid (CSF), although studies employing labeled neurotransmitter precursors (32) or neuroendocrine challenges (45) suggest alternative strategies for the future.

The major metabolites of norepinephrine in the urine are 3-methoxy-4-hydroxymandelic acid (VMA) and 3-methoxy-4-hydroxyphenylglycol (MHPG) (17). Studies of norepinephrine metabolism in a variety of species including man [reviewed in detail elsewhere (28)] indicate that although urinary VMA is derived almost entirely from peripheral sources, over half of the urinary MHPG appears to come from CNS sources, making urinary MHPG a promising indicator of central norepinephrine turnover. Dopamine is metabolized principally to 3-methoxy-4-hydroxyphenylacetic acid (HVA) and, to a lesser extent, to 3,4-dihydroxyphenylacetic acid (DOPAC) (16). The major metabolite of serotonin both centrally and peripherally is 5-hydroxyindoleacetic acid (5-HIAA) (34). It has generally been assumed that brain metabolism of both dopamine and serotonin is difficult to estimate from urinary metabolite studies because of the large peripheral contribution; therefore, studies of the CSF have provided the major avenue for direct investigation of the hypothesized dysfunction in dopaminergic and serotonergic activity in the CNS.

These CSF studies raise numerous methodological issues [reviewed in detail elsewhere (24)], such as the extent to which ventricular CSF levels of metabolites reflect brain levels, and the extent to which lumbar CSF reflects ventricular CSF. The CSF contains only a portion of the amine metabolites that originate in brain tissue; nevertheless, it has been demonstrated by a variety of techniques that changes in amine metabolism in the brain are reliably reflected in parallel changes in metabolites in the ventricular CSF [reviewed in (24)]. Regarding the extent to which lumbar CSF reflects ventricular CSF, it would seem reasonable to conclude from a series of studies [reviewed in (28)] that a substantial portion of lumbar 5-HIAA originates in spinal cord whereas the majority of HVA comes from brain. It might be emphasized, however, that even if it were to be shown that 5-HIAA reflects predominantly spinal cord metabolism, such alterations may still be clinically and biologically important since many of the serotonin terminals in the spinal cord originate in cell bodies localized in brainstem nuclei.

Aside from this issue of where the lumbar CSF metabolites originate, one should note that the metabolite levels in the CSF depend on the rate of clearance from CSF as well as the rate of production. Thus, first, the levels may not reflect accurately the rate of production of the parent amine, and second, even if it does reflect the rate of production, it is not a measure integrated over time, and is therefore subject to hour-to-hour variations.

A more recent elaboration of the CSF methodology is the use of probenecid which competitively inhibits the transport of acid amine metabolites out of the CSF, thus increasing the concentration of 5-HIAA and HVA in the CSF (39). In addition to increasing the concentration of acid metabolites in lumbar CSF and thereby reducing measurement errors, it provides a value which is integrated over time (thus, not subject to hour-to-hour variance) yielding a value somewhat analogous to turnover (namely, the rise in concentration per unit time). However, the use of probenecid has itself introduced other interesting yet potentially confounding sources of variance, described in detail elsewhere (21).

With regard to MHPG in CSF, recent studies seem to indicate that much of the MHPG in lumbar fluid comes from the spinal cord (31), and since it is not an acid metabolite, probenecid does not cause accumulation of MHPG in CSF; thus, spinal fluid measurements seem to offer no advantages, whereas urinary MHPG at least provides a measure of norepinephrine activity per unit time. Therefore, of the CSF metabolites, only 5-HIAA and HVA will be discussed in this chapter.

Although there are unanswered questions about how well metabolite studies reflect the functional state of central neurotransmitter systems, it has been demonstrated that drugs producing known changes in central monoaminergic activity also produce the predicted changes in urinary and CSF metabolites in patients. For example, CSF HVA levels after probenecid are increased by L-DOPA (a dopamine precursor) and decreased by alpha-methyl-para-tyrosine (an inhibitor of dopamine synthesis). Similarly, CSF 5-HIAA levels after probenecid are increased by L-tryptophan (a serotonin precursor) and decreased by a blocker of serotonin synthesis (para-chloro-phenylalanine) (25). These metabolite studies have to date provided our best "window" into central neurotransmitter functioning.

ARE TRADITIONAL DIAGNOSTIC GROUPS "MEANINGFUL" GIVEN CURRENT BIOLOGICAL KNOWLEDGE?

The goal of biological research is a greater naturalistic understanding of the biological substrate (etiology, pathophysiology, and anatomy) and the clinical manifestations of an illness—an understanding which may in turn permit more accurate assessments of prognosis and contribute to the development of effective prevention, prophylaxis, or treatment. The process is a dynamic one, as our early clues to biological abnormalities in psychiatric disorders came from the discovery of effective treatments: pharmacology thus provided an initial conceptual bridge between traditional clinical diagnostic groups and biology.

Since then, there has been a virtual explosion of biologically based psychiatric research, interrelating clinical, pharmacological, and biological data. This research has taken place largely within the framework of the traditional clinical diagnostic schema. We must ask whether these traditional clinical diagnoses continue to be meaningful, given our current pharmacological and biological understanding of the illnesses.

"Meaningful" Diagnoses

In medicine in general, diagnosis is a process by which an individual with a given set of historical data, symptoms, signs, behaviors, biological measures, and/or pharmacologic responses is classified into a diagnostic group. As noted earlier, traditional diagnostic schemata of the major mental illnesses are predominantly clinically based. Thus, groups are defined by the course of illness, the presence of particular symptoms, and the absence of others. The problems in establishing consistent reliability with these diagnostic approaches have been amply documented elsewhere (11,33,55), in studies that demonstrate apparent changes in criteria over time, differences from culture to culture, differences from observer to observer, and differences in clinical presentation and diagnosis from episode to episode.

To evaluate whether clinically based diagnostic schemata are "meaningful," we must first explore whether clinical diagnostic reliability can be improved. As reviewed throughout this volume, much of the recent work in psychiatric diagnosis addresses this issue directly by specifying consistent criteria for diagnoses, based on signs, symptoms, behavior, and course of illness. The Research Diagnostic Criteria (RDC) of Spitzer et al., the forthcoming *Diagnostic and Statistical Manual* of the American Psychiatric Association (DSM-III), and the Present State Examination (PSE) of Wing are prominent examples of this trend. Various studies document the improved reliability of such standardized approaches (see Spitzer and Endicott, *this volume*).

Given improved reliability of the clinical judgments, how might one explore the "meaningfulness" of the resultant diagnoses? Within the clinical realm, data showing consistency of the diagnoses over time in the same individual would help support a clinical distinction. Family studies showing distinct spectra of psychiatric disorders which seem to run in families suggest that the clinical syndromes are distinctive, provided that genetics can be implicated, rather than just social experience (e.g., patterning symptoms after observed relatives). Excellent reviews of the clinical support for the schizophrenia/schizoaffective disorders/affective illness distinctions are found in the accompanying chapters by Spitzer and Endicott, Tsuang, and Kety et al. Similarly, the evidence for clinically consistent subgroupings of affective illness (endogenous/reactive, bipolar/unipolar, etc.) is reviewed in Dunner et al. (13).

In the major psychiatric illnesses, however, the ultimate test of clinically derived diagnoses will be whether they correspond to biological and pharmacological data. The model shown in Fig. 1 helps conceptualize the relationships among the three main spheres of information about an individual patient. Clinical variables include basic physical descriptions (sex, age, height, weight), enduring traits (personality variables), current and past course of the illness (symptoms, time of onset, periods of remission), and family history (medical, psychiatric). Biological findings and pharmacologic response have provided two additional distinct areas of information.

For purposes of this discussion, the specific task would be to validate clinical subgroups (defined by, let us say, RDC criteria) by relating them to observed variance in biological findings and pharmacologic response. Individuals meeting the clinical criteria for schizophrenia would be compared to those meeting the criteria for major depressive disorder (unipolar depressed), or bipolar illness I (major depressions and mania) or bipolar illness II (major depressions and hypomania). Further diagnostic subgroupings (such as "good prognosis" and "poor prognosis" schizophrenia) and clinical states (bipolar I depressed versus bipolar II depressed versus unipolar depressed, or endogenous versus nonendogenous depressed, etc.) can also be explored using this approach to subgroup validation.

Most of the literature in psychobiologic research involves demonstrating

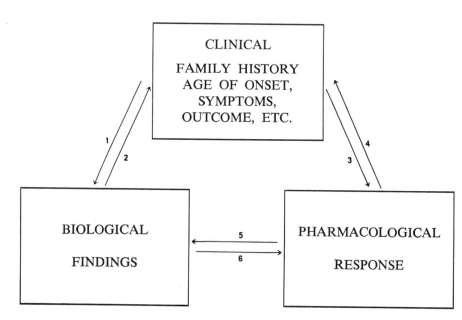

FIG. 1. Approaches to the validation of subgroups in psychiatry.

that clinical diagnostic groups differ with respect to a few biological variables or pharmacologic responses. Although such research may produce a provocative association, the meaning of the association is unclear. Such a relationship may be a spurious finding resulting from uncontrolled factors presumably extrinsic to the illness itself (such as diet). Or a relationship between diagnosis and biological finding may obscure a yet stronger association between some aspect of the clinical picture (such as anxiety) and the biological finding. Mere correlation is not particularly strong evidence.

The association would be more significant if the biological variable were nonnormally distributed, and if the groups of clustered points on the distribution corresponded well to clinically defined groups. The association would be still more meaningful if a biological change could be shown to be specific to a given clinical diagnosis.

Another pattern of findings would support the validity of extant clinical subgroups; if two variables showed a given relationship in one clinical subgroup but not in another (for example, if 5-HIAA in the CSF were strongly associated with imipramine response in unipolar depressed patients but not in bipolar), it would support the "meaningfulness" of that clinical distinction.

Biological Findings in Clinical Diagnostic Groups

In this section, we will outline significant findings which serve to support or question traditional clinical distinctions. As noted earlier, our primary focus will be the amine neurotransmitter research, and we will place particular emphasis on the findings in the affective disorders. The individual studies summarized below are discussed in detail by Goodwin et al. (24,28), and will not be individually referenced here.

Positive findings tend to support both the meaningfulness of the clinical groupings and the involvement of neurotransmitters in the disorders. Negative or inconsistent findings would suggest that (a) different diagnostic groupings are needed to demonstrate neurotransmitter abnormalities; (b) neurotransmitters do not play a key role in these illnesses; (c) our techniques for assessing neurotransmitter functioning are too crude to demonstrate a relationship; or (d) any combination of the above.

Baseline CSF Studies

Five of ten studies have found a decreased baseline level of 5-HIAA in depression compared to various "control" groups, whereas the other half found no significant difference. In the case of HVA, four of the six studies reported a deficit of HVA in depression compared to controls. In manic patients 5-HIAA has been reported as not different than controls in four studies, although not all studies agree. HVA has been found to be higher in manics than in depressed patients or controls in three out of five studies. With a few exceptions, baseline levels of 5-HIAA and HVA have not been reported as significantly different in patients with a variety of schizophrenic diagnoses compared to controls. For both metabolites much of the discrepancy in the results between investigators is related to the large differences in the values for the various "control" groups, presumably reflecting variability both in the composition of the groups and/or in the methods for obtaining the CSF.

Probenecid Studies

In relation to 5-HIAA, the two European studies report a significant deficit in accumulation in depressed patients compared to controls, whereas Bowers notes no differences in his overall group, but does find a 5-HIAA deficit in a subgroup of bipolar patients. In the NIMH study we noted a trend toward a low 5-HIAA accumulation in depressed patients compared to controls. In relation to HVA, our findings are clearly in agreement with the two European studies and with the data of Bowers for his bipolar patients in that the depressed patients are significantly lower than the controls, differences which cannot be attributed to differences in a level of probenecid found in the CSF.

With regard to schizophrenia, probenecid-induced accumulation of both 5-HIAA and HVA has not been demonstrated to be different from groups of controls or depressed patients. However, within a group of schizophrenics HVA accumulation on probenecid has been noted to be lowest in Schneiderian-positive poor prognosis schizophrenics, and the NIMH study noted a similar negative correlation between HVA accumulation and Schneiderian symptoms.

Urinary MHPG Studies

The distinctive urinary MHPG findings center on the affective disorders. Inconsistent results have been found in depressed patients, with some studies demonstrating decreased excretion and others failing to confirm this. MHPG has been reported to increase after recovery from depression and to be higher in the manic phase than in the depressed phase of bipolar affective illness.

The Question of Biologically Meaningful Subgroups Within Affective Illness

One of the striking features of amine metabolite studies in affective illness is the biochemical variability within a group of depressed patients who are apparently relatively homogeneous clinically. Several attempts have been made to explore metabolite differences in independently derived clinical subgroups of depressed patients. The unipolar-bipolar dichotomy by which patients with major depressive illness can be subdivided according to the pres-

TABLE 1. *Urinary MHPG in subgroups of depressed patients (μg/24 hr)*

	Bipolar	Unipolar	Schizo-affective	Controls	Comments
Maas et al. (36)	916[a] (N = 5)	1,070 (N = 5)	—	1,348 (N = 21)	Controls were outpatients. Means for groups computed after elimination of non-primary affective disorder patients.
Schildkraut et al. (47)	1,240 (N = 5)	1,800 (N = 6)	800 (N = 1)	—	Study reported difference between "manic-depressive depression" and "chronic characterologic depression."
Goodwin et al. (19)	1,020[a] (N = 11)	1,623 (N = 19)	880 (N = 5)	1,350 (N = 15)	

[a] Significantly lower than controls.

ence or absence, respectively of a prior history of mania has revealed significant differences between these subgroups in a wide variety of parameters including family history, age of onset, course, clinical features of the depression, biological measures, and therapeutic responses to specific drugs [reviewed in (13,15,54)]. Among the NIMH group of depressed patients subdivided according to the unipolar-bipolar dichotomy, no unipolar-bipolar differences in CSF amine metabolites were found, although some differences have been reported by others (4).

However, the unipolar-bipolar distinction does help clarify the inconsistent urinary MHPG findings noted above. Table 1 presents the data from the three major studies of urinary MHPG in depression. It can be seen that all three investigative groups report essentially the same mean values for the bipolar patients with the discrepancy being due to the unipolar group. On reflection, this is not surprising if one considers that diagnostic agreement concerning bipolar patients is more likely because these patients have a history of mania, an unusually clear and dramatic "marker." The unipolar diagnosis, on the other hand, tends to include a more heterogeneous group of patients. Unfortunately, the Research Diagnostic Criteria have not yet been available long enough to allow the collection of sufficient numbers of unipolar patients diagnosed prospectively according to its criteria.

Summary

The available data on CSF amine metabolites in affectively ill patients and normal controls do not convincingly support the concept of a straightforward biological continuum with depression at one end (deficiency), normal in the middle, and mania at the other end (excess), nor a continuum with schizophreniform psychosis at one end and the nonpsychotic state at the other. On the other hand, there is support for some significant clinical distinctions, such as the unipolar-bipolar distinction.

Similarly, the metabolite data do not support a single amine model, particularly in the case of affective illness where the most data are available. There is some evidence for alterations in dopamine, norepinephrine, and serotonin metabolism in depressive syndromes and evidence for changes in serotonin and dopamine metabolism in mania. Perhaps a disturbance originates in a single amine system subsequently producing secondary changes in interrelated systems. On the other hand, the possibility of an abnormality that would affect all amine systems should be considered. An alternative view might postulate "subgroups" corresponding to individual amines; however, in the absence of independent evidence for the existence of a subgroup (i.e., genetic, clinical, or pharmacologic evidence), such postulations remain speculations. The specificity issue becomes more broad when one conceptualizes the biology of the functional psychoses in terms of a complex and changing series of interactions between underlying (predisposing) abnormalities and more acute, superimposed dysfunctions.

Although it is clear that standardized traditional diagnostic groupings greatly facilitate the study of the major psychoses, the paucity of reproducible biological findings suggests that gross clinical groupings may not correspond well to identifiable single pathophysiologic derangements, at least as reflected in neurotransmitter studies. This is not surprising when one reflects on the multiple sources of variance in biological data, and the complex interrelationships within a functioning biological system.

Sources of Variance in Biological Data

We begin with an organism which is astoundingly complex in its natural state. It maintains a homeostatic balance, a steady *milieu internal,* through complex feedback mechanisms such as hormones, neurotransmitters, neuromodulators, enzyme induction, and changes in receptor sensitivities. These multiple compensatory changes are a prime source of interpretive difficulty for the researcher. Just as ketoacidosis is essentially a compensatory response and not the fundamental pathophysiology of diabetes, the different stages of mania (10) or of a schizophrenic episode (12) may reflect either the waxing and waning of a fundamental pathology or the intervention of compensatory mechanisms. Thus different phases of the natural history of the illness may produce radically different biological findings—yet in biological studies in psychiatry the phase of the illness is only rarely reported.

Other sources of variance may confound biological data in ways that are difficult to interpret meaningfully. Sex, age, diet, and activity are four ubiquitous, unavoidable sources of variance which must be dealt with in some way. Several illustrations of problems dealing with these sources of variance will illustrate the issue more clearly. There are sex differences in a wide variety of biological measures (enzyme activity, endocrine measures, urinary and CSF metabolites). If the sex effect is consistent from clinical group to group, then it would seem reasonable to sex standardize the data. Usually, however, the picture is far more complex. Recently Asberg and associates (2) reported a bimodal distribution of baseline 5-HIAA values in the CSF of drug-free patients with "endogenous" depression; we find a similar, apparently bimodal distribution in 5-HIAA among 78 drug-free depressed patients studied while on probenecid (26). However, in both studies males were predominant in the low 5-HIAA "subgroup." Across diagnostic groups CSF 5-HIAA is lower in males than females (43), and thus unequal sex distribution accounts for some of the bimodality in both studies. A similar question can be raised about a subsequent study of Asberg and colleagues (3) reporting a correlation between low 5-HIAA values and suicide attempts. If the sex distribution is similarly skewed, the question arises as to whether suicide attempts are related to a disorder of serotonin metabolism (manifested by low CSF 5-HIAA), to being male, or to some other biological variance correlated with sex (and thereby with low 5-HIAA).

Sometimes standardizing data can increase the power of the variable to differentiate subgroups. For example, earlier work from our group noted essentially the same modest but significant correlation between urinary MHPG and age in both the unipolar and bipolar depressed patients (19). In this instance, removing the contribution of age resulted in increasing the significance of the unipolar-bipolar differences in MHPG. On the other hand, there are two clear instances in which a variable which might be thought to have a consistent effect across subgroups (and thus be an appropriate variable to remove) turned out to be a critical means of differentiating subgroups. In depressed patients, discontinuation of a low monoamine diet resulted in significant increases in urinary MHPG (averaging 70% for the group), although this dietary alteration in normal controls studied under identical conditions on the same ward produced no change (41). Similarly, moderate exercise produced substantial increases in MHPG in bipolar depressed patients, but had no effect in normal controls (41).

An Alternate Approach to Clinical, Pharmacological, and Biological Heterogeneity

The difficulties finding clear-cut and replicable correlates of traditional diagnostic groups and the discovery of complex interrelationships among sources of biological and pharmacological variance have led to a reemphasis on careful observation of clinical heterogeneity, combined with parallel efforts to describe meaningful biological and pharmacological heterogeneity. Psychopharmacologists and clinicians have emphasized the usefulness of multidimensional diagnostic schemata which emphasize the partial independence of mood, activation, vegetative changes, and thought disorder. Corresponding multidimensional schemata of drug effects have been developed, such as neurotransmitter schemata (dopamine blockers, serotonin agonists, etc.) or behavioral schemata (drugs reducing avoidance behavior, augmenting locomotor activity, reducing excitement arousal, etc.) (29). The task then becomes one of interrelating observed variance on a variety of clinical, pharmacological, and biological dimensions, and using the observed interrelations to "control" possible sources of "extraneous" variance statistically, and to generate predictors or further hypotheses. The task becomes one necessitating multivariate techniques. The following two sections illustrate multivariate approaches to psychobiologic research which avoid the focus on correlates of traditional clinical diagnostic groupings.

MULTIVARIATE TECHNIQUES IN PREDICTIVE RESEARCH

Clinical practice provides one familiar model to illustrate this multivariate approach. Here we are concerned primarily with issues of prediction—prediction of course of illness and prediction of response to treatment. The clinician draws on history and observation of the individual and his own experience to classify the patient and choose a treatment. Particular facts, conscious or subliminal, may influence the clinician to use one drug in preference to another, and may influence his expectations of response.

Clinical research may aim to make this decision-making process more explicit and then to verify the decision-making paradigms in controlled clinical trials. Such decision making is easier if symptoms are highly specific for a given illness or drug response. Depression (a nonspecific syndrome) combined with sluggish reflexes, decreased thyroid hormones, and increased TSH (relatively specific signs) leads to a prediction of response to thyroid hormone supplementation. A fluctuating mental status with disorientation strongly suggests "organic" causes, although this observation is somewhat less specific. Unfortunately, predictors of course and response in the "functional" major psychiatric disorders seem to be far less specific and necessitate the use of relatively sophisticated multivariate techniques in order to increase predictive power.

Depressive syndromes illustrate this point. Recent articles by Murphy (40) and by Bielski and Friedel (7) review the controlled studies of clinical and biological findings which are associated with drug response. We might cast these studies in a more statistical manner by suggesting that, given someone with "depression," a broad heterogeneous syndrome, the probability of a response to imipramine, amitriptyline, phenelzine, lithium, or placebo can be calculated *a priori*. These clinical studies of drug response in depression suggest that the presence or absence of certain findings will then change the expected probability of a response to the different drugs. For example, a family history of response to a tricyclic increases the likelihood of a tricyclic response and may diminish the likelihood of response to other drugs. A history of bipolar illness increases the likelihood of lithium response. Endogenous symptoms probably increase the likelihood of response to the tricyclic antidepressants and decrease the likelihood of a placebo response.

Theoretically, one might develop equations using multivariate analytic techniques, which would predict drug response in a more objective way. Table 2 illustrates how such equations might be derived. Attempts to develop explicit probabilities of drug response based on clinical data might help ground our clinical intuition in scientific methodology.

In addition to this approach to predicting response using exclusively clinical variables, we can ask the further question of whether adding biological variables to the predictive equations improves their accuracy. For example, experimental findings, such as certain MMPI patterns (D. F. Donnelly, D. L. Murphy, I. N. Waldman, and F. K. Goodwin, *unpublished observations*), a euphoric response to amphetamine infusion (14), a reducing average evoked response pattern (M. Buchsbaum, F. K. Goodwin, and D. L. Murphy, *unpublished observations*), low urinary MHPG in a unipolar patient (5,37), and high CSF 5-HIAA in a unipolar patient (26) may be associated

TABLE 2. *Hypothetical data illustrating drug response prediction using a discriminant function approach*

Discriminant function analysis could be applied to a large-scale controlled study of clinical and biological variables and drug response. In this example, a D-score equation was generated for each drug and for placebo by choosing the clinical variables (Eq. 1) or the clinical and biological variables (Eq. 2) which contribute the most to discriminating known responders from known nonresponders. The equations might take the form:

Eq. 1 D (imipramine response) = 0.12 + 0.024 × (# of endogenous features) − 0.02 × (extent of delusions) + 0.02 × (unipolarity) + 0.01 × (psychomotor retardation) − 0.005 × (# of Schneiderian S's) . . .

Eq. 2 D (imipramine response) = 0.16 + 0.06 × (# of endogenous features) + 0.08 × (urinary MHPG) − 0.008 × (CSF 5-HIAA) + 0.014 × (unipolarity) − 0.03 × (extent of delusions) . . .

Although the multiplying factors in these equations do not necessarily reflect the relative weight that each individual variable contributes to response prediction, such relative weights (rank order of predictors) can be derived statistically.

These equations are then used to generate the probability that a given individual, with particular clinical and biological findings, will respond to a given drug.

Pharmacological agent	Hypothetical probability of response knowing only that the patient is "depressed"	Hypothetical probability of response generated from equations (like Eq. 1) using this patient's clinical data	Hypothetical probability of response generated from equations (like Eq. 2) using this patient's clinical and biological data
Lithium	0.42	0.66	0.72
Amitriptyline	0.60	0.82	0.80
Imipramine	0.55	0.76	0.89
Phenelzine	0.45	0.48	0.49
Placebo	0.33	0.20	0.19

with, and thereby increase the probability of, an imipramine response. We would then examine statistically whether using these biological tests would contribute to our ability to distinguish imipramine responders from non-responders.

Unfortunately, such multivariate equations cannot be developed from existing studies. Such multivariate techniques have prerequisites: (a) a numerically adequate and representative sample of patients, (b) thorough collection of basic observations by standardized techniques with high interrater reliability, and (c) data on most if not all of the variables studied for each of the patients contributing to the analysis. However, in studies to date, different patient populations, varying choices of relevant observations, unevenly controlled conditions of study, and disparate results make the choice and weight of variables for a given drug very difficult. The relative paucity of randomized trials and especially the lack of crossover studies make interdrug comparisons of response probabilities impossible.

Two recent studies, however, illustrate the potential of such statistical approaches. Using discriminant analytic techniques, Schildkraut et al. (49) developed a "D-type" equation employing urinary metabolites of neurotransmitters to discriminate patients with "chronic characterological depression" from bipolar depressed patients. The D-type equation "predicted polarity with 100% accuracy when applied prospectively to another group of 25 patients." In addition, the equation predicted future course of illness rather dramatically in one patient with clinically unipolar illness, who had been classified biochemically using the D-type equation as bipolar. Several months after the "prediction" was made (and not communicated to patient or therapist), he experienced his first hypomania at the age of 60. Donnelly et al. (*unpublished observations*) have developed four discriminant functions of MMPI items which predict imipramine and lithium response in males and females separately. These equations "predicted" drug response with 80 to 100% accuracy when applied to a second population of patients. Further studies with clinical, biological, and pharmacological variables are underway which may have clear relevance to clinical practice.

MULTIVARIATE APPROACHES TO FINDING "CAUSAL" CONNECTIONS

Whereas predictive research employs any variable which is associated with ("is a marker for," "predicts") a given outcome, without necessarily being concerned about the reasons for such an association, psychobiologic research ultimately aims to elucidate the causes of a given condition, the mechanisms by which these causes express themselves as an observable disorder, and the mechanisms by which treatments exert an effect on the illness. In short, the emphasis is on extracting causal relationships from among a wide variety of correlated observations.

Earlier in this chapter we discussed several sources of potentially confounding variance in biologic data, such as age, sex, diet, and activity. Although particularly problematic when the researcher is trying to demonstrate clear-cut biological differences between diagnostic subgroups, such sources of variance become potentially interesting data for the psychobiologist using multivariate concepts.

Thus, although researchers' attempts to demonstrate a single neurotransmitter abnormality in particular psychiatric disorders have yielded inconsistent results, these attempts have uncovered some preliminary but intriguing relationships between clinical, pharmacological, and biological variables. Our approach to psychobiologic research employs a relative "benign neglect" of classic clinical subgroups, with a corresponding emphasis on more discrete relationships among variables; we attempt to relate a symptom to a treatment response to a pathophysiologic mechanism, all of which may cut across traditional diagnostic groupings. In these final pages, we will illustrate several such psychobiologic approaches.

Naturalistic Studies

A direct approach involves the naturalistic study of symptoms and their relationship to demonstrable pathophysiology. Although it may not be clear whether a given biological finding is a cause of the clinical state, or is itself a consequence of the clinical state, or, like the clinical state, is caused by another more basic biological alteration, the naturalistic state remains a prime focus for research.

Two studies illustrate this naturalistic approach to define possible subgroups of depressed individuals. The first is Asberg's finding (3) of a relationship between the baseline level of 5-HIAA in the CSF of depressed patients and their overt behavior, particularly the negative correlation with the likelihood of a suicide gesture or attempt. Although there are conceptual problems with the study as we discussed earlier, such findings suggest that serotonin may be intimately involved in some depressive symptomatology, rather than being a "marker" for the entire depressive syndrome *per se*. Similarly, Goodwin et al. (18) studying a group of unipolar depressed patients found a significant relationship between anxiety and urinary MHPG excretion, apparently not accounted for by age. Assuming this is not due to confounding peripheral sources of norepinephrine metabolites, it suggests a role of central norepinephrine in anxiety associated with depression, whether causal, compensatory, or correlated.

These studies illustrate suggestive correlations between clinical and biological data; yet they are all studies of a highly limited series of variables, usually taken only two or three at a time (with some attempt to control for gross sources of variance). Larger studies using covariate techniques would allow much more powerful naturalistic explorations of psychobiologic mechanisms in psychiatric illness.

Studies Using Pharmacologic Interventions

A second approach to relating symptoms and pathophysiological mechanisms involves experimental manipulations which perturb the clinical-biochemical status quo. One manipulation which offers relative promise because of its close association with biologic mechanisms is the administration of drugs. Indeed, as noted earlier, pharmacology stimulated the original formulations of the neurotransmitter hypotheses based on known biological effects of the drugs. Drugs that increase the functional levels of one or more of the biogenic amines in the brain, such as tricyclic antidepressants and monoamine oxidase inhibitors, can alleviate some depressions when used clinically, whereas many drugs that block central dopamine receptors, such as the phenothiazines and butyrophenones, have potent tranquilizing properties and are quite useful in the treatment of the acute psychoses of schizophrenia and mania. Conversely, reserpine, a drug which decreases brain amines, can precipitate depression in some individuals, whereas amphetamine, which enhances catecholamine function, can precipitate or mimic the symptoms of acute schizophrenia.

In its conceptually pure form, a drug directly affecting only one pathophysiological mechanism is administered and its effects on the target symptoms observed. A change in the symptom indicates a causal link. In actuality, this "ideal" experiment is not possible for several reasons. First, techniques for measuring the effects of a given drug on neurotransmitter systems may give varying results. *In vitro* techniques in animals may not reflect *in vivo* drug effects in man. Second, drugs are seldom if ever specific. Although phenothiazines are predominantly blockers of dopamine receptors, they have effects on other neurotransmitter receptors, particularly those for norepinephrine. Tricyclic antidepressants generally affect the reuptake of both catecholamines and indoleamines, in degrees that vary from drug to drug. In addition, such potent drugs often have cholinergic or anticholinergic "side" effects. Finally, the direct effects of the drug may induce compensatory responses in the organism—altered activity in antagonistic pathways, feedback inhibition or excitation of the same or parallel pathways, or changed receptor functioning (e.g., hypersensitivity) (42). Nonetheless, pharmacologic response studies which seek to relate clinical response to biological mechanisms are promising; several examples drawn largely from research in the affective disorders should illustrate these relationships.

Specific Pharmacologic Actions and Specific Target Symptoms

Studies of the response of manic and depressive symptomatology to a variety of pharmacologic agents suggest that certain symptoms may be

TABLE 3. Drugs which decrease catecholamine function: clinical effects in manic patients

Drug	Relative decrease in catecholaminergic function		Effects on manic symptoms[a]		
	NE	DA	Elation grandiosity	Hyperactivity arousal	Psychosis
Reserpine	+++	+++	+++	+++	+++
Phenothiazines	++	++++	+	++++	++
Haloperidol	++	++++	+	++++	++
Pimozide	0?	++++	+	++++	++
AMPT	+++	+++	+++	+++	+++
Lithium	+++	+?	+++	+	+
Fusaric acid	+	−	+?	0	−

[a] See text for descriptions.

associated with changes in specific neurotransmitters. It has been widely known that antimanic drugs generally decrease catecholamine function at the postsynaptic receptor, through receptor blockade (phenothiazines), synthesis inhibition (alpha-methyl-para-tyrosine), or transmitter depletion (reserpine). More recently, several studies (30,44) have suggested some symptom specificity to the antimanic responses, especially in a comparison of chlorpromazine and lithium. The neurotransmitter effects noted in *in vitro* studies and the symptomatic responses most commonly seen are summarized in Table 3. Although the overlapping amine effects of drugs make clear-cut conclusions impossible, there is a suggestion of a relationship between noradrenergic functioning and the elation-grandiosity dimension. Similarly, the data suggest a possible association between dopaminergic function and the hyperactivity-arousal dimension. The correlation between dopaminergic treatment effects and psychosis is only suggestive, but would be consistent with presumed dopaminergic mechanisms in schizophrenic psychosis.

Similarly, Table 4 illustrates two interesting observations of differential symptom responses in depression. When large doses of the catecholamine precursor L-DOPA were administered to depressed patients, they showed some improvement in psychomotor retardation (activation), but not improvement in mood or cognition (20). Similarly L-tryptophan, the amino

TABLE 4. Symptom responses in depression

Agent	Presumed effects on neurotransmitters at receptor		Effects on depression	
	NE	5-HT	Psychomotor retardation	Depressed mood
L-DOPA	↑↑	0	↓↓	0
L-Tryptophan and a tricyclic	↑	↑↑↑	0	↓↓

acid precursor of serotonin, has recently been shown to potentiate the effects of a tricyclic antidepressant on depressed mood and anxiety, but not on the level of psychomotor activity or arousal (53). These and other pharmacological data suggest that there may be some relationship between specific amine changes and distinct symptoms or clusters of symptoms.

Pharmacological Activity and Biological Measurements as Predictors of Drug Response

Animal studies [reviewed in (35)] and, more recently, clinical studies (6,26) suggest that the various tricyclic compounds have different effects on the blockade of serotonin and norepinephrine reuptake. The results of these studies are summarized in Table 5. To understand the clinical implication of these findings, it is important to note that the tertiary amines (chlorimipramine, amitriptyline, and imipramine) are partially converted by the liver to the corresponding secondary amines (desmethylchlorimipramine, nortriptyline, and desipramine). Thus, after "steady-state" is achieved in a patient taking amitriptyline, both amitriptyline and nortriptyline are present in the system. The few available studies of tricyclic levels indicate that, although there appear to be considerable interindividual variations in ratios of parent drug to metabolite, the parent drug amitriptyline predominates over nortriptyline in plasma (8), suggesting drug effects which are more serotonergic than noradrenergic. In contrast to this, desipramine apparently predominates over imipramine in CSF (23), suggesting drug effects which are more noradrenergic than serotonergic. Given this spectrum of drug activity, one would hope to find a parallel spectrum of serotonergic and noradrenergic activity in the patients studied. The following amine metabolite studies provide the most direct evidence for the existence of such a spectrum.

As illustrated by the third column of Table 6, the concentration of 5-HIAA

TABLE 5. *Summary of effects of various antidepressant drugs on blockade of uptake of biogenic amines*

Drug	Biogenic amines		
	5-HT	NE	DA
Chlorimipramine	+++++	0	0
Desmethylchlorimipramine	+	++	0
Amitriptyline	++++	0?	0
Nortriptyline	++	+++	0
Imipramine	+++	++	0
Desipramine	0	++++	0

For a detailed review of the relevant literature see references 6, 26, and 35.

in the CSF of unipolar patients is significantly associated with drug response, in a way which is consistent with the spectrum of drug activity described in the preceding section. In a study of unipolar depressed patients in the drug-free state, van Praag (51) found that individuals who subsequently responded to chlorimipramine, a primarily serotonergically active drug, had lower concentrations of 5-HIAA in the CSF following probenecid than did the chlorimipramine nonresponders. In our studies of amitriptyline, a drug with somewhat less serotonergic predominance, 5-HIAA in the drug-free state was a less powerful predictor of drug response, showing only a trend toward lower levels in responders. On the other hand, both Asberg (1), using baseline CSF values, and van Praag (52), using the probenecid technique, were able to demonstrate that individuals who subsequently failed to respond to nortriptyline, a drug with greater noradrenergic properties, had 5-HIAA levels that were low compared to nortriptyline responders. Goodwin et al. (26) demonstrated a similar relationship between pretreatment 5-HIAA and response to imipramine, another drug with greater noradrenergic activity.

We then examined studies reporting relationships between urinary MHPG and drug response (see the last column of Table 6). Studies by Schildkraut (47) involving a mixed group of hospitalized depressed patients and by Beckmann and Goodwin (5) involving only unipolar patients reported that patients who failed to respond to amitriptyline (a relatively serotonergically active drug) had low pretreatment levels of urinary MHPG compared to those who subsequently responded. Conversely, Maas and his associates (37) and later Beckmann and Goodwin (5) demonstrated that responders to imipramine (a relatively noradrenergically active agent) have low pretreatment urinary MHPG levels compared to nonresponders.

Unfortunately, the opposite patterns of drug response prediction shown by 5-HIAA in CSF and MHPG in urine are derived from eight different studies, each with a different patient population. No study has reported both

TABLE 6. *Tricyclic responder nonresponder differences in unipolar depression: relation to pretreatment levels of monoamine metabolites*

	Drug	CSF 5-HIAA	Urinary MHPG
Drugs with predominantly serotonergic effects	Chlorimipramine	Responders ▼ (51)	
	Amitriptyline	Responders ▼ (29)	Responders (△ 5, 50*)
Drugs with predominantly noradrenergic effects	Nortriptyline	Responders △ (1, 55)	
	Imipramine	Responders △ (29)	Responders ▼ (5, 40*)

Responders ▼ = lower than nonresponders; responders △ = higher than nonresponders.
*The studies of Schildkraut and of Maas did not separate unipolar and bipolar depressed patients.

5-HIAA and MHPG findings in the same individuals, allowing for direct comparison of noradrenergic or serotonergic predominance in a given depressed person. However, we have studied both 5-HIAA and MHPG in another series of patients. When patients with probenecid-induced CSF 5-HIAA levels below 100 ng/ml (the "low 5-HIAA" subgroup) were compared with those patients with levels above 100 ng/ml (the "high 5-HIAA" subgroup), a significantly higher urinary MHPG level was found in the low 5-HIAA subgroup (21,26). This finding lends support to the possibility that levels of 5-HIAA show a reciprocal relationship to levels of MHPG in depressed individuals, perhaps suggesting the existence of low 5-HIAA–high MHPG and high 5-HIAA–low MHPG subgroups of depressed patients.

If this proves to be the case, it would support our assertion that biological research may result in diagnostic groupings which do not correspond well with traditional clinical distinctions, either because a given biological abnormality is common to patients with varied clinical diagnoses (e.g., a common abnormality underlying psychosis), or because a given biological abnormality explains variance within a clinical diagnostic group and yet has no known clinical correlates (e.g., the low and high 5-HIAA subgroups of unipolar depressed patients).

FUTURE DIRECTIONS

Traditional clinical diagnoses have provided a convenient framework for grouping patients, both clinically and for research. It is not yet clear, however, whether such groupings are the most meaningful way to classify illnesses. In some instances, there are substantial biological and pharmacological supports for clinical distinctions, such as schizophrenia versus affective disorder and unipolar versus bipolar affective disorder. Yet it is conceivable that a relatively rigid adherence to traditional diagnoses may obscure similarities across diagnostic groups and heterogeneities within them, which have more biological significance than the diagnoses themselves.

We have suggested that the tremendous complexity of the biological systems probably involved in psychiatric disorders may necessitate more sophisticated research designs consistent with multivariate statistical techniques. There is a need for multidimensional studies in a broadly representative group of patients—studies which will allow clearer statements about the interrelationships of symptoms, history, genetic liabilities, biological abnormality, and response to pharmacologic agents. So long as the research focuses on a few relationships between variables in one study and other relationships between variables in another study using different patients, the powerful statistical techniques of multivariate analysis will remain unavailable to us.

Progress in sorting out complex biological relationships may also result from the use of pharmacologic agents with more specific biological effects. Several of these agents are currently under investigation. With regard to the dopaminergic system, pimozide appears to have greater specificity as a dopamine blocking agent than do the commonly used antipsychotic medications. Piribedil (ET-495) is a drug with relative specificity for the dopaminergic system, apparently acting as an agonist under some conditions and an antagonist under others. Similarly, cyproheptadine may be a more specific serotonin agonist than other available agents; and zymelidine seems to have a high specificity for blockade of serotonin reuptake as opposed to norepinephrine. Such agents may help clarify the relationships between neurotransmitter systems, symptoms, and drug response.

Natually, there is also a need for improved techniques for *in vivo* assessment of physiological functioning in patients. But in spite of these shortcomings of clinical-biological research, it is not premature to suggest that, although the research to date has not clearly identified causal pathophysiological mechanisms in the major psychiatric disorders, it has begun to delineate a complex set of interrelated mechanisms associated with disturbances of activity, cognition, and mood. Several studies additionally suggest that biological data may help describe more meaningful groupings of psychiatric illnesses, and may help guide the clinician's choice of an effective treatment.

REFERENCES

1. Asberg, M., Bertilsson, L., Tuck, D., Cronholm, B., and Sjoqvist, F. (1973): Indoleamine metabolites in the cerebrospinal fluid of depressed patients before and during treatment with nortriptyline. *Clin. Pharmacol. Ther.,* 14:277–286.
2. Asberg, M., Thoren, P., Traskman, L., Bertilsson, L., and Ringberger, V. (1976): "Serotonin depression"—A biochemical subgroup within the affective disorders? *Science,* 191:478–480.
3. Asberg, M., Traskman, L., and Thoren, P. (1976): 5-HIAA in the cerebrospinal fluid. *Arch. Gen. Psychiatry,* 33:1193–1197.
4. Ashcroft, G. W., Crawford, T. B. B., Eccleston, D., Sharman, D. F., MacDougall, E. J., Stanton, J. B., and Binns, J. K. (1966): 5-Hydroxyindole compounds in the cerebrospinal fluid of patients with psychiatric or neurological diseases. *Lancet,* 2:1049–1052.
5. Beckman, H., and Goodwin, F. K. (1975): Antidepressant response to tricyclics and urinary MHPG in unipolar patients. *Arch. Gen. Psychiatry,* 32:17–21.
6. Bertilsson, L., Asberg, M., and Thoren, P. (1974): Differential effect of chlorimipramine and nortriptyline on cerebrospinal fluid metabolites of serotonin and noradrenaline in depression. *Eur. J. Clin. Pharmacol.,* 7:365–368.
7. Bielski, R. J., and Friedel, R. O. (1976): Prediction of tricyclic antidepressant response. *Arch. Gen. Psychiatry,* 33:1479–1489.
8. Braithwaite, R. A., and Widdop, B. (1971): A specific gas chromatographic method for the measurement of "steady state" plasma levels of amitriptyline and nortriptyline in patients. *Clin. Chim. Acta,* 35:461–472.
9. Bunney, W. E., Jr., and Davis, J. M. (1965): Norepinephrine in depressive reactions. *Arch. Gen. Psychiat.,* 13:483–494.
10. Carlson, G. A., and Goodwin, F. K. (1973): The stages of mania: A longitudinal analysis of the manic episode. *Arch. Gen. Psychiatry,* 28:221–228.
11. Cooper, J. E., Kendel, R. E., Gurland, B. J., Sharpe, L., Copeland, J. R. M., and Simon, R. (1972): *Psychiatric Diagnosis in New York and London.* Oxford University Press, London.
12. Docherty, J. P., van Kammen, D. P., Siris, S. G., and Marder, S. R. (1977): Stages of onset of schizophrenic psychosis. *Am. J. Psychiatry (in press).*

13. Dunner, D. L., Gershon, E. S., and Goodwin, F. K. (1976): Heritable factors in the severity of affective illness. *Biol. Psychiatry,* 11:31–42.
14. Fawcett, J., and Siomapoulos, V. (1971): Dextroamphetamine response as a possible predictor of improvement with tricyclic therapy in depression. *Arch. Gen. Psychiatry,* 25:247–255.
15. Gershon, E. (1977): The search for genetic markers in affective disorder. In: *Psychopharmacology—A Generation of Progress,* edited by M. Lipton, A. DiMascio, and K. Killam. Raven Press, New York (*in press*).
16. Goodall, McC., and Alton, H. (1968): Metabolism of 3-hydroxytryptamine (dopamine) in human subjects. *Biochem. Pharmacol.,* 17:905–914.
17. Goodall, McC., and Rosen, L. (1963): Urinary excretion of noradrenaline and its metabolites at ten-minute intervals after intravenous injection of dl-noradrenaline-2-C^{14}. *J. Clin. Invest.,* 42:1578–1588.
18. Goodwin, F. K., and Beckmann, H. (1974): Paper read at the World Congress of Psychiatry, Section on Biological Psychiatry, Munich, Germany.
19. Goodwin, F. K., and Beckmann, H. (1975): Urinary MHPG in unipolar and bipolar affective disorders. *Sci. Proc. Am. Psychiatr. Assoc.,* 128:96–97.
20. Goodwin, F. K., Brodie, H. K. H., Murphy, D. L., and Bunney, W. E., Jr. (1970): L-DOPA, catecholamines and behavior: A clinical and biochemical study in depressed patients. *Biol. Psychiatry,* 2:341–366.
21. Goodwin, F. K., Cowdry, R., and Webster, M. (1977): Predictors of pharmacological efficacy in the affective disorders. In: *Psychopharmacology—A Generation of Progress,* edited by M. Lipton, A. DiMascio, and K. Killam, pp. 1277–1288. Raven Press, New York.
22. Goodwin, F. K., and Murphy, D. L. (1974): Biological factors in the affective disorders and schizophrenia. In: *Psychopharmacological Agents, Vol. III,* edited by M. Gordon, pp. 9–37. Academic Press, New York.
23. Muscettola, G., Goodwin, F. K., Potter, W. Z., Cloeys, M. M., and Markey, S. P. (1977): Imipramine and desipramine in plasma and spinal fluid: Relationship to clinical response and serotonin metabolism. *Arch. Gen. Psychiatry* (*in press*).
24. Goodwin, F. K., and Post, R. M. (1975): Studies of amine metabolites in affective illness and in schizophrenia: A comparative analysis. In: *The Biology of the Major Psychoses,* edited by D. Freedman, pp. 299–332. Raven Press, New York.
25. Goodwin, F. K., Post, R. M., Dunner, D. L., and Gordon, E. K. (1973): Cerebrospinal fluid amine metabolites in affective illness: The probenecid technique. *Am. J. Psychiatry,* 130:73–79.
26. Goodwin, T. K., Cowdry, R., Jimerson, D., and Post, R. L. (1977): Serotonin and norepinephrine "subgroups" in depression. *Sci. Proc. Amer. Psychiat. Assoc.,* 130:108.
27. Goodwin, F. K., and Sack, R. L. (1974): Central dopamine function in affective illness: Evidence from precursors, enzyme inhibitors, and studies of central dopamine turnover. In: *Neuropsychopharmacology of Monoamines and Their Regulatory Enzymes,* edited by E. Usdin, pp. 261–279. Raven Press, New York.
28. Goodwin, F. K., Wehr, T., and Post, R. M. (1977): Clinical approaches to the evaluation of brain amine function in mental iilness: Some conceptual issues. In: *Essays in Neurochemistry and Neuropharmacology,* edited by W. Lovenberg and M. Youdim. John Wiley & Sons, London (*in press*).
29. Irwin, Samuel (1974): How to prescribe psychoactive drugs. *Bull. Menninger Clin.,* 38:1–13.
30. Johnson, G., Gershon, S., Burdock, E. I., Floyd, A., and Hekimian, L. (1971): Comparative effects of lithium and chlorpromazine in the treatment of acute manic states. *Br. J. Psychiatry,* 119:267–276.
31. Kessler, J. A., Gordon, E. K., Reid, J. L., and Kopin, I. J. (1976): Homovanillic acid and 3-methoxy-4-hydroxyphenylethyleneglycol production by the monkey spinal cord. *J. Neurochem.,* 26:1057–1061.
32. Kopin, I. J. (1976): Measuring turnover of neurotransmitters in human brain.

Presented at the Fifteenth Annual Meeting, American College of Neuropsychopharmacology, Quebec City.

33. Kreitman, N. (1961): The reliability of psychiatric diagnosis. *J. Ment. Sci.,* 107: 876–886.
34. Lovenberg, W., and Engelman, K. (1971): Assay of serotonin, related metabolites and enzymes. *Meth. Biochem. Anal.,* 19:1–34.
35. Maas, J. W. (1975): Biogenic amines and depression. *Arch. Gen. Psychiatry,* 32: 1357–1361.
36. Maas, J. W., Fawcett, J. A., and Dekirmenjian, H. (1968): 3-Methoxy-4-hydroxyphenylglycol (MHPG) excretion in depressive patients: A pilot study. *Arch. Gen. Psychiatry,* 19:129–134.
37. Maas, J. W., Fawcett, J. A., and Dekirmenjian, H. (1972): Catecholamine metabolism, depressive illness, and drug response. *Arch. Gen. Psychiatry,* 26:252–262.
38. Matthysse, S. (1977): Central catecholamine metabolism in psychosis. In: *Neurotransmission and Disturbed Behavior,* edited by H. M. van Praag. De Erven Bohn BV, Amsterdam (*in press*).
39. Moir, A. T. B., Ashcroft, G. W., Crawford, T. B. B., Eccleston, D., and Guldberg, T. C. (1970): Central metabolites in cerebrospinal fluid as a biochemical approach to the brain. *Brain,* 93:357–368.
40. Murphy, D. L., Shiling, D., and Murray, R. (1977): Psychoactive drug responder subgroups: Possible contributions to psychiatric classification. In: *Psychopharmacology—A Generation of Progress,* edited by M. Lipton, A. DiMascio, and K. Killam, pp. 807–820. Raven Press, New York.
41. Muscettola, G., Wehr, T., and Goodwin, F. K. (1976): Central norepinephrine responses in depression versus normals. Presented at the Annual Meeting, American Psychiatric Association, *New Research Abstracts,* p. 8, Miami, Florida.
42. Post, R. M., and Goodwin, F. K. (1975): Time-dependent effects of phenothiazines on dopamine turnover in psychiatric patients. *Science,* 190:488–489.
43. Post, R. M., and Goodwin, F. K. (1975): Studies of cerebrospinal fluid amine metabolites in depressed patients: Conceptual problems and theoretical implications. In: *The Psychology of Depression,* edited by J. Mendels, pp. 47–67. Spectrum Publications, New York.
44. Prien, R. F., Caffey, E. M., Jr., and Klett, C. J. (1972): Comparison of lithium carbonate and chlorpromazine in the treatment of mania. *Arch. Gen. Psychiatry,* 26:146–153.
45. Sachar, E. J. (Ed.) (1976): *Hormones, Behavior and Psychopathology.* Raven Press, New York.
46. Schildkraut, J. J. (1965): The catecholamine hypothesis of affective disorders: A review of supporting evidence. *Am. J. Psychiatry,* 122:509–522.
47. Schildkraut, J. J. (1973): Norepinephrine metabolites as biochemical criteria for classifying depressive disorders and predicting responses to treatment: Preliminary findings. *Am. J. Psychiatry,* 130:695–698.
48. Schildkraut, J. J. (1973): Depressions and biogenic amines. In: *American Handbook of Psychiatry, Vol. 4.* edited by D. Hamburg. Basic Books, New York.
49. Schildkraut, J. J., Orsulak, P. J., Gudeman, J. E., Schatzberg, A. F., Rohde, W. A., LaBrie, R. A., Cahill, J. F., Cole, J. O., and Frazier, S. H. (1977): Norepinephrine metabolism in depressive disorders: Implications for a biochemical classification of depressions. In: *Biology and Treatment of Depression,* edited by J. M. Cole, S. Frazier, and A. F. Schatzberg, pp. 75–101. Plenum Press, New York.
50. Snyder, S. H., Banerjee, S. P., Yamamura, H. I., and Greenberg, D. (1974): Drugs, neurotransmitters and schizophrenia. *Science,* 184:1243–1253.
51. van Praag, H. M. (1977): Significance of biochemical parameters in the diagnosis, treatment and prevention of depressive disorders. *Biol. Psychiatry* (*in press*).
52. van Praag, H. M., and Korf, J. (1976): 4-Chloramphetamines. In: *Psychotherapeutic Drugs,* edited by E. Usdin and I. S. Forrest. Marcel Dekker, New York.
53. Walinder, J., Skott, A., Carlsson, A., Nagy, A., and Roos, B.-E. (1976): Potentiation of the antidepressant action of clomipramine by tryptophan. *Arch. Gen. Psychiatry,* 33:1384–1389.

54. Winokur, G. (1977): Mania and depression: Family studies, genetics, and relation to treatment. In: *Psychopharmacology—A Generation of Progress,* edited by M. Lipton, A. DiMascio, and K. Killam, pp. 1213–1222. Raven Press, New York.
55. World Health Organization (1973): *Report of the International Pilot Study of Schizophrenia, Vol. 1.* World Health Organization, Geneva.

Critical Issues in Psychiatric Diagnosis,
edited by Robert L. Spitzer and Donald F. Klein.
Raven Press, New York © 1978.

Neurotransmitter-Related Enzymes and Psychiatric Diagnostic Entities

Dennis L. Murphy and Monte S. Buchsbaum

Clinical Neuropharmacology Branch and Adult Psychiatry Branch, National Institute of Mental Health, Bethesda, Maryland 20014

Various aspects of brain neurotransmitter function have been shown to be genetically influenced. Differences between rodent strains have been reported for a number of brain enzymes in biogenic amine and other neurotransmitter pathways, including tyrosine hydroxylase (96), acetylcholinesterase (90,107), aromatic *l*-amino acid decarboxylase (90), phenylethanolamine *N*-methyl transferase (16), and monoamine oxidase (MAO) (6,54,107). In addition, other aspects of neurotransmitter-related structure and function such as the number of dopamine neurons (96) and catecholamine receptor sensitivity (102) have been found to differ in various mouse and rat strains. In primates, species differences have been reported for one biogenic amine-related enzyme, monoamine oxidase (74). In man, significant monozygotic-dizygotic differences or sibling-sibling correlations have been found for MAO, dopamine-β-hydroxylase (DBH) and catechol-O-methyl transferase (COMT) activity measured in plasma or blood cells (36,67,80,97,112).

There is substantial evidence for familial and in some cases definite genetic contributions to schizophrenia, bipolar and unipolar affective disorders, alcoholism, and other psychiatric disorders, including possibly some of the neuroses (24,61). Individual differences in neurotransmitter-related enzymes would seem to provide one possible mechanism mediating genetic vulnerability for these disorders. Although considerations of how enzyme measurements might be relevant for psychiatric disorders and their diagnosis have focused most on genetic models, enzyme measurements in other areas of medicine have also proved of value in providing laboratory indices of acute organ pathology (e.g., plasma enzyme changes in various heart, liver, or brain disorders) and occasionally in predicting side effects from drugs (e.g., succinylcholine supersensitivity associated with low plasma pseudocholinesterase activity). This chapter will briefly review the present status of studies of neurotransmitter-related enzymes in psychiatric patient populations. It will also consider the models which underlie these studies, and some consequences of these models for methodology in this field.

ENZYMES MEASURED IN PSYCHIATRIC
PATIENT POPULATIONS

Most of the studies reviewed below have examined neurotransmitter-related enzymes found in plasma or blood cells, especially platelets and erythrocytes. Only a very few other tissues such as muscle have been biopsied for enzyme determinations. Post-mortem brain studies may confirm results in other tissues, but methodological problems reduce their usefulness, and they are inapplicable to problems of diagnosis or longitudinal follow-up.

Dopamine β-Hydroxylase

DBH converts dopamine to norepinephrine (50), and would seem of relevance to the various hypotheses relating these catecholamines to such psychiatric disorders as depression, mania, schizophrenia, and anxiety. DBH can be measured in plasma or serum. It is present in brain, the adrenal gland, and tissues with sympathetic nervous system innervation. DBH in plasma is not known to differ in its properties from DBH in other tissues, and it is thought that plasma DBH is released from vesicles in noradrenergic nerve terminals. Factors regulating its release into plasma and its removal from plasma are incompletely understood. Several reviews of plasma DBH studies have been published recently (1,44).

In studies in patients with psychiatric disorders, no differences in plasma or serum DBH have generally been found when depressed, manic, or schizophrenic patient groups were compared with controls (22,34,46,113). There is one recent report of decreased serum DBH activity in psychotically depressed unipolar patients (59) and another recent report of increased serum DBH activity in a large number of patients with various psychiatric and neurological disorders, including schizophrenia, depression, and alcoholism but not mania (55). In patients with neurological or other medical disorders, higher plasma or serum activities of DBH have been found associated with torsion dystonia (118,123), neuroblastoma (33), Huntington's disease (51), hypothyroidism (81), and the Lesch-Nyhan syndrome (95). Decreased DBH activity has been reported in Down's syndrome (26), Parkinson's disease (51), hyperthyroidism (81,82), familial dysautonomia (27, 111), and primary orthostatic hypotension (124).

Among the factors which have been evaluated as possible contributors to individual differences in plasma DBH activity, no male versus female enzyme activity differences have been observed (84,97,111–113) with the exception of one study which reported higher values in women (42). Plasma DBH activity is lower in children but generally has not been found to vary appreciably with age in adults (27,84,97,111–113), although in two other studies small correlations (both positive and negative) with age have been observed (27,84). Although DBH activity remains quite stable over time in individuals studied repetitively, small elevations have been observed in response to diurnal activity changes, exercise, and other stimuli which activate the sympathetic nervous system (25,30,49,83,85,88,105,117). A number of drugs including a specific inhibitor, fusaric acid (56), and haloperidol (55) reduce plasma DBH activity. Increases in DBH activity have been reported during treatment with imipramine (92), methylphenidate (92), amphetamine (55), and electroshock (45).

Erythrocyte Catechol-O-Methyl Transferase

This cytoplasmic enzyme catalyzes an important step in the degradation of dopamine, norepinephrine, epinephrine, and their deaminated metabolites. It acts sequentially with monoamine oxidase to yield homovanillic acid (HVA), vanylmandelic acid (VMA), 3-methoxy, 4-hydroxyphenylglycol (MHPG), and other catecholamine metabolites measured in the urine and cerebrospinal fluid in many studies of psychiatric patients. In addition to its localization in brain, liver, and other tissues, it is also found in human erythrocytes and leukocytes (2,3). Erythrocyte COMT has been most often investigated in clinical studies; the properties of this enzyme appear similar to those found in studies of COMT in other tissues (2,18).

In studies of COMT in psychiatric patient groups, this enzyme was originally reported to be reduced in activity in female unipolar (12,18,21) and bipolar (18,21) depressed patients, but normal in male patients (18,21). More recently, contradictory studies have appeared, with one investigation finding no differences in female unipolar depressed patients (114), and one finding slightly higher COMT activity in unipolar and bipolar patients of both sexes (32). In the latter study, a similar difference from controls was not seen in well relatives of these patients. In schizophrenic patients, no difference from controls was observed in three studies (18,21,57), whereas one other study reported a significant increase in COMT activity (114). Different assay procedures were used by three of the four different laboratory groups. In nonpsychiatric patient populations investigated, parkinsonian patients had normal activity (29) whereas children with Down's syndrome had elevated activities (37).

No sex or age differences in COMT activity have been noted in these studies, with the exception that higher activities were found in males included in one study (32). The enzyme has been described as stable over time in individuals studied repetitively (21). Although L-DOPA and estrogens reduce COMT activity (12,29), most psychotropic drugs investigated have been said not to influence erythrocyte COMT activity. Some of the variations in activity found with the different assays for COMT may be related to a recently reported activation of the enzyme by calcium (91).

Platelet Monoamine Oxidase

This enzyme is located in mitochondria and catalyzes the oxidative deamination of many biogenic amines. Although most tissues in most species contain both the A and B forms of MAO, the human platelet enzyme exhibits properties of the B form only (20,69). Recently, nonhuman primate brain has been demonstrated to contain predominantly MAO-B activity in contrast to the nearly equal amounts of MAO-A and MAO-B found in the many studies of rat and mouse brain MAO; less complete data have also suggested that human brain might possess relatively more MAO-B activity than is found in most other species (69,70,104). In all characteristics studied, platelet MAO activity appears essentially identical to MAO-B in brain and other tissues (20,69). Both the MAO-A and MAO-B types are sensitive to the MAO-inhibiting drugs used as antidepressant and antihypertensive drugs.

In studies of patients with psychiatric disorders, platelet MAO activity has generally been found to be reduced in chronic schizophrenic patients in comparison to controls [for a recent review, see (71)]. Paranoid schizophrenic patients, in particular, exhibit reduced MAO activity (89,100), whereas acute schizophrenic patients in various studies showed no reduction or a lesser reduction in enzyme activity (14,60). Chronic schizophrenic patients maintained without antipsychotic drugs in a research setting for a minimum of 6 months showed markedly lower MAO activity (with no overlap with controls) in one study (19), whereas in another, larger study of chronic schizophrenic patients selected for treatment without drugs, no differences from controls were observed (86).

In patients with affective disorders, comparisons of hospitalized bipolar and unipolar depressed patients have revealed reduced MAO activity in bipolar patients (75) and their families (48), but no differences from controls in unipolar patients, although not all studies are in agreement (7,47). One study reported higher platelet MAO activity in a mixed group of depressed patients (79). Individuals with alcoholism have also been reported to have reduced platelet MAO activity (106).

Reduced MAO activity would not seem to be a result of being ill, as first-degree, well relatives of patients with bipolar affective disorders and schizophrenia (48,119) and the well twins in a study of monozygotic twins discordant for schizophrenia (120) all manifested equivalent reductions in MAO activity when compared to their ill relatives. In addition, comparisons of patients with depression, mania, or acute schizophrenia studied at the time of hospital admission and again at discharge did not yield greater differences than found for normals studied repetitively (66,77). It has been suggested that MAO functions in a regulatory fashion for several components of neurotransmitter amine metabolism, and that reduced MAO activity may represent one contributing factor predisposing to the affective disorders, chronic schizophrenia, and other forms of psychopathology (63,64,67,75).

Iron deficiency anemia (122), Down's syndrome (9), and migraine (99) have also been reported to be associated with reduced MAO activity; other investigations of patients with Down's syndrome (52) and muscular dystrophy (53) have demonstrated normal MAO activities.

Among various factors evaluated for possible influences on platelet MAO activity, sex differences have been reported in several studies, with females having higher activities (76,94). A tendency for platelet MAO activity to increase with age was found in one (94) but not several other investigations (47,76). Small changes occur during the human menstrual cycle (8). Various drugs in addition to the MAO inhibitors may affect platelet MAO activity, including the tricyclic antidepressants (23) and epinephrine (31). Contradictory results have been reported for lithium carbonate (10,87), whereas the phenothiazines do not appear to affect the enzyme (67) or may increase it slightly (86). Although animal studies have suggested that some hormones may affect the activity of the enzyme, reduced MAO activity in chronic schizophrenic patients does not appear to be accompanied by alterations in testosterone or thyroid hormone levels (66).

Platelet MAO activities measured over various time intervals in the same individual remain generally stable (66,76). Variations as great as those observed during the menstrual cycle (15 to 20%) are observed with repeated samplings in both sexes, but these differences are of relatively small import when contrasted with the 20-fold differences between individuals (76).

Other Enzymes

A number of enzymes which function in neurotransmitter pathways or which may affect the metabolism of neurotransmitter substances have begun to be studied in psychiatric patient groups. Only one or two reports are available for each of these enzymes, and generally the assessment of the effects of psychoactive drugs and of other factors which may affect the activity of these enzymes is limited. Among these enzymes are a plasma amine oxidase, an indoleamine *N*-methyl transferase which forms triptolines, a catecholamine-responsive adenyl cyclase, Mg- and Na-K-adenosine triphosphatases which are components of membrane cation pumps, histamine *N*-methyl transferase, a methanol-forming enzyme, ITP phosphohydrolase, and purine phosphoribosyl transferase (4,15,18,40,41,62,72,73,78,108–110,121). Two siblings with schizophrenic-like behavior and deficient 5,10-methylenetetrahydrofolate reductase activity have been reported, and provide one recent plausible example of a specific genetic disorder leading to symptoms resembling schizophrenia (28; J. M. Freedman, *personal communication*). Of additional interest, platelet MAO activity was reduced in one of the siblings studied during a period of psychosis, and platelet MAO activities tended to be low in other family members as well (28).

DISCUSSION

As reviewed above, differences in the activities of over 10 different enzymes between psychiatric patient groups and controls have been reported in the last few years. These findings have generated wide attention, as differences in enzyme function and structure constitute the mechanisms by which many of the well-known genetic disorders found in other areas of medicine are expressed. In addition, many of the enzymes reported to differ in psychiatric patient populations function in the metabolic pathways of the brain neurotransmitter systems, rendering likely the possibility that these enzyme alterations might be directly associated with behavioral differences.

There have been speculations that one or another of the enzyme differences might prove to be a biological "cause" for psychiatric diagnostic entities like schizophrenia or alcoholism. Alternatively, the possibilities that enzyme differences either might represent genetic markers or at least provide laboratory tests helpful in the diagnosis of certain disorders have been suggested.

The data now available, however, generally do not strongly support any of these speculations, and certainly none of these speculations has been proved. In part this could reflect a demonstratively inadequate data base, with too few individuals from the needed different patient groups and control groups studied to reasonably evaluate these questions. Enzyme studies are still a frontier area in psychiatry, with many methodologic issues incompletely resolved (77). The lack of support for these speculations may also reflect on problems in the models or expectations on which these hypotheses are based.

Enzymes and Heterogeneity Within Clinical Diagnostic Syndromes

If "schizophrenia" (or, similarly, other psychiatric disorders) is comprised of groups of disorders—e.g., "the schizophrenias," as has often been suggested (5)—and is not a distinct disease entity in itself, then it may be expected that only a particular subgroup of patients with a diagnosis of "schizophrenia" possessing each specific genotype would demonstrate a particular enzyme difference. Although such possible heterogeneity within psychiatric syndromes has explicitly been accepted in many quarters, it obviously is not an operational element in the many studies of enzymes in psychiatric patients which include a small number of subjects identified only by a diagnostic label and which report only group means and not individual values for patients and controls.

Enzymes as Vulnerability or Risk Factors in Clinical Syndromes

A less discussed concept of relevance to speculations about enzymes, genetics, and psychiatric diagnosis is the psychiatric disorder spectrum hypothesis. Implicit in such diagnostic terms as "schizoaffective" and "borderline," the concept has appeared most directly in various studies of the biological relatives of schizophrenic patients. Not only schizophrenia but, more commonly, "schizophrenic spectrum disorders," including chronic, latent, and acute schizophrenia, borderline (uncertain) schizophrenia, and inadequate or schizoid personality in the family studies of Kety et al. (43), and schizophrenia, antisocial personality, and mental retardation in the studies of Heston (38,39) have been found among the family members of schizophrenic individuals. A spectrum of disorders has also been described for the affective disorders (115,116) and for sociopathy (17). If these associations are biologically based, it would seem conceivable that some of our diagnostic classifications may be overly specific or restrictive in terms of actual genetic contributions to such syndromes.

It seems necessary to consider that some more general factors in psychopathology might be inherited, rather than the clinical entities *per se*. Heston has suggested that "schizoidia" might be one such factor; other variables might be as broad as anxiety, psychomotor activity differences, or reward-related behavior characteristics (38,39). Such factors need not be explicit psychopathologic characteristics in themselves, but rather might summate with other genetic or environmental variables to produce vulnerability to manifest psychopathology, as suggested in Fig. 1. The application of this vulnerability or risk factor concept to an enzyme, as in the case of platelet MAO, requires exploration of enzyme activities in different psychiatric patient populations, their relatives, and nonpatient groups as well, and not just comparisons of one psychiatric diagnostic group with normal controls.

Enzymes as Laboratory Indicators of Psychiatric Disorders

Enzyme differences in patients may also be epiphenomena which are not directly connected with an etiologic component of a psychiatric disorder. Just as the activities of certain enzymes in plasma rise in association with tissue injury in myocardial infarction or hepatitis, so also may some changes in enzymes like creatine phosphokinase (CPK) be elevated in the early phases of acute psychotic episodes in patients with both schizophrenia and affective disorders (58). Enzyme changes such as these are thought to be primarily clinical state-related phenomena, and hence different from some of the enzyme differences discussed above, which have been suggested to represent relatively stable, heritable characteristics of individuals. Enzymes in plasma (such as DBH and CPK) which are released from cells and whose measured activities in plasma are functions not only of synthesis but also of rates of release and removal from the circulation may be relatively more

Clinical Manifestation   Causal Factors

I.   One disorder-one enzyme

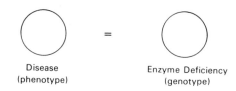

Disease   Enzyme Deficiency
(phenotype)   (genotype)

II.   One syndrome-many etiologies

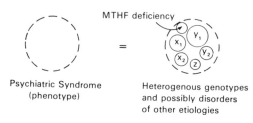

Psychiatric Syndrome   Heterogenous genotypes
(phenotype)   and possibly disorders
                            of other etiologies

III. One syndrome-contributing vulnerabilities

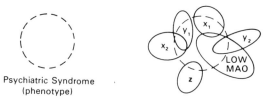

Psychiatric Syndrome
(phenotype)

FIG. 1. Three models for mechanisms by which differences in enzyme function might contribute to behavioral disorders.

Model I. According to the classic genetic model, an enzyme abnormality in an important metabolic pathway results in a specific disorder (*solid circle*). Although no behavioral disorders are yet known to fit this model of a one-to-one relationship between an enzyme deficiency and a clinical state, phenylketonuria (PKU) is an example of disorder resulting from a deficiency in a specific enzyme, phenylalanine hydroxylase. False positives or false negatives may be due to errors in enzyme analysis or failure to apply stringent enough diagnostic criteria to the patient population.

Model II. Commonly, psychiatric disorders are thought to represent syndromes (*dashed circle*) composed of heterogenous groups of discrete disorders. These disorders may have different etiologies, including one or more genotypes with simple enzyme deficiency states. For example, individuals with PKU comprise one subgroup within the syndrome of mental retardation. An example in the behavioral area is methylene tetrahydrofolate (MTHF) deficiency, which yields a schizophreniform syndrome, as discussed in the text. Other schizophrenic individuals may develop a schizophrenia subtype on the basis of psychosocial difficulties (X_1, X_2), other yet unidentified enzyme deficiencies (Y_1, Y_2) or a hypothesized slow virus infection (Z). Among the "schizophrenias" with a potential enzyme basis, it would be postulated that each specific entity would be contributed to by one enzyme deficiency which results from one specific gene abnormality. Typical examples of this model are found among the anemias, a group of disorders with common features which result from various enzyme deficiencies (e.g., G-6PD deficiency, thalassemia, and other hemoglobinopathies) as well as infections (malaria) and even behavioral differences (choosing a vegetarian diet).

Model III. Alternatively, psychiatric syndromes may represent the summative interaction of several vulnerability or risk factors. A difference in enzyme activity may place the individual at greater risk for being influenced by deleterious environmental factors (X_1, X_2) or, of course, other genetic influences (Y_1, Y_2). In this model, the enzyme activity difference itself does not alone result in the complete expression of particular psychiatric syndrome, although it may be associated with some characteristic behavioral or personality features. Thus, individuals with the enzyme difference but without other interacting factors are found among the normal population. Individuals possessing several interacting factors may have a more severe form of the syndrome.

These three models are not mutually exclusive, since, as discussed in the text, in certain known disorders risk factors of both environmental and genetic origin interact with classic enzyme deficiency states to yield maladaptive or, occasionally, superadaptive states.

susceptible to multiple clinical state influences. Nonetheless, DBH and CPK manifest some evidence of stability and genetic influence, as well as evidence that other factors may modulate their activity. Assessment of the relative contributions of "trait" or "state" factors for a particular enzyme requires fairly extensive evaluation of the many differences in drug treatment, diet, physical activity, and other features which may be different in patient groups compared to controls. It also requires twin and family studies and studies of the same individuals over periods of time.

Platelet MAO Studies as a Model for Biological Risk Factor Investigations in Psychopathology

These issues of (a) possible differences between psychiatric diagnostic entities and actual enzyme-related genotypes or risk factor characteristics representing either subgroups or supergroups, and (b) state versus trait differences in enzyme activities, have generally been incompletely addressed in studies of enzymes of psychiatric interest. Additional data from various psychiatric and medical patient groups and additional control groups as well as studies of the many factors which affect these enzymes [as discussed above and in previous reviews (63,77)] are required. On the basis of data on hand, however, we have focused our studies of platelet MAO activity on the hypothesis that it may represent a vulnerability factor for psychopathology which is not specific to any one psychiatric diagnostic entity, at least as these are currently described. Our interest is to define how MAO activity differences might contribute or correspond to behavioral and psychological differences between individuals, particularly individuals exhibiting psychopathology.

Models for our attempts to understand how the available data on platelet MAO activity might relate to behavioral differences and psychopathology are available from other areas of medicine. A number of genetic disorders have some features which provide intriguing examples for imagining how complex and apparently different behavioral maladaptations ranging from long-standing personality problems to acute psychotic episodes might still be ascribable, in part, to the effects of a postulated risk factor such as reduced MAO activity. This conceptualization is based on much evidence that MAO functions as a regulatory enzyme and that reductions in MAO activity are associated with alterations in the synthesis, storage, release, and metabolism of monoamine neurotransmitters and "false" neurotransmitters. In particular, reduced MAO activity has been shown to lead to impaired handling of a wide variety of amines and their precursors, including L-DOPA, L-tryptophan octopamine, phenylethylamine, and others, which may enter monoamine pathways as exogenous metabolic loads or in response to other stimuli which increase amine synthesis. If MAO is inhibited, these amines, their precursors, or other stimuli which ordinarily may not alter behavior or other physiologic functions become capable of yielding marked behavioral changes, as in certain models for hyperactivity or depression (35,64). Changes in monoamine metabolism and behavior similar to those studied in animals may also occur in man (68).

Glucose-6-phosphate dehydrogenase (G-6PD) deficiency, a disorder which can lead to anemia, provides one well-studied genetic problem with some features analogous to those postulated for MAO activity and behavior. G-6PD deficiency constitutes only one relatively uncommon subtype found in the many individuals presenting with clinical features of anemia. Structural abnormalities in the enzyme protein are associated with enzyme activity differences, but these activity differences (at least as measured under optimal assay conditions *in vitro*) only partially correlate with clinical symptoms. It is now understood that different modulating characteristics within the cell may enhance or diminish the consequences of G-6PD structural abnormalities; these cellular characteristics are not examined in routine studies of the cellular characteristics of the enzyme by activity measurements or electrophoresis approaches. G-6PD deficiency may present either as a chronic low-grade anemia, or as an acute hemolytic crisis with massive destruction of blood cells and severe clinical symptoms. Some individuals with the same genetic components may never experience a hemolytic crisis, since these principally occur in response to environmental changes produced by certain drugs, the ingestion of fava beans, or as a response to infections. An evolutionary selective advantage for G-6PD deficiency has been postulated on the basis of this deficiency having a possible protective effect against malaria.

Many similar parallels can be drawn among other disorders such as diabetes, porphyria, and gout where varying contributions from genetic factors, other familial contributions, and exogenous events (e.g., cultural as well as individual dietary preferences or drug use) act in combination to yield initially mild, chronic impairments which may appear clinically only under some conditions, or only as laboratory test abnormalities ("prediabetic" hypoglycemia, increased urinary porphobilinogen excretion, hyperuricemia), or which may appear fulminantly as syndromes with different clinical features (diabetic coma, an acute intermittent porphyric episode, or acute gouty arthritis). If indeed similar situations prevail among the behavioral disorders, we need to anticipate not only diverse genotypes contributing heterogeneity within each psychiatric diagnostic entity but also the presence of risk factors, including enzyme function differences such as reduced MAO activity, possibly contributing to more than one psychiatric disorder. It should also be noted that hypoglycemia and porphyria may appear clinically as psychiatric disorders with anxiety, paranoia, and even frank psychosis, further suggesting the importance of biological heterogeneity. Multigene interaction may also be important in determining clinical symptomatology. Thus, for example, individuals with thalassemia or sickle cell disease in the heterozygous form may not be symptomatic, whereas individuals heterozygous for both thalassemia and sickle cell disease may be quite symptomatic. One deficit may also ameliorate another, as in the combination of homozygous thalassemia and hemoglobin D disease in which the manifestations of the latter are diminished. Possible examples of disorders in which MAO activity differences might interact with other enzyme deficiency states include methylene tetrahydrofolate deficiency (discussed above) (28) and hypoxanthine-guanine phosphoribosyltransferase deficiency. The latter deficiency, which can result in the Lesch-Nyhan syndrome, has recently been reported to be associated with markedly reduced MAO activity in neuroblastoma and glioma clones (11,103) and also in fibroblasts from patients with the Lesch-Nyhan syndrome (11,98). A possible example of a protective interaction might be the sex steroid-related differences in MAO activity (8), which could interact with other factors to account for some of the sex-specific differences in the behavioral and psychological correlates of reduced platelet MAO activity discussed below.

To evaluate these possibilities in regard to reduced MAO activity, we have chosen to examine normal populations first, in order to avoid sampling difficulties and secondary illness effects among patient populations. A preliminary study in 95 college students yielded evidence that reduced MAO activity was associated with elevated MMPI profiles suggestive of an overall increase in psychopathology and also with increased sensation-seeking behavior in males (65). In a subsequent, more extensive study of 375 individuals screened to select those at the extremes in platelet MAO activity, interview data revealed more frequent psychiatric or psychologic counseling in the 10% of individuals within the lowest MAO activities compared to the 10% with highest MAO activities (13). Low-MAO males in this study also had significantly more convictions for non-traffic legal offenses, and their relatives had an eightfold increase in the incidence of suicide or suicide attempts over those found in the high-MAO sample. Further investigations in student groups have led to successful replications of the sensation-seeking personality differences and the MMPI psychopathology findings (101). In addition, preliminary data from an item analysis of the MMPI suggest that low MAO activity in normals is associated with such personality features as high social contact and interpersonal concern. These MMPI findings corroborated other self-report data demonstrating increased time spent socializing and increased club and organizational membership in low MAO subjects. Behavioral items reflecting activity and social contact were also found to be inversely correlated with MAO activity in an earlier study in rhesus monkeys (93). Although such cross-species comparisons are difficult, the patterns of behavior in these primates were stable over a 4-month period and the socialization/MAO relationship was statistically significant in both males and females tested independently.

These attempts to identify behavioral and psychological characteristics associated with MAO activity differences need much additional work and eventually will need to be extended to patient groups. They do appear to represent a new strategy in the identification of biological processes associated with psychopathology, which may provide a model for the study of other enzymes and other biological factors in psychiatric disorders, and which perhaps may eventually aid in the delineation, classification, and possibly treatment of these disorders.

REFERENCES

1. Axelrod, J. (1972): Dopamine-β-hydroxylase: Regulation of its synthesis and release from nerve terminals. *Pharmacol. Rev.,* 24:233–243.
2. Axelrod, J., and Cohn, C. K. (1971): Methyltransferase enzymes in red blood cells. *J. Pharmacol. Exp. Ther.,* 176:650–654.
3. Baldessarini, R. J., and Bell, W. R. (1966): Methionine-activating enzyme and catechol-O-methyl transferase activity in normal and leukemic white blood cells. *Nature,* 209:78–79.
4. Barchas, J. D., Elliott, G. R., DoAmaral, J., Erdelyi, E., O'Connor, S., Bowden, M., Brodie, H. K. H., Berger, P. A., Renson, J., and Wyatt, R. J. (1974): Triptolines: Formation from tryptamines and 5-MTHF by human platelets. *Arch. Gen. Psychiatry,* 31:862–867.
5. Bellak, L., and Loeb, L. (Eds.) (1969): *The Schizophrenic Syndrome.* Grune & Stratton, New York.
6. Bellin, I. S., and Sorrentino, J. M. (1974): Kinetic characteristics of monoamine oxidase and serum cholinesterase in several related rat strains. *Biochem. Genet.,* 11:309–317.
7. Belmaker, R. H., Ebbsen, K., Ebstein, R., and Rimon, R. (1976): Platelet monoamine oxidase in schizophrenia and manic-depressive illness. *Br. J. Psychiatry,* 129:227–232.
8. Belmaker, R. H., Murphy, D. L., Wyatt, R. J., and Loriaux, D. L. (1974): Human platelet monoamine oxidase changes during the menstrual cycle. *Arch. Gen. Psychiatry,* 31:553–556.
9. Benson, P. F., and Southgate, J. (1971): Diminished activity of platelet monoamine oxidase in Down's syndrome. *Am. J. Hum. Genet.,* 23:211–214.
10. Bockar, J., Roth, R., and Heninger, G. (1974): Increased human platelet monoamine oxidase during lithium carbonate therapy. *Life Sci.,* 15:2109–2118.
11. Breakefield, X. O., Castiglione, C. M., and Edelstein, S. G. (1976): Monoamine oxidase activity decreased in cells lacking hypoxanthine phosphoribosyltransferase activity. *Science,* 192:1018–1020.
12. Briggs, M. H., and Briggs, M. (1973): Hormonal influences on erythrocyte catechol-O-methyl transferase activity in humans. *Experientia,* 29:279–280.
13. Buchsbaum, M., Coursey, R. D., and Murphy, D. L. (1976): The biochemical high risk paradigm: Behavioral and familial correlates of low platelet monoamine oxidase activity. *Science,* 194:339–341.
14. Carpenter, W. T., Murphy, D. L., and Wyatt, R. J. (1975): Platelet monoamine oxidase activity in acute schizophrenia. *Am. J. Psychiatry,* 132:438–441.
15. Cho, H. W., and Meltzer, H. Y. (1974): Mg^{++}-dependent adenosine triphosphatase activity in erythrocyte ghosts of schizophrenic patients. *Biol. Psychiatry,* 9:109–116.
16. Ciaranello, R. D., and Axelrod, J. (1973): Genetically controlled alterations in the rate of degradation of phenylethanolamine N-methyltransferase. *J. Biol. Chem.,* 248:5616–5623.
17. Cloninger, C. R., Reich, T., and Guze, S. G. (1975): The multifactorial model of disease transmission: III. Family relationship between sociopathy and hysteria. *Br. J. Psychiatry,* 127:23–32.
18. Cohn, C. K., Dunner, D. L., and Axelrod, J. (1970): Reduced catechol-O-methyl-

transferase activity in red blood cells of women with primary affective disorder. *Science,* 170:1323–1324.

19. Domino, E. F., and Khanna, S. S. (1976): Decreased blood platelet MAO activity in unmedicated chronic schizophrenic patients. *Am. J. Psychiatry,* 133:323–326.

20. Donnelly, C. H., and Murphy, D. L. (1977): Substrate- and inhibitor-related characteristics of human platelet monoamine oxidase. *Biochem. Pharmacol.,* 26:853–858.

21. Dunner, D. L., Cohn, C. K., Gershon, E. S., and Goodwin, F. K. (1971): Differential catechol-O-methyltransferase activity in unipolar and bipolar affective illness. *Arch. Gen. Psychiatry,* 25:348–353.

22. Dunner, D. L., Cohn, C. K., Weinshilboum, R. M., and Wyatt, R. J. (1973): The activity of dopamine-beta-hydroxylase and methionine-activating enzyme in blood of schizophrenic patients. *Biol. Psychiatry,* 6:215–220.

23. Edwards, D. J., and Burns, M. O. (1974): Effects of tricyclic antidepressants upon platelet monoamine oxidase. *Life Sci.,* 15:2045–2058.

24. Fieve, R. R., Rosenthal, D., and Brill, H. (1975): *Genetic Research in Psychiatry.* Johns Hopkins University Press, Baltimore.

25. Freedman, L. S., Ebstein, R. P., Parks, D. H., Levitz, S. M., and Goldstein, M. (1973): The effect of cold pressor test in man on serum immunoreactive dopamine-β-hydroxylase and on dopamine-β-hydroxylase activity. *Res. Commun. Chem. Pathol. Pharmacol.,* 6:873–878.

26. Freedman, L. S., Goldstein, M., and Coleman, M. (1974): Serum dopamine-β-hydroxylase activity in Down's syndrome: A familial study. *Res. Commun. Chem. Pathol. Pharmacol.,* 8:543–549.

27. Freedman, L. S., Ohurchi, T., Goldstein, M., Axelrod, F., Fish, I., and Dancis, J. (1972): Changes in serum dopamine-β-hydroxylase with age. *Nature,* 236:310–311.

28. Freeman, J. M., Finkelstein, J. D., and Mudd, S. H. (1975): Folate responsive homocystinuria and "schizophrenia." *N. Engl. J. Med.,* 292:491–496.

29. Frere, J. M., and Barbeau, A. (1971): Blood catechol-O-methyltransferase activity in Parkinson's disease. *Lancet,* 2:269–270.

30. Frewin, D. B., Downey, J. A., and Levitt, M. (1973): The effect of heat, cold, and exercise on plasma dopamine-β-hydroxylase activity in man. *Can. J. Physiol. Pharmacol.,* 51:986–989.

31. Gentil, V., Greenwood, M. H., and Lader, M. H. (1975): The effect of adrenaline on human platelet MAO. *Psychopharmacologia,* 44:187–194.

32. Gershon, E. S., and Jonas, W. Z. (1975): Erythrocyte soluble catechol-O-methyl transferase activity in primary affective disorder. *Arch. Gen. Psychiatry,* 32:1351–1356.

33. Goldstein, M., Freedman, L., Bohuan, A. C., and Guerinot, F. (1972): Serum dopamine-β-hydroxylase activity in neuroblastoma. *N. Engl. J. Med.,* 286:1123–1125.

34. Goldstein, M., Freedman, L. S., Ebstein, R. P., and Park, D. H. (1974): Studies on dopamine-β-hydroxylase in mental disorders. *J. Psychiatr. Res.,* 11:205–210.

35. Green, A. R., and Grahame-Smith, D. G. (1976): Effects of drugs on the processes regulating the functional activity of brain 5-hydroxytryptamine. *Nature,* 260:487–491.

36. Grunhaus, L., Ebstein, R., Belmaker, R., Sandler, S. G., and Jonas, W. (1976): A twin study of human red blood cell catechol-O-methyl transferase. *Br. J. Psychiatry,* 128:494–498.

37. Gustavson, K.-H., Wetterberg, L., Backstrom, M., and Ross, S. B. (1973): Catechol-O-methyltransferase activity in erythrocytes in Down's syndrome. *Clin. Genet.,* 4:279–280.

38. Heston, L. L. (1966): Psychiatric disorders in foster home reared children of schizophrenic mothers. *Br. J. Psychiatry,* 112:819–825.

39. Heston, L. L. (1970): The genetics of schizophrenic and schizoid disease. *Science,* 167:249–256.

40. Hokin-Neaverson, M., Spiegel, D. A., and Lewis, W. C. (1974): Deficiency of erythrocyte sodium pump activity in bipolar manic-depressive psychosis. *Life Sci.,* 15:1739–1748.

41. Hokin-Neaverson, M., Spiegel, D. A., Lewis, W. C., Burckhardt, W. A., and

Jefferson, J. W. (1976): Erythrocyte sodium pump activity in different psychiatric disorders. *Res. Commun. Psychol. Psychiatr. Behav.*, 1:391–403.

42. Horwitz, D., Alexander, R. W., Lovenberg, W., and Keiser, H. R. (1973): Human serum dopamine-β-hydroxylase: Relationship to hypertension and sympathetic activity. *Circ. Res.*, 32:594–599.

43. Kety, S. S., Rosenthal, D., Wender, P. H., and Schulsinger, F. (1968): The types and prevalence of mental illness in the biological and adoptive families of adopted schizophrenics. In: *The Transmission of Schizophrenia,* edited by D. Rosenthal and S. S. Kety, pp. 345–362. Pergamon Press, Oxford.

44. Kopin, I. J., Kaufman, S., Viveros, H., Jacobowitz, D., Lake, R., Ziegler, M. G., Lovenberg, W., and Goodwin, F. K. (1976): Dopamine-β-hydroxylase. Basic and clinical studies. *Ann. Intern. Med.*, 85:211–223.

45. Lamprecht, F., Ebert, M. H., Turek, I., and Kopin, I. J. (1974): Serum dopamine-beta-hydroxylase in depressed patients and the effect of electroconvulsive shock treatment. *Psychopharmacologia*, 40:241–248.

46. Lamprecht, F., Wyatt, R. J., Belmaker, R., Murphy, D. L., and Pollin, W. (1973): Plasma dopamine-beta-hydroxylase in identical twins discordant for schizophrenia. In: *Frontiers in Catecholamine Research,* edited by E. Usdin and S. Snyder, pp. 1123–1126. Pergamon Press, New York.

47. Landowski, J., Lysiak, W., and Angielski, S. (1975): Monoamine oxidase activity in blood platelets from patients with cyclophrenic depressive syndromes. *Biochem. Med.*, 14:347–354.

48. Leckman, J., Gershon, E., Nichols, A., and Murphy, D. L. (1977): Reduced MAO activity in first degree relatives of individuals with bipolar affective disorders. *Arch. Gen. Psychiatry,* 34:601–606.

49. Leon, A. S., Thomas, P. E., Sernatinger, E., and Canlas, A. (1974): Serum dopamine-β-hydroxylase activity as an index of sympathetic activity. *J. Clin. Pharmacol.*, 14:354–362.

50. Levin, E. Y., and Kaufman, S. (1961): Studies on the enzyme catalyzing the conversion of 3,4-dihydroxyphenylethylamine to norepinephrine. *J. Biol. Chem.*, 236:2043–2049.

51. Lieberman, A. N., Freedman, L. S., and Goldstein, M. (1972): Serum dopamine-β-hydroxylase activity in patients with Huntington's chorea and Parkinson's disease. *Lancet,* 1:153–154.

52. Lott, I. T., Chase, T. H., and Murphy, D. L. (1972): Down's syndrome: Transport, storage and metabolism of serotonin in blood platelets. *Pediatr. Res.*, 6:730–735.

53. Lott, I. T., Murphy, D. L., and Chase, T. H. (1972): Down's syndrome: Central monoamine turnover in patients with diminished platelet serotonin. *Neurology (Minneap.)*, 22:967–972.

54. MacPike, A. D., and Meier, H. (1976): Genotype dependence of monoamine oxidase in inbred strains of mice. *Experientia*, 32:979–980.

55. Markianos, E. S., Nystrom, I., Reichel, H., and Matussek, N. (1976): Serum dopamine-β-hydroxylase in psychiatric patients and normals. Effect of d-amphetamine and haloperidol. *Psychopharmacology,* 50:259–267.

56. Matta, R. J., and Wasten, G. F. (1973): The pharmacology of fusaric acid in man. *Clin. Pharmacol. Ther.*, 14:541–546.

57. Matthysse, S., and Baldessarini, J. (1972): S-adenosylmethionine and catechol-O-methyltransferase in schizophrenia. *Am. J. Psychiatry,* 128:1310–1312.

58. Meltzer, H. Y. (1975): Neuromuscular abnormalities in the major mental illnesses. I. Serum enzyme studies. In: *Biology of the Major Psychoses: A Comparative Analysis,* edited by D. X. Freedman, pp. 165–188. Raven Press, New York.

59. Meltzer, H. Y., Cho, H. W., Carroll, B. J., and Russo, P. (1976): Serum dopamine-β-hydroxylase activity in the affective psychoses and schizophrenia. *Arch. Gen. Psychiatry,* 33:585–591.

60. Meltzer, H. Y., and Stahl, S. M. (1974): Platelet monoamine oxidase activity and substrate preferences in schizophrenic patients. *Res. Commun. Chem. Pathol. Pharmacol.*, 7:419–431.

61. Miner, G. D. (1973): The evidence for genetic components in the neuroses. *Arch. Gen. Psychiatry,* 29:111–118.

62. Moskowitz, J., Harwood, J. P., Reid, W. D., and Krishna, G. (1971): The interaction of norepinephrine and prostaglandin El on the adenyl cyclase system of human and rabbit blood platelets. *Biochim. Biophys. Acta*, 230:279–285.
63. Murphy, D. L. (1976): Clinical, genetic, hormonal and drug influences on the activity of human platelet monoamine oxidase. In: *Monoamine Oxidase and Its Inhibition*, edited by G. E. W. Wolstenholme and J. Knight, pp. 341–351 (Ciba Foundation Symposium 39). Elsevier, Amsterdam.
64. Murphy, D. L. (1976): The behavioral toxicity of monoamine oxidase inhibiting antidepressants. *Adv. Pharmacol. Chemother.*, 81:178–202.
65. Murphy, D. L., Belmaker, R. H., Buchsbaum, M., Martin, N. F., Ciaranello, R., and Wyatt, R. J. (1977): Biogenic amine-related enzymes and personality variations in normals. *Psychol. Med.*, 7:149–157.
66. Murphy, D. L., Belmaker, R., Carpenter, W. T., and Wyatt, R. J. (1977): Monoamine oxidase in chronic schizophrenia: Studies of hormonal and other factors affecting enzyme activity. *Br. J. Psychiatry*, 130:151–158.
67. Murphy, D. L., Belmaker, R., and Wyatt, R. J. (1974): Monoamine oxidase in schizophrenia and other behavioral disorders. *J. Psychiatr. Res.*, 11:221–247.
68. Murphy, D. L., Brand, E., Goldman, T., Baker, M., Wright, C., van Kammen, D., and Gordon, E. (1977): Platelet and plasma amine oxidase inhibition and urinary amine excretion changes during phenelzine treatment. *J. Nerv. Ment. Dis.*, 164:129–134.
69. Murphy, D. L., and Donnelly, C. H. (1974): Monoamine oxidase in man: Enzyme characteristics in platelets, plasma and other human tissues. In: *Neuropsychopharmacology of Monoamines and Their Regulatory Enzymes*, edited by E. Usdin, pp. 71–85. Raven Press, New York.
70. Murphy, D. L., Donnelly, C. H., Baulu, J., and Redmond, D. E., Jr. (1977): Monoamine oxidase activity in brain and other tissues of the rhesus monkey. (*In preparation.*)
71. Murphy, D. L., Donnelly, D. H., Miller, L., and Wyatt, R. J. (1976): Platelet monoamine oxidase in chronic schizophrenia: Some enzyme characteristics relevant to reduced activity. *Arch. Gen. Psychiatry*, 33:1377–1381.
72. Murphy, D. L., Donnelly, C., and Moskowitz, J. (1973): Inhibition by lithium of prostaglandin El and norepinephrine effects on cyclic adenosine monophosphate production in human platelets. *Clin. Pharmacol. Ther.*, 14:810–814.
73. Murphy, D. L., Donnelly, C. H., and Moskowitz, J. (1974): Catecholamine receptor function in depressed patients. *Am. J. Psychiatry*, 131:1389–1391.
74. Murphy, D. L., Redmond, D. E., Jr., Baulu, J., and Donnelly, C. H. (1977): Platelet monoamine oxidase activity in 116 normal rhesus monkeys: Relationships between enzyme activity and age, sex and genetic factors. *Comp. Biochem. Physiol.* (*in press*).
75. Murphy, D. L., and Weiss, R. (1972): Reduced monoamine oxidase activity in blood platelets from bipolar depressed patients. *Am. J. Psychiatry*, 128:1351–1357.
76. Murphy, D. L., Wright, C., Buchsbaum, M., Nichols, A., Costa, J. L., and Wyatt, R. J. (1976): Platelet and plasma amine oxidase activity in 680 normals: Sex and age differences and stability over time. *Biochem. Med.*, 16:254–265.
77. Murphy, D. L., and Wyatt, R. J. (1975): Enzyme studies in the major psychiatric disorders: I. Catechol-O-methyl-transferase, monoamine oxidase in the affective disorders, and factors affecting some behavior-related enzyme activities. In: *The Biology of the Major Psychoses: A Comparative Analysis*, pp. 277–288. Raven Press, New York.
78. Naylor, G. J., Reid, A. H., Dick, D. A. T., and Dick, E. G. (1976): A biochemical study of short-cycle manic-depressive psychosis in mental defectives. *Br. J. Psychiatry*, 128:169–180.
79. Nies, A., Robinson, D. S., Harris, L. S., and Lamborn, K. R. (1974): Comparison of monoamine oxidase substrate activities in twins, schizophrenics, depressives, and controls. In: *Neuropsychopharmacology of Monoamines and Their Regulatory Enzymes*, edited by E. Usdin, pp. 59–79. Raven Press, New York.
80. Nies, A., Robinson, D. S., Lamborn, K. R., and Lampert, R. P. (1973): Genetic control of platelet and plasma monoamine oxidase activity. *Arch. Gen. Psychiatry*, 28:834–838.

81. Nishzawa, Y., Hamada, N., Fujii, S., Moril, H., Okuda, K., and Wada, M. (1974): Serum dopamine-β-hydroxylase activity in thyroid disorders. *J. Clin. Endocrinol. Metab.*, 39:599–602.

82. North, R. H., and Spaulding, S. W. (1974): Decreased serum dopamine-β-hydroxylase in hyperthyroidism. *J. Clin. Endocrinol. Metab.*, 39:614–617.

83. Ogihara, T., and Nugent, C. A. (1974): Serum dopamine-β-hydroxylase in three forms of acute stress. *Life Sci.*, 15:923–930.

84. Ogihara, T., Nugent, C. A., Shen, S.-W., and Goldstein, S. (1975): Serum dopamine-β-hydroxylase activity in parents and children. *J. Lab. Clin. Med.*, 85:566–573.

85. Okada, T., Fujita, T., Ohta, T., Kato, T., Ikuta, K., and Nagatsu, T. (1974): A 24-hour rhythm in human serum dopamine-β-hydroxylase activity. *Experientia*, 30:605–607.

86. Owen, F., Bourne, R., Crow, T. J., Johnstone, E. C., Bailey, A. R., and Hershon, H. I. (1976): Platelet monoamine oxidase in schizophrenia. *Arch. Gen. Psychiatry*, 33:1370–1373.

87. Pandey, G. N., Dorus, E. B., Dekirmenjian, H., and Davis, J. M. (1975): Effect of lithium treatment on blood COMT and platelet MAO in normal human subjects. *Fed. Proc.*, 34:778.

88. Planz, G., Wiethold, G., Appel, E., Bohmer, D., Palm, D., and Grobecker, H. (1975): Correlation between increased dopamine-β-hydroxylase activity and catecholamine concentration in plasma: Determination of acute changes in sympathetic activity in man. *Eur. J. Clin. Pharmacol.*, 8:181–188.

89. Potkin, S. G., Cannon, H. E., Murphy, D. L., and Wyatt, R. J. (1977): Paranoid schizophrenia: A different disorder? *New Engl. J. Med.* (*in press*).

90. Pryor, G. T., Schlesinger, K., and Calhoun, W. H. (1966): Differences in brain enzymes among five inbred strains of mice. *Life Sci.*, 5:2105–2111.

91. Quiram, D. R., and Weinshilboum, R. M. (1976): Catechol-O-methyltransferase in rat erythrocyte and three other tissues: Comparison of biochemical properties after removal of inhibitory calcium. *J. Neurochem.*, 27:1197–1203.

92. Rapoport, J. L., Quinn, P. O., and Lamprecht, F. (1974): Minor physical anomalies and plasma dopamine-β-hydroxylase activity in hyperactive boys. *Am. J. Psychiatry*, 131:386–390.

93. Redmond, D. E., Jr., and Murphy, D. L. (1975): Behavioral correlates of platelet monoamine oxidase (MAO) activity in rhesus monkeys. *Psychom. Med.*, 37:80.

94. Robinson, D. S., Davis, J. M., Nies, A., Ravaris, C. L., and Sylwester, D. (1971): Relation of sex and aging to monoamine oxidate activity of human brain, plasma, and platelets. *Arch. Gen. Psychiatry*, 24:536–539.

95. Rockson, S., Stone, R., van der Weyden, M., and Kelley, W. N. (1974): Lesch-Nyhan syndrome: Evidence for abnormal adrenergic function. *Science*, 186:934–935.

96. Ross, R. A., Judd, A. B., Joh, T. H., Pickel, V. M., and Reis, D. J. (1976): Strain dependent differences in tyrosine hydroxylase in inbred mice are due to differences in number of dopaminergic neurons. *Neurosci. Abstr.*, p. 473.

97. Ross, S. B., Wetterberg, L., and Myrhed, M. (1973): Genetic control of plasma dopamine-β-hydroxylase. *Life Sci.*, 12:529–532.

98. Roth, J. A., Breakefield, X. O., and Castiglione, C. M. (1976): Monoamine oxidase and catechol-O-methyltransferase activities in cultured human skin fibroblasts. *Life Sci.*, 19:1705–1710.

99. Sandler, M., Youdim, M. B. H., and Hanington, E. (1974): A phenylethylamine oxidizing defect in migraine. *Nature*, 250:335–337.

100. Schildkraut, J. J., Herzog, J. M., Orsulak, P. J., Edelman, S. E., Shein, H. M., and Frazier, S. H. (1976): Reduced platelet monoamine oxidase activity in a subgroup of schizophrenic patients. *Am. J. Psychiatry*, 133:438–439.

101. Schooler, C., Zahn, T. P., Murphy, D. L., and Buchsbaum, M. S. (1977): Psychological correlates of monoamine oxidase activity in normals. *J. Nerv. Ment. Dis.* (*in press*).

102. Segal, D. S., Geyer, M. A., and Weiner, B. E. (1975): Strain differences during

intraventricular infusion of norepinephrine: Possible role of receptor sensitivity. *Science,* 189:301–303.

103. Skaper, S. D., and Seegmiller, J. E. (1976): Hypoxanthine-guanine phosphoribosyltransferase mutant glioma cells: Diminished monoamine oxidase activity. *Science,* 194:1171–1172.

104. Squires, R. J. (1972): Multiple forms of monoamine oxidase in intact mitochondria as characterized by selective inhibitors and thermal stability: A comparison of eight mammalian species. *Adv. Biochem. Psychopharmac.,* 5:335–370.

105. Stone, R. A., Kirshner, N., Gunnells, J. C., and Robinson, R. R. (1974): Changes of plasma dopamine-β-hydroxylase activity and other plasma constituents during the cold pressor test. *Life Sci.,* 14:1797–1805.

106. Sullivan, J. L., Stanfield, C. N., and Dackis, C. (1977): Low platelet monoamine oxidase activity in chronic alcoholics. *Am. J. Psychiatry (in press).*

107. Tunnicliff, G., Wimer, C. C., and Wimer, R. E. (1973): Relationships between neurotransmitter metabolism and behaviour in seven inbred strains of mice. *Brain Res.,* 61:428–434.

108. Vanderheider, B. S., and Zarate-Mogano, C. (1976): Erythrocyte ITP phosphohydrolase deficiency in a psychiatric population. *Biol. Psychiatry,* 11:755–765.

109. Wang, Y.-C., Pandey, G. N., Mendels, J., and Frazer, A. (1973): Effect of lithium on prostaglandin El-stimulated adenylate cyclase activity of human platelets. *Biochem. Pharmacol.,* 23:845–855.

110. Wang, Y.-C., Pandey, G. N., Mendels, J., and Frazer, A. (1974): Platelet adenylate cyclase responses in depression: Implications for a receptor defect. *Psychopharmacologia,* 36:291–300.

111. Weinshilboum, R. M., and Axelrod, J. (1971): Reduced plasma DBH activity in familial dysautonomia. *N. Engl. J. Med.,* 285:938–942.

112. Weinshilboum, R. M., Raymond, F. A., Elveback, L. R., and Weidman, W. H. (1973): Serum dopamine-B-hydroxylase activity: Sibling-sibling correlation. *Science,* 181:943–945.

113. Wetterberg, L., Aberg, H., Ross, S. B., and Froden, O. (1972): Plasma dopamine-β-hydroxylase activity in hypertension and various neuropsychiatric disorders. *Scand. J. Clin. Lab. Invest.,* 30:283–289.

114. White, H. L., McLeod, M. N., and Davidson, J. R. (1976): Catechol O-methyltransferase in red blood cells of schizophrenic, depressed, and normal human subjects. *Br. J. Psychiatry,* 128:184–187.

115. Winokur, G. (1974): The division of depressive illness into depression spectrum disease and pure depressive disease. *Int. Pharmacopsychiatry,* 9:5–13.

116. Winokur, G., Cadoret, R., Baker, M., and Dorzab, J. (1975): Depression spectrum disease versus pure depressive disease. *Br. J. Psychiatry,* 127:75–77.

117. Wooten, G. F., and Cardon, P. V. (1973): Plasma dopamine-β-hydroxylase activity. *Arch. Neurol.,* 28:103–106.

118. Wooten, G. F., Eldridge, R., Axelrod, J., and Stern, R. S. (1973): Elevated plasma dopamine-β-hydroxylase activity in an autosomal dominant torsion dystonia. *N. Engl. J. Med.,* 288:284–288.

119. Wyatt, R. J., Belmaker, R., and Murphy, D. L. (1975): Low platelet monoamine oxidase and vulnerability to schizophrenia. In: *Genetics and Psychopharmacology,* edited by J. Mendlewicz, pp. 38–56. S. Karger, Basel.

120. Wyatt, R. J., Murphy, D. L., Belmaker, R., Cohen, S., Donnelly, C. H., and Pollin, W. (1973): Reduced monoamine oxidase activity in platelets: A possible genetic marker for vulnerability to schizophrenia. *Science,* 179:916–918.

121. Wyatt, R. J., Saavedra, J. M., and Axelrod, J. (1973): A dimethyltryptamine-forming enzyme in human blood. *Am. J. Psychiatry,* 130:754–760.

122. Youdim, M. B. H., Grahame-Smith, D. G., and Woods, H. F. (1976): Some properties of human platelet monoamine oxidase in iron-deficiency anaemia. *Clin. Sci. Mol. Med.,* 50:479–485.

123. Ziegler, M. G., Lake, C. R., Eldridge, R., and Kopin, I. J. (1976): Plasma norepinephrine and dopamine-β-hydroxylase in dystonia. *Adv. Neurol.,* 14:307–318.

124. Ziegler, M. G., Lake, C. R., and Kopin, I. J. (1977): The sympathetic-nervous-system defect in primary orthostatic hypotension. *N. Engl. J. Med.,* 296:293–297.

Discussion

Morris A. Lipton

*Department of Psychiatry, University of North Carolina School of Medicine,
Chapel Hill, North Carolina 27514*

As a discussant I did not write a chapter in advance and will limit myself
to a consideration of the preceding chapters, and of the thoughts they have
generated.

Let me begin with the information about mental retardation mentioned by
Dr. Gottesman. He told us that McKuskick from Hopkins has reported that
there are now 263 phenotypes associated with mental retardation. Of these,
3% are autosomal dominants, 19% are autosomal recessives, and 15% are
sex linked. The remainder, almost two-thirds, have an unknown and probably complex form of inheritance. Equally important is the fact that with
today's information, all of these together account for only 11% of the cases
of retardation. The causes of the remainder are not known and so they are
called idiopathic. There have been no major breakthroughs in determining
the etiology of this large heterogeneous group, but there is a constant chip-
ping away and their number is diminishing.

I focused on mental retardation because it raises important questions with
regard to schizophrenia. We all agree that there is probably more than one
schizophrenia, but how many? If we use only inclusion criteria, i.e., we include all patients who show schizophrenic symptomatology even though they
may have other manifest defects such as porphyria, nutritional deficiencies,
or metabolic errors, then the number will be very high. If, as we properly
do, we use exclusion criteria as well, eliminating all cases with known illness
that may contribute to schizophrenic symptoms, the number will certainly
be smaller, but may still be large. We cannot really say at this time whether
there are a few schizophrenias or many.

Genetic studies seem to bear this out. The transmission of schizophrenia,
like that of most forms of mental retardation, does not follow the classic
Mendelian ratios for either autosomal dominant or autosomal recessive
disease. Instead, the work of Heston, Rosenthal, Gottesman, and others
suggests that the inheritance pattern best fits a polygenic model or that alternatively there may be a single gene whose expression is modified by many
other factors, some of them genetic. The genetic modifiers may themselves
be polygenic like intelligence, which seems to be inversely correlated with
the occurrence and severity of the disease.

Regardless of whether the illness turns out to be polygenic or a single gene having interaction with modifying genes, the problem of specifying the biological defect with laboratory methods is clearly difficult and is not likely to yield simple answers. The axiom that one gene equals one protein has been productive in stimulating biochemical research in both bacteria and higher organisms, especially when the proteins are readily identifiable like enzymes are. But when they are repressors or structural proteins the task is more difficult. To illustrate this difficulty it is worth noting that McKusick in 1975 listed 2,500 known Mendelian traits and pointed out that among these only 7% have an identified biochemical mechanism. For example, we know nothing of the biochemistry of club foot or cleft palate. It may amuse you to learn that the oldest of all Mendelian traits, the wrinkled pea from which Mendel derived his theory, still has an unknown biochemistry. The chemistry of the wrinkling is not known. McKusick's data must be kept in mind as we continue to investigate the biology of mental illness and try to develop laboratory tests. Although ultimately we may be able to express the pathogenesis in biochemical language, it is today as likely that we may find the answers from noninvasive electrophysiological, neurophysiological, and perhaps even anatomical experiments. Investigations in all of these disciplines are worthwhile and will become more so as new technologies are developed. The advances in computerized EEG technology that permit spectral analyses of the EEG and the increasing use of evoked potential techniques in differing clinical states described by Dr. Sutton hold a good deal of promise. Dr. Fink's suggestion that electrophysiological response to drugs be used to study the correlation with clinical response is also very sound.

There is good reason to believe that neurotransmitters and their receptors are involved in mental illness because pharmacological manipulations of these are our most powerful methods for generating models of illness in animals and for treating the illness as it occurs in man. Hence the study of the enzymes involved in their metabolism is logical. This can be done directly by enzyme measurements, but unfortunately the enzymes of the central nervous system are not directly accessible and we must use those of the blood or peripheral tissues. Alternatively, we may measure the metabolic products of these enzymes in peripheral tissues or fluids, but here we have the problem of trying to determine whether these low molecular weight metabolites are formed in the brain or in peripheral tissues.

The studies described by Dr. Murphy on DBH, MAO, and COMT reflect a strategy that should be followed. DBH is a synthetic enzyme for norepinephrine which is extruded from synaptic vesicles, and it is, therefore, measurable in plasma. MAO and COMT are degrading enzymes. DBH levels have been shown to be elevated in some neurological or metabolic diseases and down in others. The lack of specificity is disappointing. COMT is a cytoplasmic enzyme found in brain, liver, and blood cells. The study of enzyme levels in different clinical populations has led to inconsistent and contradictory results.

In summary, it is clear that we are still far from having a single reliable laboratory test for the diagnosis of specific mental illnesses. Much exciting work is in progress not only in biochemistry but in endocrinology, neurophysiology, electrophysiology, and neuropsychology, and all of this is promising. In the meantime it is worth recalling that few medical illnesses are diagnosed by a single pathognomonic laboratory finding. In most major medical illnesses, many of which are heterogeneous, diagnosis is still made by a careful history plus results from a battery of diverse laboratory tests which reveal a constellation from which the diagnosis is made.

Critical Issues in Psychiatric Diagnosis,
edited by Robert L. Spitzer and Donald F. Klein.
Raven Press, New York © 1978.

Diagnosis and Psychiatry

Richard Jed Wyatt

Laboratory of Clinical Psychopharmacology, Division of Special Mental Health Research, IRP, NIMH, Saint Elizabeths Hospital, Washington, D.C. 20032

The last few chapters have contained thoughtful presentations on psychiatric diagnosis. In earlier chapters psychological tests were reviewed. These tests were examined for their ability to determine to what extent a selected person is like a class of individuals and to what extent he or she is different.

Attempts at dividing patients by diagnoses are derived from our notion of what a person with a certain diagnosis should look like. However, these notions may produce problems when defined by psychological tests. We will surely find physiological phenocopies which are not dissectable by traditional psychological tools. Indeed, a seemingly pure sample defined by conventional psychological tests might be impure. For example, if our test were to define all things that fly, then birds, bees, airplanes, and balloons would be in the same classification. On the other hand, and of perhaps worse consequence, by attempting to purify our diagnoses, we might omit individuals. Just as, for example, we might leave out flightless, aquatic birds, such as penguins, from the bird category, we might omit individuals who do not manifest a thought disorder from the paranoid schizophrenic category. The sin of omission can be as grave as the sin of commission.

Dr. Winokur earlier elegantly peeled concentric rings off his diagnostic onion, concluding, "I will peel no more—this is paranoia." Was he overly inclusive or exclusive? How can we determine this?

Dr. Donald Goodwin raised another problem. When two disciplines (e.g., psychology and psychiatry) disagree, how do we determine which is correct? In theory this can be answered by follow-up studies, treatment studies, family studies, adoption studies, and so on. In practice, however, when all else fails, we revert to an artificial hierarchy. We ask the Rorschach or TAT to objectify something these tests are probably not capable of doing. Fortunately, we are now using tools such as structured interviews which increase reliability. What about their validity, however? Are we confident of what they have told us? Do we know what they will contribute?

A unique way of using the Rorschach was discussed by Dr. Margaret Singer. From blind assessment of Rorschach protocols, she examines the communication between the tester and the person being tested and demonstrates communication deviance in schizophrenics and their families. In Dr.

Singer's hands this methodology has had a long tradition of reliability. Recently, it has been shown to have high reliability in at least one other investigator's hands (8). This skill remains an art, however, until it can be easily transferred to others.

Dr. Edward Donnelly (*personal communication*) of our laboratory has demonstrated the use of the MMPI to predict drug response in affective disorders. He identified two empirically derived subscales which predicted imipramine and lithium response above 90%. This tool requires validation in other laboratories.

This section of the volume was dedicated to other kinds of tools. These tools are aimed primarily at understanding basic processes that might be related to a disorder; as yet no one is willing to say that what we are finding are not simply epiphenomena.

Do the host of abnormal EEG patterns listed by Dr. Fink have an important meaning that only future studies will determine? His suggestion that we use the EEG abnormalities for diagnoses rather than trying to correlate them with the traditional psychological diagnosis is an excellent one. Recently a young investigator in our laboratory, Dr. Steven Potkin (7), found that a subgroup of chronic schizophrenics who had low platelet monoamine oxidase (MAO) activity also had a high incidence of abnormal EEGs compared to a group of chronic schizophrenics with high platelet MAO. This could mean that any abnormal chemistry produced by low MAO induces an abnormal EEG or that the physiology that produces the abnormal EEG also decreases MAO activity. Another possibility is that abnormal EEGs and low platelet MAO activity are independent but, when they are present together in an individual, they produce a subgroup of schizophrenia.

Drs. Sutton and Tueting reviewed the literature on evoked potentials and diagnosis. I have a particular interest in the augmenting/reducing phenomena and how they relate to schizophrenia. Buchsbaum and collaborators (1,5) have been able to subdivide schizophrenics and use them as their own controls. When schizophrenics are put into paranoid and nonparanoid divisions, this group finds that the paranoid and the bipolar patients are augmenters. Dr. Dennis Murphy has found that bipolar patients have lower than normal platelet MAO. Perhaps there is a relationship between EEG augmenting and bipolar and schizophrenic patients with low platelet MAO activity.

If we are to progress, however, in our understanding of the etiology of psychological disorders and grow in our use of the tools to which I have referred, we must understand them on a physiological level. We have been remiss in this respect. What does it mean physiologically to say an individual is an augmenter? Does this mean, for example, that as a signal passes from the ear to the cortex, augmenters have increased neuronal firing? If this is so, at what level? This question should be easily tested in animals. One could probably even find a strain of animals that augments and another that reduces—giving leverage for elegant genetic studies.

Some areas of electrophysiology that were not covered and are of interest are sleep, reaction time, and eye tracking. Kupfer (3), for example, has documented that a shortened rapid eye movement (REM) latency is more likely to be associated with primary rather than secondary depression. Since only a few nights of sleep recording are required to make this determination and since this can be done in almost any hospital, these findings, if confirmed by other laboratories, may facilitate the selection of proper therapy. Delayed reaction times have differentiated schizophrenics from other groups for many years (6). Recently, disruption in the eye tracking has been associated with deficits in some schizophrenic and affective disorder patients (2).

Dr. Frederick Goodwin summarized some of our current understandings of affective disorders and schizophrenia. It is striking how much further ahead the affectologists are than the schizophreniologists. Researchers of affective disorders have had testable hypotheses for a dozen or more years, hypotheses which were developed when methodology was becoming more powerful. The number of excellent groups studying affective disorders is large—many of them have been working together for considerable time periods. By contrast, the number of groups studying schizophrenia over a long period of time is small.

Besides the availability of testable hypotheses, why are there fewer groups examining schizophrenia? First, for many years we have had a good idea how the tricyclics and monoamine oxidase inhibitors might work; on an absolute scale, these drugs for affective disorders work better than the neuroleptics do for schizophrenia. This is particularly true of lithium. Second, patients with affective disorders, as well as their families, are more cooperative (and consequently easier to study) than patients with schizophrenia, who are by definition ambivalent. Third, mood (the primary disturbance of affective disorders) is easier to understand than cognition. And fourth, animal models are available for affective disorders and not for schizophrenia. No one is willing to say a cat, dog, or monkey hallucinates.

Recently we have tried to make meaningful subdivisions in schizophrenia using platelet MAO activity as a discriminator. We initially found that schizophrenics as a group had lower enzyme activity than normals. Subsequently, we found the difference seemed to be present only in chronic schizophrenics—acute patients being essentially the same as normals. Dr. Potkin has been trying to see if low platelet MAO activity segregates with any conventional subdiagnosis of chronic schizophrenia. In two studies, a retrospective chart analysis and another study in which each patient was interviewed, chronic paranoid schizophrenics as a group had lower platelet MAO activity than nonparanoid patients. These data are similar to those of Schildkraut et al. (4) who found schizophrenic patients with low platelet MAO activity were more likely to have auditory hallucinations and delusions, usually of an accusatory and persecutory nature, than those without low platelet MAO activity.

Tools for making meaningful diagnostic and therapeutic discussions may be in our hands. We will only know this when we can demonstrate that we can prevent illness and make our patients recover more quickly by using those tools.

REFERENCES

1. Buchsbaum, M. (1975): Average evoked response augmenting/reducing in schizophrenia and affective disorders. In: *Biology of the Major Psychoses: A Comparative Analysis,* edited by D. X. Freedman, pp. 129–142. Raven Press, New York.
2. Holzman, P. S., Proctor, L. R., Levy, D. L., Yasillo, N. J., Meltzer, H. J., and Hurt, S. W. (1974): Eye tracking dysfunctions in schizophrenic patients and their relatives. *Arch. Gen. Psychiatry,* 31:141–151.
3. Kupfer, D. J. (1976): REM latency: A psychobiologic marker for primary depressive disease. *Biol. Psychiatry,* 11 (2): 159–174.
4. Schildkraut, J. J., Herzog, J. M., Orsulak, P. J., Edelam, S. E., Shein, H. M., and Frazier, S. H. (1976): Reduced platelet monoamine oxidase activity in a subgroup of schizophrenic patients. *Am. J. Psychiatry,* 133(4):438–440.
5. Schooler, C., Buchsbaum, M., and Carpenter, W. (1976): Evoked response in kinesthetic measures of augmenting/reducing in schizophrenics: Replications and extensions. *J. Nerv. Ment. Dis.,* 163:221–232.
6. Shakow, D. (1971): Some observations on the psychology (and some fewer on the biology) of schizophrenia. *J. Nerv. Ment. Dis.,* 153 (5):300–316.
7. Wyatt, R. J., Potkin, S. G., Walls, P. D., Nichols, A., Carpenter, W., and Murphy, D. (1977): Clinical correlates of low platelet monoamine oxidase in schizophrenic patients. In: *Psychiatric Diagnosis: Exploration of Biological Predictors,* edited by H. Akiskal and W. Webb. Spectrum, New York.
8. Wynne, L. C., Singer, M. T., and Toohey, M. (1976): Communication of the adoptive parents of schizophrenics. In: *Schizophrenia 75. Psychotherapy, Family Studies, Research,* edited by J. Jorstad and E. Ugelstad, pp. 413–451. University of Oslo Press, Oslo.

Discussion

Dr. Salzinger: I would like to raise a more general question, one that concerns this conference as a whole.

We began this conference by discussing a phenomenological description of the abnormal behavior of individuals, and we are finishing by discussing the substrates of behavior.

What we skipped, of course, is what happens in between. It is fine to talk about biological mechanisms. I think it is fine also to talk about phenomenological descriptions as well as we can, but we are lacking the specification of behavioral mechanisms. That is where the biochemical deficit or excess manifests itself. The biochemical fault has to manifest itself through behavioral interaction with the environment.

To demonstrate what I mean by "behavioral mechanism," I would like to briefly describe my hypothesis of schizophrenia, the immediacy hypothesis. I have been talking about that since 1964, when I received an award by this august organization for talking about it, and it certainly shows the effectiveness of reinforcement.

That hypothesis states, very simply, that the stimuli most immediate in the environment are those that generally govern the behavior of schizophrenic patients.

On the basis of that hypothesis, I was able to talk about behavioral mechanisms, as, for example, that extinction will be more rapid in schizophrenics than in normals, which was, in fact, what we found, and that the speech of a schizophrenic patient will be more difficult to understand, which we also found.

One can relate this behavioral mechanism to a biochemical hypothesis; one can hypothesize the absence or reduced activity of some inhibitory mechanism so that stimuli keep influencing an individual so afflicted; one can talk about the destruction of catecholamine fibers in rats and show that avoidance conditioning is absent, etc.

The point is that we have to bridge the gap between biochemistry and behavior by measuring them rigorously and delineating both behavioral as well as biochemical mechanisms.

Dr. Rieder: I am going to say something that struck me as this went on. I don't really expect an answer in any way, for this is more a thought than a question.

There are a multitude of things that we can measure in people. Dr. Fink examines five or six things that he can measure with the EEG and he thinks they are important. Dr. Salzinger is interested in certain things; he just mentioned extinction. How do we know what is important?

Earlier Tsuang stated that paranoid or nonparanoid symptoms are important in schizophrenia. One reason he felt they are important is that there is a transmission within families of the paranoid schizophrenia subtype. Drs. Wyatt and Murphy have looked at platelet MAO and found that it is a genetic factor, and, indeed, that it is related to another genetic factor, paranoid schizophrenia.

This struck me as a way of answering the question about what is important. Dr. Fink says, "I have five EEG measures and even though they cut across clinical syndromes, I still think they are important."

We can ask him, well, do they run in families?

The same way with Dr. Salzinger, we can ask him about extinction, does it run in families? If so, it is important for us to begin to correlate these measures with other things, such as behaviors, that we know are inherited.

It does not mean that we should focus only on things that run in families, but I see things in this perspective. I have begun to divide things that seem to be transmissible in families from things that are not, and then to take the two groups and see the intercorrelations between them.

I would be interested in any response, but it is more just a thought that I had.

Dr. Fink: The question just raised is whether or not there are EEG parameters which may have diagnostic value. There are many, for whenever scientists have examined electrophysiological phenomena, particularly their response to a defined stress, and related these to clinical phenomena, it has been of some use. Epilepsy is a well-defined example.

As to the question about phenomena occurring in families, there are some examples. Fourteen and six positive spikes is a pattern which has been reported to run in families in some studies. Bcause it is found to occur in family members, it is said to be of little clinical significance, since only the index case has the symptom picture. Maybe fourteen and six positive spiking is not the specific phenomenon which is in a specific pathogenic pathway for a defined group of symptoms, yet it may be part of the mechanism, and examination of these populations should continue to see what commonalities can be found.

In response to the discussion of the speakers following me, I have a feeling of being in a distinct minority—a minority calling for greater emphasis on objective, hopefully genotypic, measures, rather than descriptive and historical phenotypic characteristics. Two decades ago we were interested in the drug treatment response as a classificatory device. For example, in studies of EST, we found subjects who responded to four to seven treatments, and another group that required more than twelve treatments. In psychological tests, as the California F Scale and the Rorschach response, the two groups were separable. In a sense, we were operationally defining psychotic depressive and schizophrenic disorders (*Arch. Gen. Psychiatry*, 5:30–36, 1961). Similar relationships were defined in patient responses to chlorpromazine (*Arch. Gen. Psychiatry*, 7:449–459, 1962) and imipramine (*Am. J. Psychiatry*, 119:432–438, 1962) in studies with Don Klein. For EST in particular, we believed we had worked out test criteria which were useful to separate the two different EST-responsive samples.

I came to this meeting to introduce response measures and laboratory test procedures for classification of populations. I think the APA Task Force has ignored these data and selected phenomenological aspects primarily. Phenomenology marked the many earlier classification systems, and the fact that the system is revised again is evidence enough that such a strategy is expedient but inherently of limited value. Maybe we ought to emphasize and include in the next classification scheme other classification devices, such as treatment response or drug response, which may reflect the pathologic processes in the brain which seem to be the basis for most mental disorders.

Dr. Spitzer: One of the problems, as I see it, is that the purpose of a diagnosis is to help you have a plan for action, to make a prediction about what is likely to happen in the future, and to suggest a course of treatment that might be successful. In making that judgment, it seems to me that the whole purpose of a diagnosis would be confused if one were to use external validating criteria to make the diagnosis. I think it makes sense to look at patients who respond differentially to a particular kind of treatment, and then to ask if they have different clinical characteristics which may then define a subgroup, which can be the basis for a new classification. But if one includes in the defining criteria for a diagnostic category knowledge of the presence of a family member who also has the condition, or the fact that the patient has in the past responded to EST, this would lead one into a totally circular kind of reasoning which would also make future research studies virtually impossible. For example, if family data are used as a basis for making a diagnosis, how does one test the relationship of the diagnosis to family data?

My understanding of the history of classification is that most of the biological studies now being done are reconfirming clinical distinctions that have been recognized in the past. We now refer to primary affective disorders, but this is probably not very different from what used to be called Melancholia. It would be nice in the future if knowledge about behavioral characteristics of certain patients with certain biological characteristics might be the basis for a new nosological group. However, I am not aware of any new clinical categories based on biological data that were not recognized before on purely clinical grounds. Am I wrong?

Dr. Dunner: What about the studies of alcoholism?

Dr. Spitzer: Those studies merely deal with a severe form of what we call alcoholism. They do not identify a different kind of alcoholism.

Dr. Fink: It is easy to say that symptoms and history provide a basis for different classifications, and to emphasize that psychiatrists in the nineteenth century used them. But let us see how an objective test changes diagnosis and provides the basis for therapy decisions.

An individual comes into a clinic with a history of episodic behavior, marked by acting-out and aggressivity. On the basis of history and psychological and medical examination, he may be classed as an example of neurotic behavior pattern or a personality disorder. If he is given an EEG test and burst activity is found, immediately the clinicians' response is different. No matter how he was described before, after the EEG he is classed as a case of epilepsy and is treated with specific medications.

The same is true for an individual with an organic mental syndrome. If a serologic test of the spinal fluid is positive, then the diagnosis, regardless of symptom and history, is made and a specific treatment is recommended.

By excluding laboratory data and response to stimuli in the classification, I think you are artificially limiting the clues available to the psychiatrist, and indicating that the only thing the psychiatrist should do is talk, listen, write, and interview. In recent psychiatry the importance of laboratory data has been emphasized, and we should encourage psychiatrists in their classification and practice to use laboratory tools even if they are imprecise at present.

Dr. Spitzer: I would be delighted if there were laboratory tests which we could use in psychiatry, as we can in the rest of medicine, in order to make a diagnosis. I just do not believe that any laboratory tests currently available can be used in a way that is comparable to their use in the rest of medicine. For that reason I think it would be premature and not useful to include laboratory procedures as part of the operational criteria for making a diagnosis in DSM-III.

Dr. Fink: I do not think we can do it now either. But by excluding the concept, by artificially, saying that the purpose of DSM-III (or RDC) is only for research purposes, implies that laboratory tests are dependent phenomena.

If DSM-III is going to be used for classification purposes by the APA membership, why not include all the techniques available and encourage their use?

Dr. Spitzer: Let's say we recommended that an EEG be performed when one is considering schizophrenia. What help would that be?

Dr. Fink: It would be of great help. First, if the EEG shows seizure activity or diffuse slowing, then the diagnosis may have to be changed, and the treatment also. If a group of patients with schizophrenia are shown to have B-mitten patterns, perhaps they will show different treatment responses. As a descriptive marker, it will be more objective and allow better classifications in the years to come. Such data collection should be encouraged by DSM-III, not discarded. Or else your committee will be rewriting DSM-IV in 1984.

Subject Index

Abnormality, defined, 49
Acetylcholinesterase, 305
Adenosine triphosphatases, 309
Adenyl cyclase, 309
Adoption studies
  of antisocial personality, 195–199
  of schizophrenia spectrum, 213–223,
    240
Affect, shallowness of, 78
Affective disorders
  amine neurotransmitters and, 281–
    304
  cooperation of patient as factor, 329
  delusional disorder's relationship to,
    118–121
  enzymes, neurotransmitter-related,
    305, 308–309, 311
  eye tracking tests and, 329
  familial subtyping of, 203–211
  in defining mental disorder, 23, 35
  MMPI and, 328
  validity with genetic family studies,
    238–246
Aggression, in children, determined by
    projective testing, 144–146,
    149–150, 155, 160
Alcoholism
  adoption studies on, 196–200, 228–
    236
  classification of, 333
  in defining mental disorder, 19, 20,
    22, 23, 88
  enzymes in, neurotransmitter-
    related, 305–306, 310
  family studies of, 194–195
  historical review of, 225–228
  validity of genetic studies, 238–239
Allergy, in children: projective testing,
    150–151
American Psychiatric Association
    Diagnostic Manual, see Diag-
    nostic and Statistical Manual
American Psychiatric Association's
    Task Force on Nomenclature
    and Statistics, 15–39, 41, 125,
    333

Amine neurotransmitters, See also
    Neurotransmitters
  psychiatric diagnosis and, 281–304
  related enzymes, 305–321
Amine oxidase, 309
Amitriptyline, 292–293, 299
Amphetamine, 296, 307
Anemia, 314
Anhedonia
  construct validity studies and, 186
  in test for schizotypy, 172–174
  "trait" or "state" related, 180, 181
Anorgasmia, 20, 25, 26, 32–33
Anthropology, and recognition of psy-
    chosis in non-Western societies,
    1–13
Antisocial personality
  in defining mental disorder, 88, 91
  enzymes and, 311
  genetic studies of, and related disor-
    ders, 193–202
Anxiety
  a. neuroses in children: projective
    testing in, 155
  in defining mental disorder, 23, 31
  neurotransmitter-related enzymes in,
    306, 311, 314
Aphasia Screening Test, 189
Arctic hysteria, 4, 10
Aromatic l-amino acid decarboxylase,
    305
Articulation problems, projective test-
    ing in children with, 150
Asthma
  in children: projective testing and,
    150–151
  in defining mental disorder, 35
Attention, evoked potentials and, 269,
    271–272, 275
Attention deficit disorder, in defining
    mental disorder, 21, 27

Beck Inventory of Depression, 172–173
Behavior
  behavioral analysis of diagnosis,
    73–84, 106–107, 331

Behavior (*contd.*)
  behavioral deviance, as mental illness, 58
  behavior modification, projective testing and, 133
  cultural relativity and, 1–3
  vs. psychological symptoms, 91
Bender-Gestalt test, in children, 142–145, 152, 156–159
Benton visual retention test, 189–190
Biochemical factors
  amine neurotransmitters and, 281–304
  behavioral mechanisms and, 331
  enzymes, neurotransmitter-related, 305–321
  evoked potentials and, 271
  hormones as, 307, 309, 315
  in schizophrenia, 174
Bipolar affective disorder, *See also specific disorder*
  amine neurotransmitters and, 281–304
  EEG and, 328
  enzymes, neurotransmitter-related, 305–308
  evoked potentials in, 271, 274–275
  familial subtyping study of, 207–210
Blacky test, 148
Body image, in children, validity of projective testing for, 146–148
Body Image Aberration Scale
  "state" or "trait," 180, 181
  in test for schizotypy, 172–174
Brain disorders
  diagnostic tests for, 131, 189–191
  EEG to diagnose, 254–263
  resemblance to schizophrenic protocols, 182
Briquet's syndrome, *See also* Hysteria
  adoption studies, 196–200
  family studies of, 194–195

Calcium, enzyme activity related to, 307
California F Scale, 332
CAPPS structured interview, 273
Catatonic, as subtype of schizophrenia, familial study of, 207
Catecholamines
  enzymes related to, 305–321
  in psychiatric diagnosis, 281–304
  and related enzymes, 305

Catechol-O-methyl transferase (COMT) 305, 307, 324
Cerebrospinal fluid studies, of amine neurotransmitters, 283–284, 287–289, 291, 293, 298–300
Chemotherapy, for paranoia, 116–117, 119
Childhood disorders, *See also specific disorder*
  EEG responses in, 258
  validity of projective testing for, 141–166, 184
Children's Apperception Test, 142, 148–150, 154, 158
Chlorimipramine, 298–299
Chlorpromazine, 297, 332–333
Coffee drinking, 33
Communication Deviance Manual, 128
Computerized diagnostic assessment, 210
  as supplement to EEG, 255, 257
  tomography scans and MMS for diagnosing brain damage, 189
Conditioning, as factor in method of interview for diagnosing, 78
Conjugal paranoia, 109
Conversion disorders, 30
Course, defined, 46
Creatine phosphokinase (CPK), 311–313
Criminality
  adoption studies on, 196–200
  and alcoholism, 232
  criminal guilt: involuntary vs. voluntary behavior, 43
  in defining mental illness, 34, 59–62, 67, 87–88
  twin studies on, 193–194
Critical flicker function test, 187
Culture, and personality, 105
Cultural relativity, and recognition of psychosis in non-Western societies, 1–3, 10–13
Cyproheptadine, 301

Délires chroniques paranoiaques, 109, 120
Délires chroniques passionnels et de revendication, 109
Delta Percentage Index Score, 128, 173
Delusional disorder, *See also* Paranoia
  definition of, from clinical findings, 109–121

Delusional monomania, 109
Depressive disorders, *See also* Affective disorders
  amine neurotransmitters and, 282–301
  in children: validity of projective testing, 150–151
  EEG in diagnosing, 256
  enzymes in, neurotransmitter-related, 305–308
  evoked potentials in, 269–276
  in defining mental disorder, 21, 28, 29, 31
  REM in, 329
  in subtyping affective disorders, 208
  in tests for schizotypy, 172
Desipramine, 298
Desmethylchlorimipramine, 298
Diagnostic and Statistical Manual of Mental Disorders (DSM)
  in behavioral analysis of diagnosing, 74, 80
  in defining mental disorders, 15–39, 41, 86, 89, 94, 96, 142, 167, 197, 204, 246, 285, 334
  in defining stereotypes, 125
  in subtyping schizophrenia, 214–216, 220
3,4-dihydroxyphenylacetic acid (DOPAC), 283
Disability, as criteria for defining mental disorder, 20–24, 28–31, 32, 34–46, 87–89, 92–93
Disadvantage, as criteria for defining mental disorder, 20–25, 28–31, 34, 37, 92–94
Disease, concept of, 63
  evolution and, 50–52
  in defining mental disease, 53, 97
  functional illness, abnormality, dysfunction, and, 49–50
  vs. term "illness," 48
Disorder vs. illness, 179–180
Distress, as criteria in defining mental disorder, 20–24, 28–37, 92–93
Dobuans, 2
Dopamine
  in psychiatric diagnosis, 281–284, 287–288, 290, 292, 296–301
  related enzymes, 305–307
Dopamine-β-hydroxylase (DBH), 305–307, 311–313, 324
Down's syndrome, *See also* Mental retardation, 239, 306, 307, 309

Draw-A-Person Test
  illusory correlations in judging patient's response, 168–170
  in psychodiagnosis, 167, 177
  validity of, in children, 142–148, 152–153, 156–160
Drug addiction
  adoption studies of, 196–200
  in defining mental disorder, 88
  family studies of, 194–195
Drug therapy, 332, 333
  EEG responses and, as diagnostic method, 257–259, 273, 324
  enzymes and, neurotransmitter-related, 308
  evoked potentials and, 272–275
  MMPI and, 328
  neurotransmitter studies and, in diagnosing, 281–304
  paranoia and, 116–117, 119
Dynamic harmony theory, 47
Dysfunction, concept of
  defined, 48–52, 97
  ego-dystonic and ego-dystonic putative disorders related to, 54–58
  related to defining mental illness, 53, 101–106
Dyshomophilia, 32
Dysphoric affective dysregulation, EEG responses in, 258
Dysthymics, EEG responses in, 258

Ego-dystonic disorders, 54–55
Ego-syntonic disorders, 55–58
Electroencephalography (EEG)
  drug effects on, 273
  response strategies of, in diagnosing, 253–263, 324, 328, 331–332, 334
Electroshock, 307
Emotionally disturbed children, *See also* Childhood disorders
  Rorschach to diagnose, 184
Environment, observations used in diagnosing affected by, 76–77
Enzymes, neurotransmitter-related, 305–321, 324–325
Epinephrine, 307, 309
Epilepsy, EEG and, 254–255, 258
Electrophysiology, 328–329, 332
  EEG in diagnosing, 253–263
  evoked potentials in diagnosing, 265–279
EST, 332–333

Estrogens, 307
Evoked potentials, and diagnosis, 265–279, 293, 328
Evolutionary theory, and concepts of disease, 50–53, 69, 102–103
Eye tracking, 329
Exploitation, in role theory, 42

Familial dysautonomia, 306
Family studies, 285
  of alcoholism, 225–235
  of antisocial personality, 194–195
  neurotransmitter-related enzymes and, 305, 313–314
  of schizophrenia and affective disorders, 203–211, 292
  validity of, relating to psychiatric taxa, 237–247, 332, 333
Fear responses, in children, in projective testing, 150
Fetal alcohol syndrome, 225–226
Fetishism, in defining mental disorder, 20, 26
Forced choice methods, 187
Functional analysis, 97–101
Functional illness, defined, 48–50, 101–103
Fusaric acid, 297, 307

Gambling, pathological, 20, 26, 93
Genetic studies, 332
  of alcoholism, 225–235
  of antisocial personality and related disorders, 193–202
  EEG responses in subpopulations, 256–257, 259
  evoked potentials and, 274
  family studies relating to psychiatric taxa, 237–247, 285
  neurotransmitter-related enzymes and, 305, 309–315
  in Rorschach testing of schizophrenia, 172
  of schizophrenia spectrum, 213–223, 323–324, 331–332
Gilles de la Tourette's disorder, 30
Glucose-6-phosphate dehydrogenase deficiency, 314
Grief, 21, 31, 95

Habits, bad habits as "dysfunction," 56–58

Hallucinations
  enzyme activity and, 329
  of paranoia, 109
Haloperidol, 297, 307
Halstead-Reitan battery test, 189, 191
Hand Test, 146, 160
Healers, in non-Western societies, in defining insanity, 4–12
Hearing disorders, projective testing in children with, 150
Hebephrenia
  familial study of, 207
  paranoid schizophrenia and, 120
Hippocrates, in defining illnesses, 46
Homosexuality
  in defining mental disorder, 15, 16, 23, 24, 26, 32, 41, 60, 68, 86–87, 89, 93
  as ego-syntonic deviant pattern, 58
  latent or borderline schizophrenia and, 215
Homovanillic acid (HVA), 283, 287–288, 307
Hormone activity, enzymes and, 307, 309, 315
Human Figure Drawing Test, *See also* Draw-A-Person test
  validity of, in children, 142, 144–145
Huntington's disease, 238, 306
5-hydroxyindoleacetic acid (5-HIAA), 283–284, 287–288, 291, 295, 298–300
Hyperkinetic child syndrome
  adoption studies of, 198–200
  EEG to diagnose, 257
  evoked potentials and, 275
  family studies of, 194–195
Hyperthyroidism, 306
Hypochondriasis, 21, 27
Hypoglycemia, 314
Hypothyroidism, 306
Hypoxanthine-guanine phosphoribosyltransferase, 315
Hysteria (Briquet's syndrome)
  Arctic *h.*, 4, 10
  adoption studies of, 196–200
  family studies of, 194–195
Hystericopsychopaths, EEG responses in, 258

Illness, concept of
  "syndrome" and "course" defined, 46

Illness, concept of (*contd.*)
  vs. "disorder," 179–180
  vs. term "disease," 48
Imipramine, 287, 292–294, 298–299,
  307, 332–333
Inadequate personality, adoption
  studies and, 197, 216–222
Indoleamine, *see* Serotonin
Information processing, evoked potentials and, 267
Information for diagnosing
  behavioral analysis of, 77–84
  effect of environment on, 76–77
  patient's verbal behavior, 81–82
  reliability of, 73–76, 81
Insanity, defined in non-Western
  societies, 5–11
Intelligence testing, 185, 190
  IQ and projective testing, 143, 149,
  151–156, 159
  and mental retardation, 239
International Classification of Diseases, 41
Interpersonal relationship problem, in
  defining mental disorder, 20, 31,
  94
Interview, 106–107
  behavior theory and, 73–84
  in diagnosing schizophrenia, 174
  projective testing and, 124, 127, 132,
  177, 190–191
  structured, 178–179, 185, 186, 204,
  209, 273, 275
Iowa Structured Psychiatric Interview,
  204
Iowa 500 Project, 245
  in subtyping schizophrenia and affective disorders, 203–210, 242
ITP phosphohydrolase, 309

Kleptomania, 20, 26, 34, 93
Kwakiutl Indians, 2

Laboratory tests, 334
L-DOPA
  enzymes and, 313
  evoked potentials and, 271
  and neurotransmitter studies in diagnosing, 284, 297, 307
Legal considerations, in defining mental disorder, 87–88

Lesch-Nyhan syndrome, 306, 315
Lithium, 292–294, 297, 309, 329
Loss, themes of, in children, determined by projective testing,
  148–149

Manic disorders
  amine neurotransmitters and, 282
  in defining mental disorder, 20, 23
  familial subtyping of affective disorders, 207–208
  tests to diagnose, vs. schizophrenia,
  189–190
Manic-depressive episodes
  amine neurotransmitters and, 282–
  301
  enzymes in, neurotransmitter-
  related, 305–306, 308
  evoked potentials and, 274
  familial subtyping of affective disorders, 207–208, 213
Masturbation, in defining mental disorder, 24, 93
Medical approach to treatment, defining "mental disorder" to
  legitimize, 90
Medical disorder, mental disorder defined as subset of, 15–39
Melancholia, 333
Mendelian traits, 238–241, 323–324
Menninger Health Sickness Rating
  Scale (MHSRS), used conjointly
  with adoption studies, 197
Mental disorders, *See also* Mental illness, and *specific disorder*
  children with, projective testing in,
  141–166
  difficulty in diagnosis of, 179
  legal considerations, 87–88
  proposed definition and criteria of,
  15–39
  discussion of, 85–107
Mental illness
  alternative definitions, 63–69
  classification and causation of, 46–48
  cultural relativity and, 1–3
  definition proposed, 41–71
  discussion of, 66–69, 97–107
  functional illness, disease, abnormality, and dysfunction, 48–50
  historical and evolutionary concepts
  of, 46–52

Mental illness (*contd.*)
  ideological problems, 69
  in non-Western societies, 1–13
  vs. physical illness, 91
  role theory in defining, 42–46
  social deviance and, 58–62
  unhappiness and, 62–63
Mental retardation
  in defining mental disorder, 21, 30
  enzymes and, 311, 312
  genetic studies of, 238–239, 323
3-methoxy-4-hydroxymandelic acid
    (VMA), 283–284
3-methoxy-4-hydroxyphenylacetic acid
    (HVA), 283, 287–288, 307
3-methoxy-4-hydroxyphenylglycol
    (MHPG), 283–284, 288–289,
    291, 293, 295, 299, 300, 307
5,10-methylenetetrahydrofolate reduc-
    tase, 309
Methylene tetrahydrofolate (MTHF),
    312, 315
Methylphenidate, 307
N-methyl transferase, 309
Migraine, 309
Mini-Mental State Test, for brain dam-
    age, 189
Minnesota Multiphasic Personality In-
    ventory, 157, 162, 293–294
  accuracy in diagnosing with, 170
  enzyme activity correlations with,
    315
  failure to relate to diagnosis, 179
  to predict drug response in affective
    disorders, 328
  use as interview, 185
Missouri Children's Picture Series, 154
Monoamine neurotransmitters, *See*
    Amine neurotransmitters
Monoamine oxidase, 271, 305, 307–
    311, 313–316, 324, 328, 329,
    inhibitors of, 296
Muscle tension, evoked potentials and,
    271–272

Need achievement, in children, project-
    ive testing and, 149
Nervousness, in defining mental disor-
    der, 21
Neuroblastoma, 306
Neurological diseases, evoked poten-
    tials and diagnosis of, 275

Neurophysiological tests, *See also spe-
    cific test*, 189–190, 328
Neuroses
  EEG to diagnose, 256
  neurotransmitter enzymes and, 305
  projective testing and, 130–131, 133,
    155
  vs. psychosis diagnosis, using
    MMPI, 170
Neurotics, anxious, EEG responses in,
    258
Neurotransmitters
  and psychiatric diagnosis, 281–304,
    324–325
  related enzymes, in diagnosing,
    305–321
Norepinephrine
  enzyme activity and, 306, 307
  in psychiatric diagnosis, 281–284,
    288–291, 293, 295–298, 300–301
Nortriptyline, 298–299

Obsessions, in children, projective test-
    ing and, 155
Octopamine, 313
Organic disorders
  diagnostic test for, 189, 191
  organic model of, as basis for
    classification strategy, 253–263,
    334
"Organic" vs. "functional" tests, 191
Organismic dysfunction, in defining
    mental disorder, 18, 23, 37, 91,
    92, 95, 102
Orthostatic hypotension, primary, 306

Pain, evoked potentials and, 271
Panic disorder, in defining mental dis-
    order, 21, 29
Paranoia, *See also* Delusional disorder,
    91, 109–121
Paranoid schizophrenia
  delusional disorder vs., 109–121
  EEG and, 328
  enzymes in, neurotransmitter-
    related, 308, 314, 329
  evoked potentials in, 268, 271
  familial subtyping of, 206–207, 209,
    331–332
Paraphrenias, vs. paranoia syndrome,
    109

Parental test behavior, 135
Parkinson's disease, 306, 307
Passive-aggressive disorder, validity of
    projective testing in children for,
    155
Peabody Picture Vocabulary Test,
    189–190
Personality
  assessment by projective testing, 133
  enzymes and, 313, 315
  evoked potentials related to, 270
  in diagnosing mental disorder, 179–
    180, 184, 186
  role of social conditioning and rein-
    forcement in production of, 105
  Rorschach testing and variables of,
    129
Personality disorders, *See also specific*
    disorder
  antisocial *p.d.*, 20, 23, 34–35
  in defining mental disorders, 23,
    34–35, 65–67
  hysterical *p.d.*, 20, 26
  narcissistic *p.d.*,, in defining mental
    disorder, 20, 26
  Rorschach Prognostic Rating Scale
    and, 133
Personality tests, *See also specific test*
  usefullness of, 185
  validity of projective tests in chil-
    dren, 141–166
Phenelzine, 292–293
Phenothiazine drug therapy
  evoked potentials and, 273
  neurotransmitter studies and, 296–
    297
  for paranoia, 117
Phenylanine, 284
Phenylalanine hydroxylase, 312
Phenylethanolamine *N*-methyl trans-
    ferase, 305
Phenylethylamine, 313
Phenylketonuria (PKU), 237, 238, 312
Phobic disorder
  EEG responses and, 259
  in defining mental disorder, 20, 22, 23
Physical defects, in children, projective
    testing relating to, 150
Pimozide, 297, 300–301
Piribedil, 301
Placebo, in neurotransmitter study,
    292–293

Porphyria, 314, 323
Possession, 7–9
Present State Examination, 285
Probenecid, 284, 291, 299–300
Prognostic tests, 180–182, 186
Projective testing
  in children, 141–166
  role in psychiatric diagnosing, 123–
    139, 177–187
  useful as interview, 177
  vs. interview, 191
Proverbs testing, 134, 135
Psychological testing, *See also specific*
    test or testing genre, 167–175,
    177–187, 327
  vs. interview technique, 191
Psychology vs. psychiatry, 327
Psychometry, for diagnosing brain
    damage, 189
Psychoneuroses, in children, validity of
    projective testing in, 155
Psychopathic personality
  adoption studies of, 195–200
  in defining mental illness, 65–67
Psychose hallucinatoire chronique,
    109, 120
Psychoses, *See also specific psychosis*
  amine neurotransmitters and, 281–
    304
  in children, validity of projective
    testing in, 155–157
  chronic hallucinatory *p.* vs. delu-
    sional disorder, 109, 120
  EEG responses in, 258
  enzymes in, neurotransmitter-
    related, 305–321
  evoked potentials and, 266–272
  vs. neurosis diagnosis, using MMPI,
    170
  in non-Western societies, 1–13
  psychological testing and, 332
  symptoms classified, 174
Psychotherapy
  for paranoia, 116–117, 119
  rational-emotive *p.*, projective test-
    ing and, 133
  verbal responses of patient in, 81–82
Purine phosphorirobosyl transferase,
    309
Putative disorders, indications of dys-
    function relevant to, 54–58
Pyromania, 34

Rapid eye movement, 329
Raven's Matrices test, 189–190
Reaction time, in diagnosing, 329
Reading developmental disorder
   in defining mental disorder, 21, 27
   validity of projective testing for, 155
Reinforcement contingency, in be-
      havioral analysis of diagnosing,
      77–83
Reliability concept, in diagnosis, 73–84
Research Diagnostic Criteria, 178–179,
   285, 286
Research Diagnostic System, 281
Reserpine, 296–297
Role theory, 41–46, 48, 53, 58–63, 97
Rorschach test
   for children: validity of, 141–143,
      145, 148–153, 155–156, 158–160
   in diagnosing schizophrenia, 171–174
   in psychodiagnosis, 167, 177, 180–
      184, 191, 327–328, 332
   validity of, 181
Rosenzweig Picture-Frustration Study,
   157

Sadism, sexual, 20, 26, 93
Schedule for Affective Disorders and
   Schizophrenia, 127, 174
Schizoid personality
   adoption studies and, 197, 216–222
   enzymes and, 311
   schizotypal personality, 172–173,
      220–222
   validity of genetic family studies and,
      242
Schizophrenia, *See also* Paranoid
   schizophrenia
   amine neurotransmitters and, 282,
      288, 289, 290, 296–297, 300
   behavioral mechanisms in, 78, 331
   in children, projective testing and,
      151, 15–156
   in defining mental disorder, 23, 31, 35
   delusional disorder vs., 109–121
   EEG in diagnosing, 256–259, 328,
      334
   enzymes and, 305–312, 328, 329
   evoked potentials and, 266–273,
      275–276, 328
   eye tracking tests, 329
   familial subtyping of, 203–211
   genetic studies of, 213–223, 238–246

   mental retardation and, 323
   in non-Western societies, 6, 9, 10
   vs. paranoia syndrome, 109
   process *s.* vs. reactive *s.*, using
      Rorschach, 171–172
   projective testing and, 132, 151,
      155–156
   psychological testing for, 170–172
   reason for fewer investigative
      groups, 329
   schizophrenic-like test result, 183
   types of, from testing, 173–174
      subdivisions of, defined, 214–216
Self-esteem and self-image, in children,
   projective testing, 146–148
Self-ratings, in psychological testing,
   148
Senile dementia, 30
Sentence Completion test, 133
Serotonin, 282–284, 287–288, 290–292,
   295–296, 298, 300–301
Sexual behavior, 20, 23–26, 30–33,
   67–68, 93–94
Shaman, 4–5, 7–9
Siberian Eskimos, 3–13
Signal detection theory, 187
Sleep, EEG responses in, 257–259, 329
Social labeling, 2–3, 10–11
Social roles, in non-Western societies,
   3, 7–10
Sociopathy, 58–63
   genetic family studies in, 237
Speech defects, *See* Articulation prob-
   lems
Stanford-Binet, in children, validity of
   projective testing and, 152
States'' of behavior, defined, vs.
   "trait," 180, 184, 186
Stereotypes, in diagnosing, 125–126
Structured Clinical Interview of Bur-
   dock and Hardesty, 178
Suicidal
   EEG responses and, 259
   enzymes and, 315
   in interview, reinforcement con-
      tingencies of, 80–81, 82
   in neurotransmitter studies, 291, 295
   ritual type, 4
Sydenham, in defining illnesses, 46–47
Symptoms
   behavioral analysis of, in diagnosing,
      77–81

Symptoms (*contd.*)
"psychological" vs. "behavioral," 91
Syndrome
defined, 46
as evidence of mental illness, 53

Thematic Apperception Test
in children, 144–146, 148–150, 155–156, 158–160
role in psychiatric diagnosing, 133–135, 177, 327
Thomas-Chess-Birch temperament items, 198
Thought disorder, evoked potentials and, 267–268, 270
Tobacco dependence, in defining mental disorder, 22, 33
Torsion dystonia, 306
"Trait" vs. "state," defined, 180, 184, 186
Tricyclic antidepressants
enzymes and, neurotransmitter-related, 309
and neurotransmitter studies to diagnose, 282, 292–293, 296–299, 329
Twin studies
on adult criminality, 193–194
of alcoholism, 227
drawback of, 195
enzymes in, neurotransmitter-related, 308, 313

validity of, relating to psychiatric taxa, 240–242
Tyrosine, 284, 297
Tyrosine hydroxylase, 305
L-tryptophan, 284, 297, 313

Unipolar affective disorder
amine neurotransmitters and, 282–301
enzymes in, neurotransmitter-related, 305–307
evoked potentials in, 271, 275
familial subtyping of affective disorders, 207–210

Vanylmandelic acid, 307
Virus infection, 312

WAIS, 189–190
Wechsler Intelligence Scale for Children, 135, 142–143, 152, 157
World Health Organization Psychiatric Assessment Schedules, 15, 127

Yorubas, 3–13

Zuni Pueblo Indians, 1–3
Zymelidine, 301